ESTABLISHING BETTER STANDARDS OF CARE IN DOPPLER ECHOCARDIOGRAPHY, COMPUTED TOMOGRAPHY AND NUCLEAR CARDIOLOGY

Edited by **Richard M. Fleming**

Establishing Better Standards of Care in Doppler Echocardiography, Computed Tomography and Nuclear Cardiology
Edited by Richard M. Fleming

Published by InTech

Janeza Trdine 9, 51000 Rijeka, Croatia

Publishing Process Manager Mia Devic

Technical Editor Teodora Smiljanic

Cover Designer InTech Design Team

Additional hard copies can be obtained from orders@intechopen.com

Establishing Better Standards of Care in Doppler Echocardiography, Computed Tomography and Nuclear Cardiology
Edited by Richard M. Fleming
p. cm.
ISBN 978-953-307-366-8

For EU product safety concerns:
IN TECH d.o.o., Prolaz Marije Krucifikse Kozulić 3, 51000 Rijeka, Croatia,
info@intechopen.com or visit our website at intechopen.com.

Meet the editor

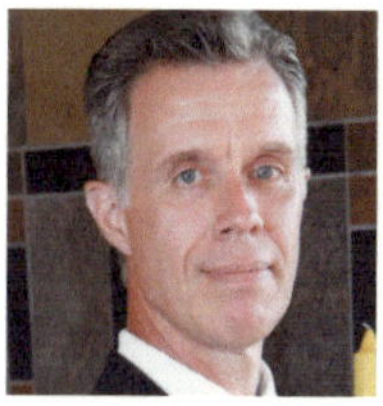

Dr. Richard M. Fleming is a Nuclear and Preventive Cardiologist, born and raised in Waterloo, Iowa, USA. He attended the University of Northern Iowa and has degrees in Physics, Biology, Psychology and Chemistry. He attended the University of Iowa College of Medicine, Creighton University and the University of Texas Health Science Center in Houston. In addition to training in Cardiology he has special Certifications in Positron Emission Tomography. He was Board Certified in Internal Medicine in 1990 and Nuclear Cardiology in 1996. He developed both the Unified Theory of Vascular Disease establishing "Inflammation" as the cause of coronary and peripheral vascular disease and the Quadratic Blood Flow Equation for Coronary Flow Reserve in the early to mid-1990s. He has published more than 50 papers in peer review medical journals, over 50 presentations at scientific conferences throughout the U.S., Europe and Asia, has authored 8 chapters in Medical Textbooks and written 3 independent books on Health Care. He has served as Faculty and a Professor at various Universities and in 2003 received a Physician of the Year award. His current work on SPECT Cardiac imaging promotes the detection of Vulnerable Inflammatory Plaques (VIPs) through reductions in radiation dosage by using principles similar to the detection of black holes and dark matter.

Contents

Preface

In 1986, I graduated from the University of Iowa College of Medicine. On the day, I entered Medical School, the Dean told us that 90% of what we would be taught was wrong, he simply did not know what that 90% was. He encouraged us to strive to determine what was wrong and what was right, allowing us to take better care of our patients. To do that would require a lifetime commitment to research, education, reading and building upon our clinical experiences. For that reason, we can never stop learning, growing or questioning what we know or think we know. When I was a Medical Student, Color Flow Doppler echocardiography had not even hit the clinical setting and when I was first introduced to it as a Cardiology Fellow, it made little sense to me as the "doppler shift" phenomena, something I knew well from my days as a physics student, meant, "red is moving away" from you, while "blue is moving toward you." (Actually, I knew this in Junior High.) Unfortunately, for Doppler echocardiography, this is the opposite as "red" is toward and "blue" is away from the transducer. This presents the classic example of mistakes in the field and the need to learn the terminology. Medicine does not stand still; however, improvements, corrections in misunderstandings and breakthroughs are constantly fighting their way to the surface of science where they can be discussed at meetings, conferences, journals and eventually books, such as this one. To that end, we present this book to the reader as s/he continues to learn and acquire new knowledge on this lifelong quest for improvement.

Recent changes in the fields of Doppler Echocardiography, Computed Tomography and Nuclear Cardiology have improved the detection and treatment of countless individuals over the last decade. This book introduces the reader to some of those improvements and provides an informative and useful framework, upon which both clinician and researcher alike can use to improve the quality of care provided to patients and their work. Hence, it establishes better standards of care and understanding in these non-invasive areas of Cardiology. We have broken this book into six main sections, with the first four sections looking at Doppler Echocardiography including (1) the right heart and its special considerations, (2) the influence of pulmonary factors which will influence doppler evaluations, (3) evaluation of left heart function, and (4) a special considerations section which will address the use of contrast agents in addition to factors which influence Doppler studies, the effects of timing and aging as seen with Doppler, evaluation of hepatic transplants and even the effects of rheumatoid arthritis. The remaining two sections include (5) Nuclear Cardiology, where dramatic shifts in understanding have significantly improved the detection of ischemic heart disease, including the detection of Vulnerable Inflammatory Plaques (VIPs), building upon the "Inflammation and Heart Disease" theory proposed by the Editor in 1995 and finally (6) the impact that Coronary CT may play in the detection of coronary artery disease. After reading this book, we believe the reader will not only have a better understanding of how to go about utilizing these unique tools in the treatment and diagnosis of individuals with heart disease; but, also be encouraged to participate in the process of constantly striving to improve patient care and management and to actively seek answers to questions yet unanswered.

The development of diagnostic methods used to Non-Invasively diagnose and aid in the treatment of Heart Disease has evolved the three separate yet equally important fields; viz. echocardiography, computed tomography and nuclear cardiology. The pioneers of these fields Inge Edler (Echocardiography), Godfrey Hounsfield (Computed Tomography) and Hermann Blumgart (Nuclear Cardiology) presented ideas, which in their day were considered controversial; yet they became the basis of today's Non-Invasive Cardiology and this book. Each breakthrough in history has been received with less than enthusiastic response as it questioned the"Traditions of the Day". Galileo Galilei's efforts to explain that the solar system was heliocentric and not geocentric was received with indignation and house arrest, particularly after emphasizing that an intelligent individual could determine this by themselves without depending upon others. Ignaz Semmelweis was reprimanded when he proposed that "germs" not "humours" were the primary cause of infant mortality. Joseph Lister was less than warmly received when he questioned the belief that Miasma (bad air) was responsible for infections in wounds and Archie Cochran showed that failure to question what we have been taught can result in the repetition of the same old mistakes. Insanity, it has been said, is repeating the same action over and over again and expecting a different result. As Max Planck once said, "A new scientific truth does not triumph by convincing its opponents and making them see the light, but rather because its opponents eventually die, and a new generation grows up that is familiar with it." This book presents those concepts, not just for future generations but also for ours. Science, like mankind keeps moving forward. When we first proposed the theory of "Inflammation and Heart Disease" in 1995, it too met with great resistance. At that time, cholesterol alone was viewed as the sole cause of coronary artery disease; yet with time, "The Fleming Unified Theory of Vascular Disease" not only stood the test of time; but, become the explanation for much of what we see today. We find this encouraging, because, it shows that today's physicians are capable of embracing paradigm shifts that they once would have resisted allowing medicine to improve at unprecedented rates.

This book is dedicated to all of those men and women before us who encouraged us to question what we think and strive to leave the world a better place as well as those who read this book in an effort to improve the care of their patients through the utilization of the use of Doppler echocardiography, Coronary Computed Tomography and Nuclear Cardiology. I dedicate the book to Gallileo, Edler, Blumgart, Lister, Hounsfeld, Semmelweis, Cochran and Planck. Lastly, I would like to thank and dedicate this book to the following individuals who have directly influenced my life and encouraged me to continue my scientific endeavors. To President J.F. Kennedy, whose scientific programs placed me on an accelerated science pathway beginning in 7th grade and who understood the importance of training future scientists. To my parents, Joseph and Margaret who encouraged me to become whatever I wanted to be; but, to be the best at whatever I chose to be. They never doubted me. To my children (Stephanie, Christian and Matthew), who have watched their father work endless hours taking care of patients, teaching students, residents and fellows, all the time working on multiple research projects over the years in an effort to improve Medicine and the treatment of patients; but, who remind me daily that the greatest gift in the world is to be a father, to my wife Susan and last but certainly never least to Gordon M. Harrington, who apart from any other individuals has persevered our endless struggles to change the paradigms that weigh down science and humanity. Gordon unlike any other has encouraged and supported me on this journey and to Dorothy Forsberg-Harrington for her loving support of Gordon and myself. To all those who have supported and believed, this book is dedicated to you.

Richard M. Fleming
Critical Care and Cardiology, Department of Internal Medicine,
Sierra Nevada Veterans Affairs Health Care System, Reno, Nevada,
USA

Part 1

Right Heart Doppler

1

Superior Vena Cava Doppler Flow Changes in Superior Vena Cava Syndrome

Yun You Duan and Li Jun Yuan
Fourth Military Medical University
China

1. Introduction

Two major topics were covered in this chapter. The first was to explore a method of establishing a rabbit model of SVCS by injecting VX2 tumor cell suspension transcutaneously under ultrasound guidance, and to observe the radiotherapeutic effects by SVC Doppler flow changes. The establishment of this model would offer an experimental evidence for better diagnosis, treatment and follow-up observation of SVCS. The second was to investigate the evolution of the SVC Doppler flow changes in patients with SVCS and its value in assessing clinical therapeutic effects in these patients.

An animal SVC obstruction model would be of use in further studies directed at optimizing the therapeutic strategies for original tumors causing SVC syndrome in patients, yet no detailed information about the establishment of an animal SVC obstruction (SVCO) model can be found in the literature. It has been reported that VX2 tumor cell could be successfully inoculated into multiple organs to induce malignant tumors in rabbits (De Crespigny et al, 1999; Goldberg et al, 1999; Ishida et al, 2000), and various imaging modalities has been adopted to assess the effect of this inoculation (Kim et al, 2000; Liu et al, 2001). We hypothesize that a rabbit model with SVCO could be established by inoculating VX2 tumors cells into the areas around the SVC.

Superior vena cava syndrome (SVCS) is a clinical expression of obstruction of blood flow through the SVC, and more than 80% cases are caused by malignant tumors. Though contrast-enhanced spiral or multi-slice CT is now able to identify accurately the site of occlusion or stenosis, it has been greatly limited by its high cost and radiation and thus is not appropriate for follow-up observations. In contrast, ultrasound is safe, reproducible, and relatively inexpensive. Doppler ultrasonography has been successfully used to assess the rabbit SVC obstruction model. We hypothesize that Doppler flow patterns of SVC could be applied for assessing the severity of SVCS and its therapeutic effects.

2. Objective

There are three objectives for the animal study. The first is to study the feasibility of establishing a model of SVCO in rabbits by infusing VX2 tumor cell suspension transcutaneously with ultrasound guidance, and to evaluate the applications of this animal model. The second is to study morphologic and hemodynamic changes of superior vena cava (SVC) in rabbits with SVCO using two-dimensional and Doppler ultrasound and to

explore the relationship between the tumor size in specimen and the two-dimensional and Doppler ultrasonographic characteristics. The third is to analyze the ultrasonographic characteristics and histopathological changes after radiotherapy in rabbits with SVCO, and to provide useful information for assessing the SVC syndrome therapeutic effect in clinic.
The objective of the human study was to evaluate the Doppler SVC's flow patterns and their value in assessing SVCS.

3. Materials and methods

3.1 Animals model establishment

Fifteen adult healthy New Zealand White rabbits were enrolled in this study. Anesthesia was performed by injecting Ketamine Hydrochloride into the posterior leg muscles of rabbits at a dose of 30mg/kg. The VX2 tumor cell suspension was prepared under the sterile condition. About 0.1ml tumor cell suspension was infused transcutaneously in front of SVC and close to its anterior wall guided by ultrasound. The SVC morphology and hemodynamics as well as the tissues around SVC were examined with two-dimensional and Doppler ultrasonography once every 3 days from the 9th day after the injection of tumor cell suspension till the natural death of the rabbits. These findings were compared with those by CT and digital subtraction angiography (DSA).

3.2 Ultrasonographic examinations

One rabbit did not develop tumor after the injection of VX2 tumor cell suspension and thus excluded. The rest of the fourteen rabbit models of SVCO were examined by two-dimensional and Doppler ultrasonography using Sequoia 512 computed ultrasonograph with the probe of 7v3c.
The sizes of the tumor and the SVC morphology and hemodynamics were observed with the transducer placed in the right supraclavicular region view using Sequoia 512 computed ultrasonograph once every 3 days from the 12th day after the injection, and compared with the ultrasonographic findings before injection. The ultrasonographic findings were also compared with those of CT and autopsy findings, respectively.

3.3 Radiotherapy for rabbits with SVCO due to VX2 tumor injection

Thirteen survived rabbits with SVCO due to VX2 tumor were enrolled in this study. The tumors in mediastina were exposed one minute with 2gy everyday by SIEMNS MEVATRON 6745, which was 10 times in all. Before the radiotherapy and On the 10, 17 and 24 day after radiotherapy, the sizes of the tumor and SVC, SVC velocities and echo characteristics in the 13 rabbits were detected with the transducer placed in the right supraclavicular region using Sequoia 512 computed ultrasonograph. The mediastina neoplasm tissue before and after radiotherapy were sampled for HE staining and TUNEL for analysis of the number of the apoptotic cells.

3.4 Patients

Forty-two patients (26 females and 16 males) with SVCS caused by neoplasm (34 with right upper lung cancer and 8 with mediastinal tumor), aged from 22 to 56 years old were included in this study when they were scheduled for radiotherapy and/or chemotherapy treatment from January 2000 to June 2005. All the patients had upper extremity and facial swelling at initial diagnosis. Twenty volunteers (15 males and 5 females) aged 23-52 years with no history of cardiac and pulmonary diseases were recruited as controls. All informed consents of the patients were acquired.

3.5 Methods of human study

Acuson Sequoia 512 ultrasonograph equipped with7V3C transducer was used. Electrocardiogram and respiratory curve were recorded simultaneously. The following procedures were in accordance with the ethical standards of the committee on human experimentation of the institution and approved by Tangdu Hospital committee.

Right supraclavicular approach. Patients took a supine position. With the transducer placed in the fossa between the sterna and clavicular heads of the sternomastoid muscle, the upper part of the SVC and its adjacent structures were fully displayed.

Subcostal approach. Patients took a supine position. With the transducer placed in the subcostal region, the lower part of SVC was displayed.

The SVC spectra were recorded. The flow velocities of the two forward waves, systolic wave (S) and diastolic wave (D) and the two reversed waves during ventricular and atrial contraction (VR and AR), were measured. The variation of these flow velocities with cardiac cycle and respiration was analyzed with SPSS software. All the patients were followed up for more than 11 months.

4. Results

4.1 The success rate of establishing SVCO rabbit models

Fourteen rabbits were found to have the tumors para-SVC and/or in the SVC cavity by ultrasonography. One rabbit dropped off because no tumor grew until 42nd day after the infusion. The success rate of developing rabbit SVCO model was about 93.33%.

4.2 Two-dimensional ultrasonographic findings of SVCO

The diameters of the tumors were (80.70±4.28) mm. With the tumor growing, the lumen of SVC was deformed and narrowed, and the wall of SVC was disrupted shown by two-dimensional ultrasonography (Figure 1 and 2). The tumor size growth was linearly correlated with time, and the correlation coefficient was 0.9855 (Figure 3). The tumor diameter by ultrasound was similar to the diameter by autopsy ((80.70±4.28mm vs. 82.16±3.41mm, t=0.998, P=0.327405).

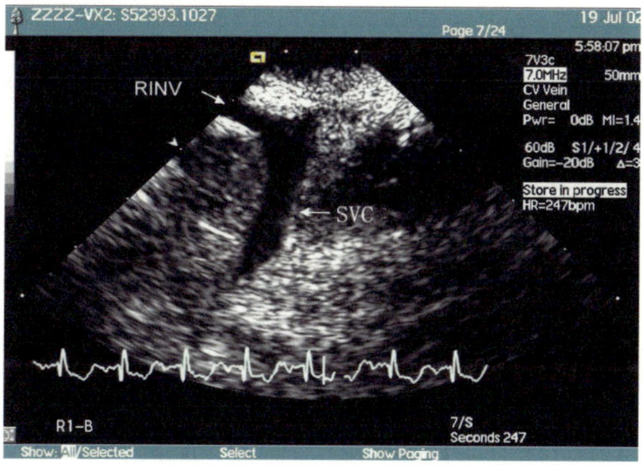

Fig. 1. Two-dimensional ultrasonography of normal SVC

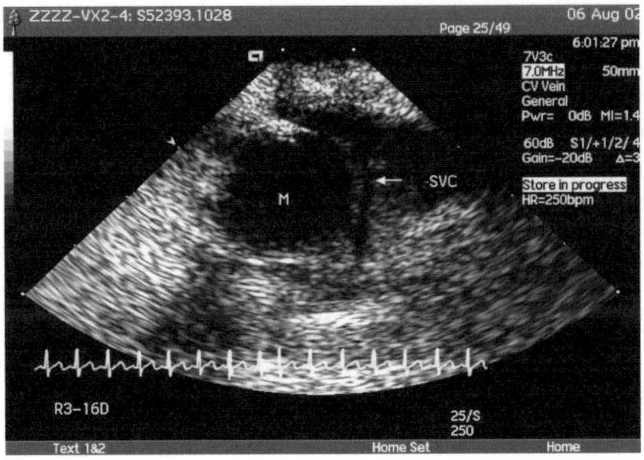

Fig. 2. Two-dimensional ultrasonography of a rabbit with SVCO

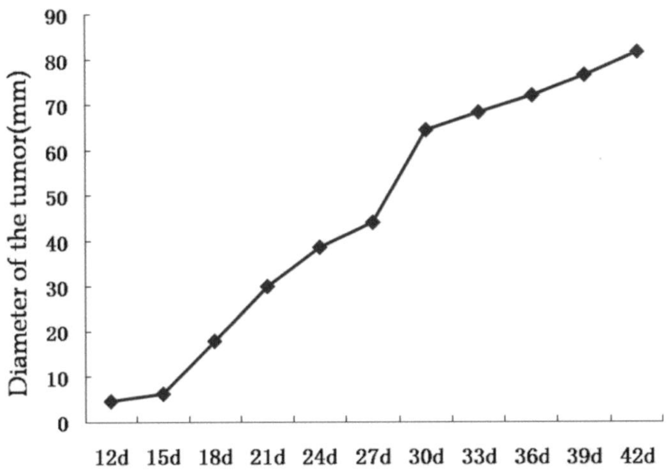

Fig. 3. Tumor growing with time

4.3 SVCO development

All the 14 rabbits developed SVCO. In eight rabbits, SVC was found to be oppressed by two-dimensional ultrasonography on the 15th day after infusion, Aliasing mosaic flow signals and high flow velocity spectra in SVC were demonstrated by Doppler ultrasonography. In another 4 rabbits, the stenotic blood flow velocities were displayed on the 18th day after infusion. In the last 2 rabbits, the abnormal blood flow was seen on the 21st and the 24th day, respectively.

4.4 The different stages of SVCO

The development of SVCO could be divided into three stages. Early stage: About 1 week after. The tumor area was 0.5 cm^2~3cm^2. The echotexture was hpyoechoic and evenly distributed, the shape of the tumor was regular with pseudocapsule. SVC was compressed, but the SVC wall was relatively intact (Figure 4). Mid stage: the tumor area was 3.1 cm^2~6.0

cm^2. Most of the tumors still were hypoechoic echotexture. Hyperechoic textures could be seen within some tumors. T shape of the tumor was not regular. At this stage, the SVC was oppressed and its course became abnormal; the lumen of SVC was narrowed, and the wall was infiltrated by tumors (Figure 5). Late stage: The tumor area reached more than 6.1 cm^2, and the shape was dramatically irregular. Mixing echotexture was seen, but was mainly hypoechoic. SVC was severely oppressed and correlated well with the size of the tumor (Figure 6). The ultrasonographic findings of SVCO at the late stage correlated well with those findings by CT and the autopsy.

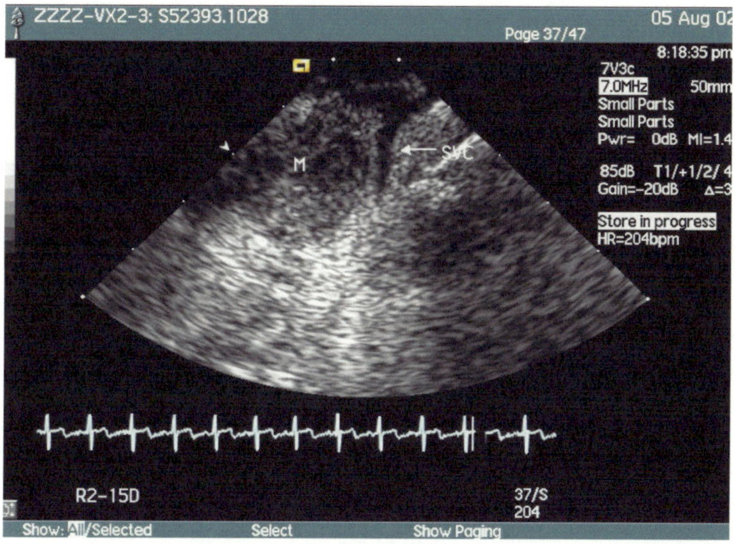

Fig. 4. SVC being compressed by a mass (M) in a rabbit with SVCO. The wall of SVC is intact

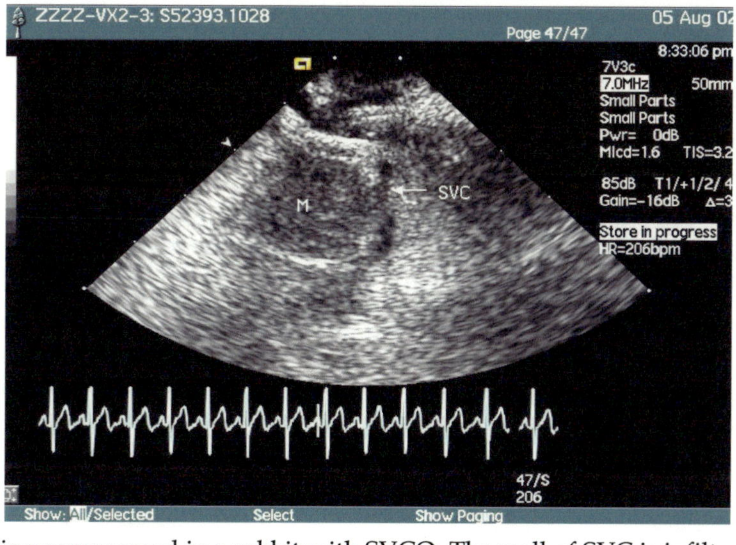

Fig. 5. SVC being compressed in a rabbit with SVCO. The wall of SVC is infiltrated by the mass (M)

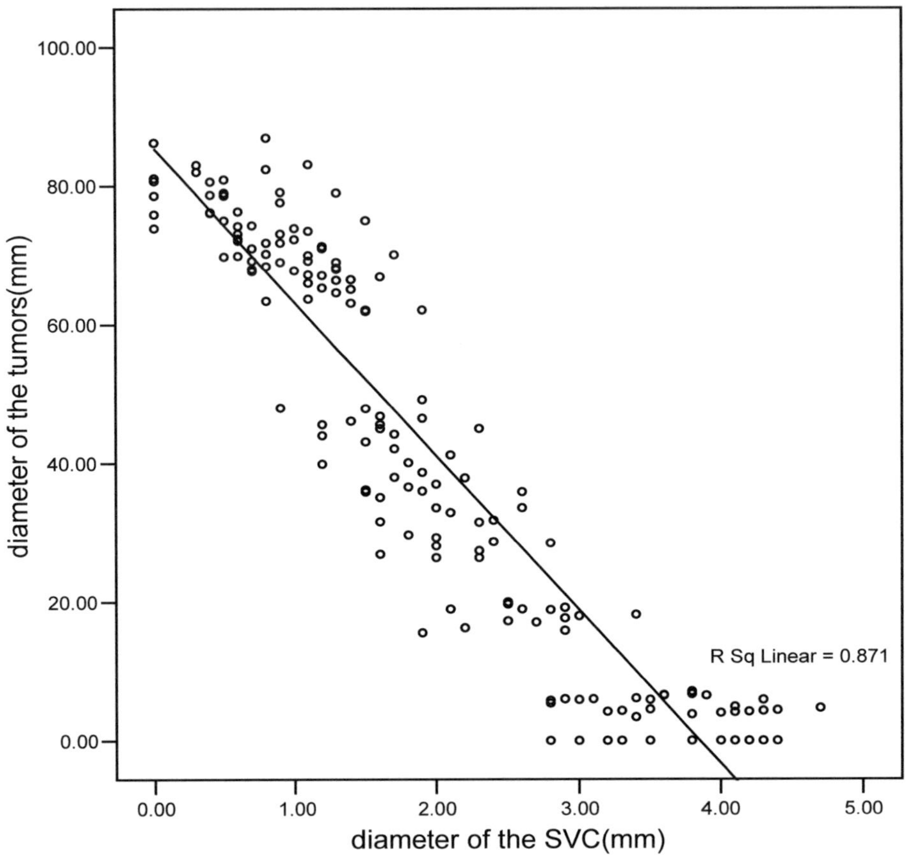

Fig. 6. Relationship between the tumor size and the SVC diameter

4.5 Doppler ultrasonographic findings of SVCO

In SVCO, the color Doppler ultrasound showed mosaic or weak or even no flow signals within SVC (Figure 7). In normal rabbits, the pulsed Doppler ultrasound showed laminar flow in SVC (Figure 8); while in rabbits with SVCO, the SVC flow was turbulent and the spectral window was disappeared (Figure 9). The peak flow velocities of SVC waves were less influenced by respiratory cycle in SVCO compared to normal (Figure 10). SVC flow velocities significantly increased during early and mid stages of SVCO (Table 1).

	S	D	VR	AR
Early and middle stages	78.25±14.97	59.68±13.16	19.22±4.99	17.44±2.67
Late stage	33.71±18.90	33.55±20.03	10.53±3.27	9.33±1.58
T	6.912	4.079	5.450	9.781
P	<0.0001	0.0004	<0.0001	<0.0001

Table 1. SVC flow velocities changes at different stages of SVCO（$\bar{x} \pm s$, cm/s)

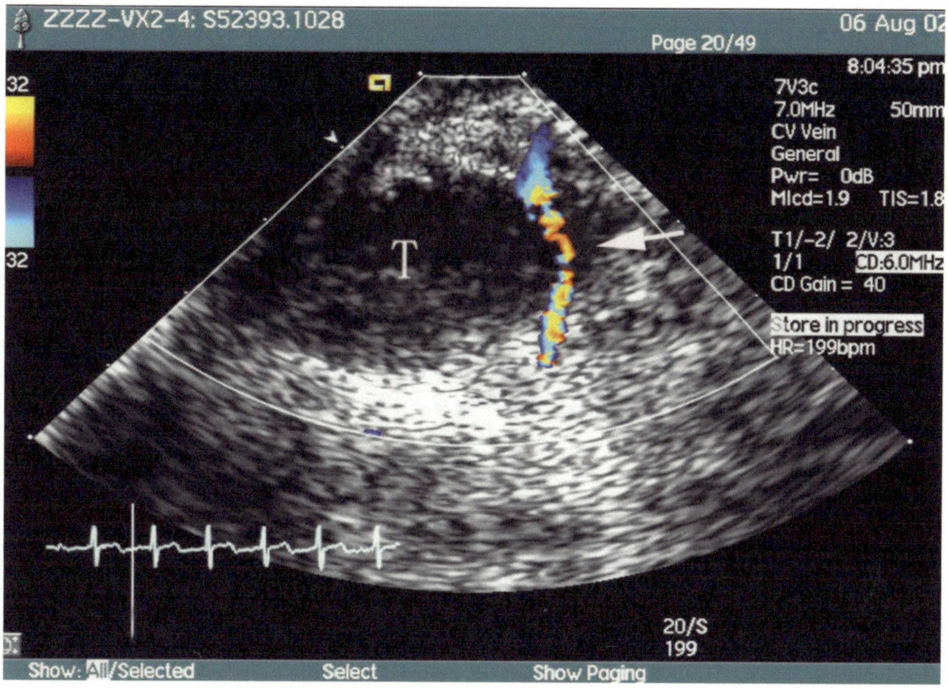

Fig. 7. Mosaic and thread-like color Doppler flow signals were seen in SVC in a rabbit with SVCO by color Doppler ultrasonography. T: tumor

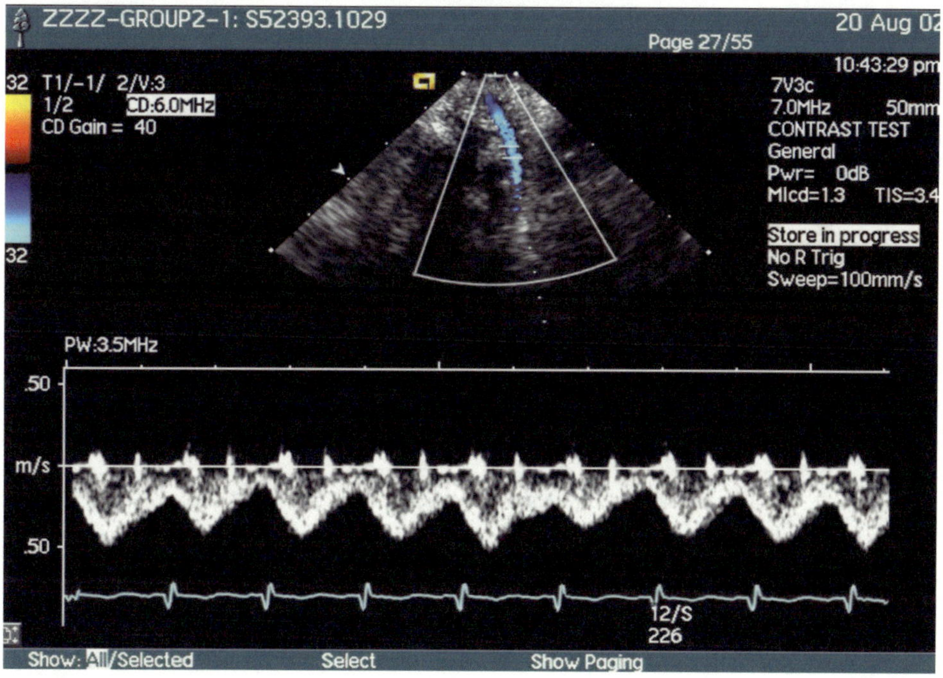

Fig. 8. Normal SVC Doppler flow

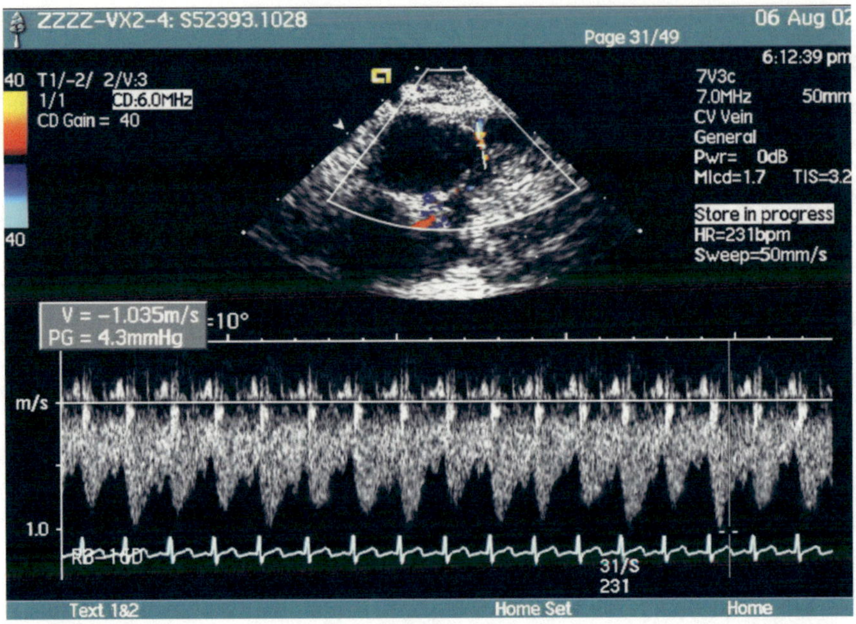

Fig. 9. Increased SVC Flow velocities in the same rabbit as shown in figure 7

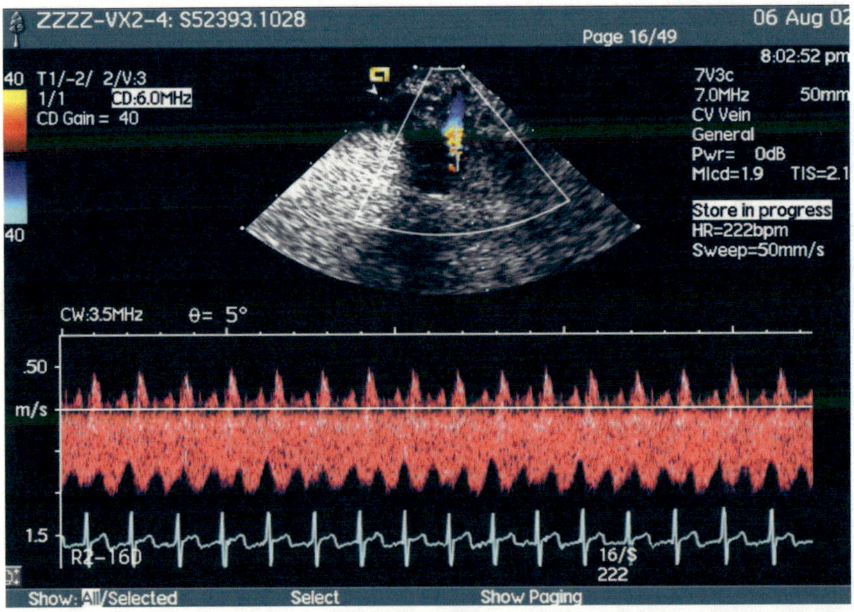

Fig. 10. Peak velocities of SVC waves were less influenced by respiratory cycle than normal

4.6 Evaluation of radiotherapeutic effect in SVCO rabbits

The tumor showed a tendency to get smaller after radiotherapy. The echotexture of the tumor partly turned to be hyperechoic. The diameter of SVC become bigger and the flow velocities decreased at the site of tumor compared with that before the radiotherapy (Figure

11 and 12). The tumor diameter, SVC diameter and velocity changes after radiotherapy were shown in table 2.

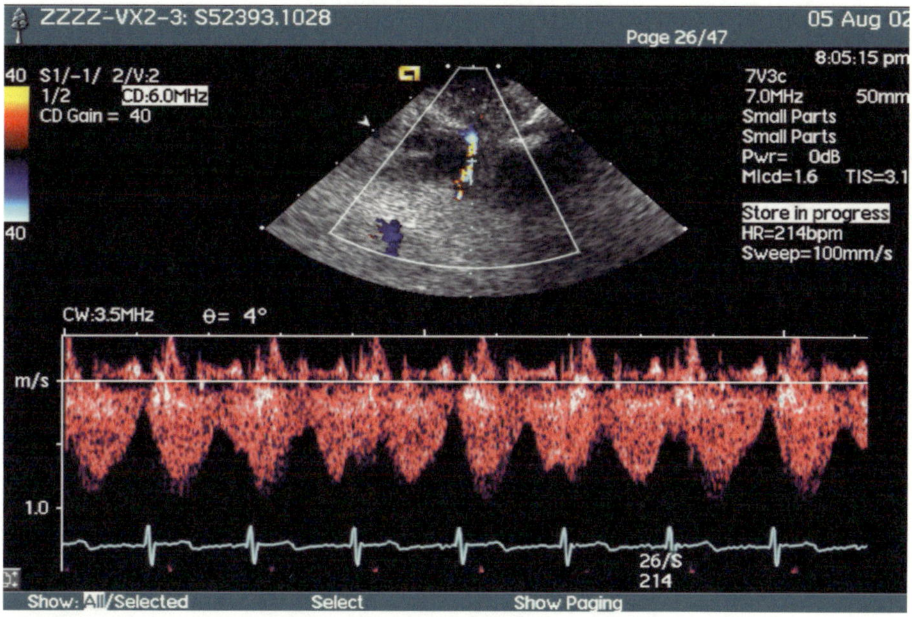

Fig. 11. SVC Doppler flow waveforms before the radiotherapy

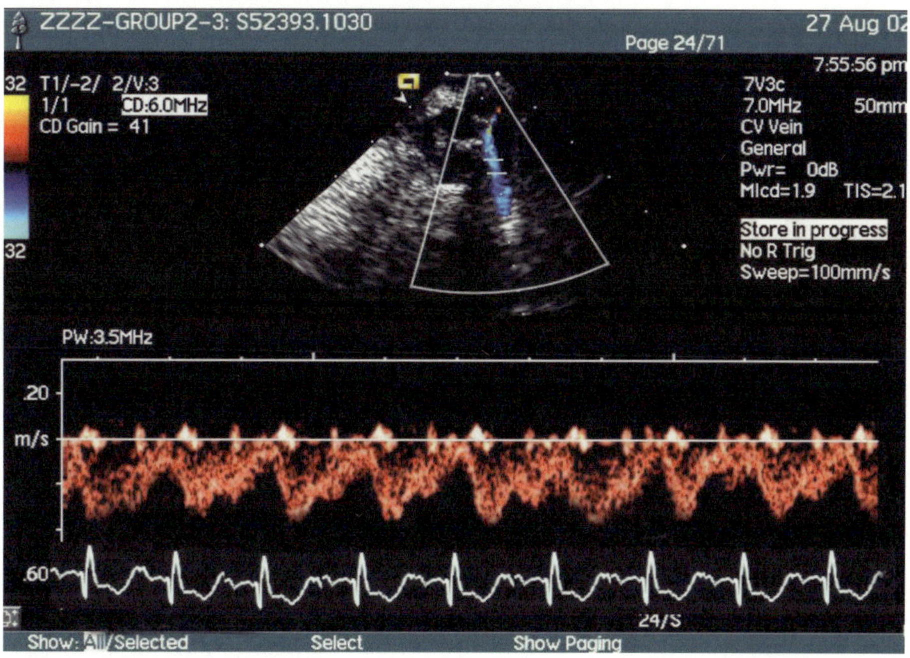

Fig. 12. SVC Doppler flow velocities decreased after radiotherapy from the same patient shown in figure 11

	D1 (mm)	D2(mm)	SysVmax (cm/s)
Before radiotherapy	17.86±1.12	2.65±0.32	87.38±12.94
10d after radiotherapy	17.64±1.08	2.78±0.37	84.65±11.46
17d after radiotherapy	17.13±1.18	2.94±0.93	81.37±11.50
24d after radiotherapy	16.38±1.60	3.23±0.28	77.55±12.34

Table 2. Tumor diameter (D1), SVC diameter (D2) and systolic maximal flow velocity (SysVmax) changes after radiotherapy

HE staining and TUNEL assay showed that the number of apoptotic cells in the tumor was much more than that before the radiotherapy (Figure 13& 14) ($P<0.01$).

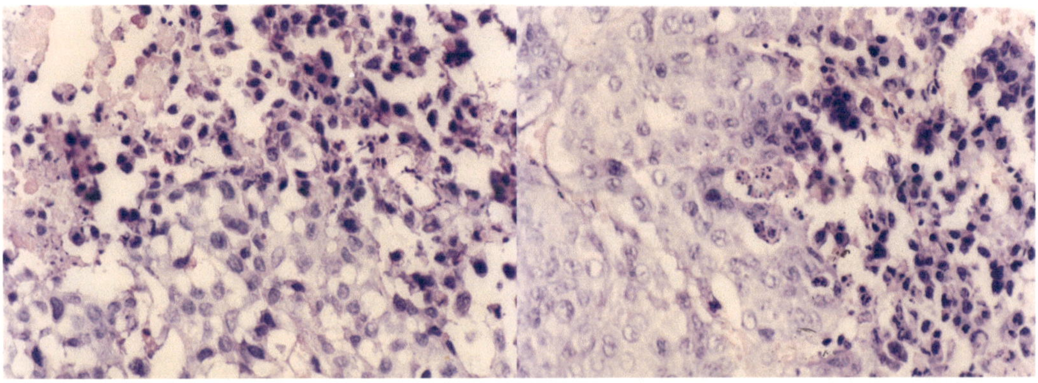

Fig. 13. HE staining showing that the apoptotic cells increased after radiotherapy (Right) compared to those before (Left)

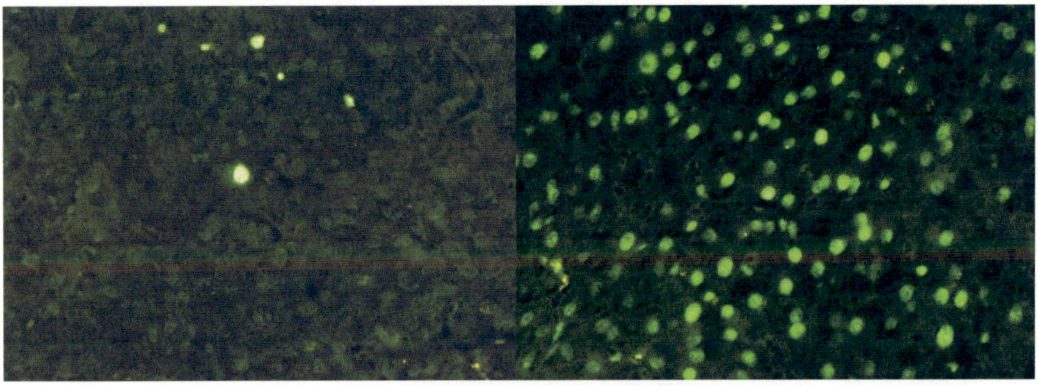

Fig. 14. TUNEL assay showing that the apoptotic cells increased after radiotherapy (Right) compared to those before (Left)

4.7 SVC Doppler flow in patients with SVCS

Different from healthy subjects, where laminar flow was demonstrated (Figure 15), the SVC flow spectra in patients with mild SVCS showed turbulent flow (Figure 16) and the spectral window was disappeared. In patients with moderate degree of SVCS, the distinct biphasic forward waves (S- and D-waves) of SVC were lost (Figure 17). In addition, we found that the smaller of the VR- and AR-waves were, the farther the oppressed segment of SVC was away from the right atrium.

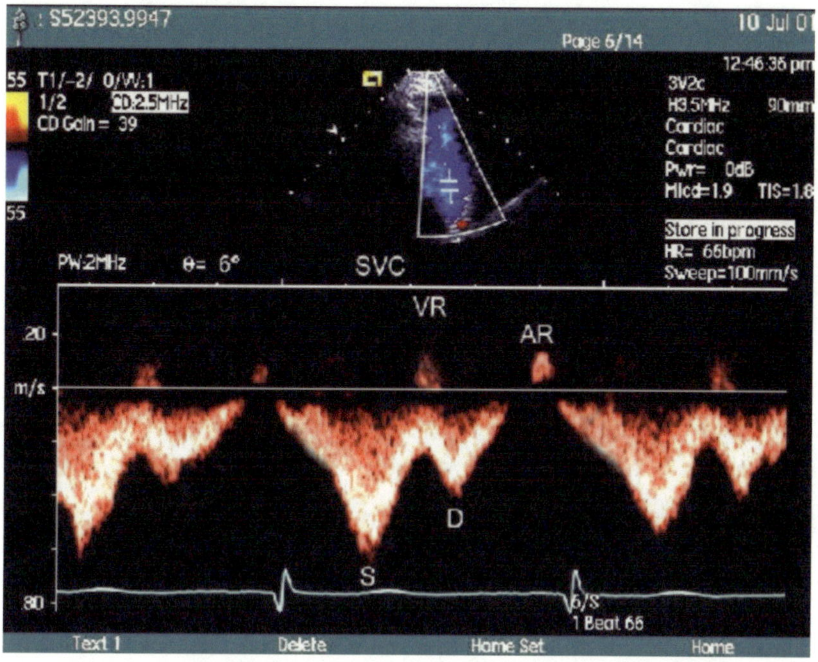

Fig. 15. SVC Doppler flow spectra in healthy subjects. Doppler interrogation of the SVC shows systolic and diastolic phases of flow (S- and D-waves) toward the heart and late ventricular systolic and atrial systolic phases of backward flow (VR- and AR-waves)

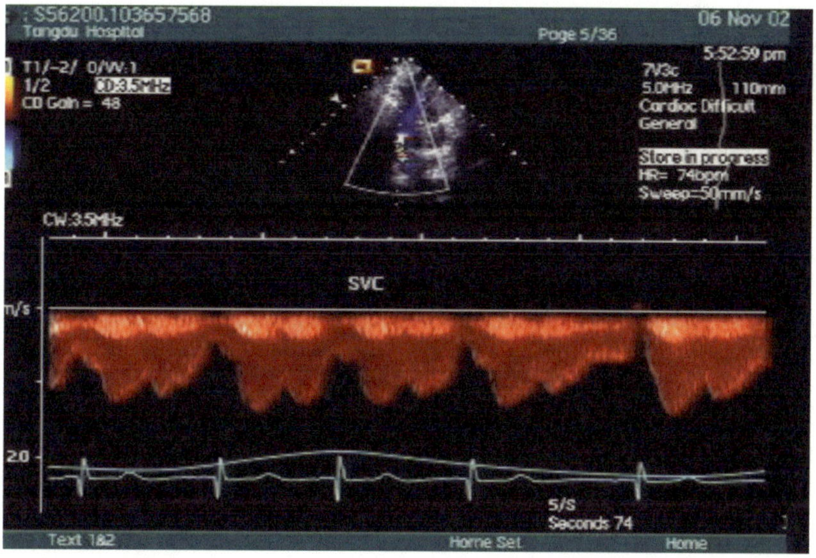

Fig. 16. SVC Doppler flow spectra in mild SVCS. The forward waves showed high velocity and no distinct spectral window

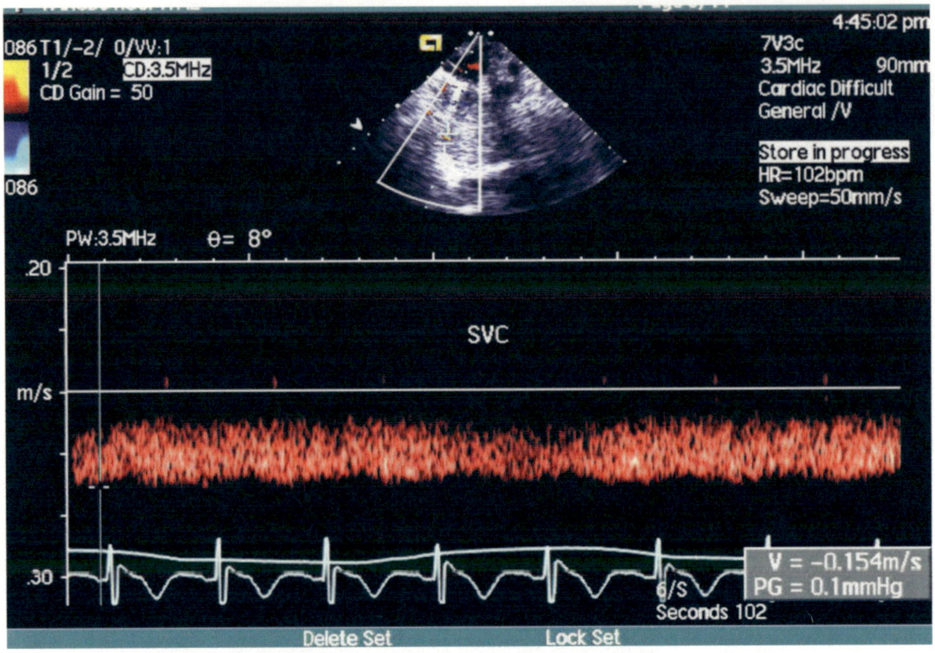

Fig. 17. SVC Doppler flow spectra in severe SVCS. The S, D AR, and VR waves could not be identified

The RVI in SVCS group were much lower than those in the control group (S-wave: 1.9±3.6 % vs.16.34±8.96%, P = 0.0003; D-wave: 2.80±1.23% vs. 26.32±42%, P =0.0087). After treatment, the flow velocities of SVC decreased significantly with each month and the RVI was significantly increased compared to those before the treatment.

5. Comments

The animal study demonstrated that SVCO rabbit model could be easily established transcutaneously with the guidance of ultrasound. With VX2 tumor growing, SVC was oppressed and/or infiltrated by the tumor tissues and ultimately resulted in the blockage of the SVC, and developed SVCO. The pathogenesis of SVCO in rabbits was similar to that of SVCO in humans, indicating that this rabbit model of SVCO caused by VX2 tumor could be an ideal model of SVCO.

Two-dimensional ultrasonography could be used to demonstrate the morphologic changes of the tumor and SVC. Color Doppler could sensitively detect the abnormal blood flow of SVC in rabbits with SVCO. It could be mosaic, weak or even no flow signals depending on the different stages and severity of SVCO. Doppler flow spectra of SVC showed less respiratory influences on the flow velocities in rabbits with SVCO.

Linear accelerator radiotherapy could lead to cell apoptosis of the VX2 tumor transplanted besides SVC. HE staining and TUNEL assay showed increased number of apoptotic cells of the tumor tissue compared to that before radiotherapy. With the apoptosis of the tumor cells, the echotexture of the tumor partly turned to be hyperechoic and the tumor itself was getting smaller. Thereby the oppression severity of the SVC was decreased, the diameter of SVC was getting bigger, and finally the obstruction was getting resolved.

With the release of the obstruction after radiotherapy, the respiratory variation of the SVC Doppler flow velocities could be recovered and the peak flow velocities of SVC decreased gradually after the treatment shown by Doppler ultrasonography. However, the tumor size, SVC diameter and the flow velocity could not completely get back to normal after treatment. This suggests that Linear accelerator radiotherapy could not inactivate VX2 tumor completely, which might be related to the high grade of malignancy, poor proliferation of the VX2 tumors.

The human study demonstrates that respiratory variations of SVC Doppler flow velocities are significantly decreased in patients with SVCS, but could be recovered gradually after treatment, indicating that respiratory variations of Doppler flow changes of SVC correlate well with the severity of SVCS, and may be used to assess the therapeutic effects of SVCS.

The SVC Doppler flow patterns in patients with SVCS were characterized with fill-in and broaden spectra, nondistinct outlines. The D-wave was unable to return to the baseline at end diastole, which was consistent with previous studies (Yano&Shimada, 1997). When the patients' condition improved after treatment, , the pressure gradient at the stenotic segment of SVC also decreased, indicating that SVC hemodynamic changes was in accordance with the clinical courses of SVCS (Behar et al., 2001; Tighe et al., 2000).

It has been well known that, respiration had significant influence on SVC flow velocities in healthy subjects. The S- and D-wave peak velocities are much greater on inspiration compared with those on expiration because the decreased intrathoracic pressures during inspiration causes increased venous return (Jellinek et al., 2000; Vieillard et al., 2001). In patients with SVCS, However, the obstruction prevents the conduction of the intrathoracic pressure changes into the right atrium and to SVC, resulting in decreased or even diminished respiratory variations of S- and D-wave flow velocities. Once this obstruction is released after treatment, the SVC Doppler flow velocities would decrease and the respiratory variations of these flow velocities would be back.

6. Conclusions

Rabbit model of SVCO caused by VX2 tumor could be an ideal model of SVCO for clinical study. Doppler ultrasound is the first method of choice for assessing the hemodynamics of SVCO.

Normally, respiration had significant influence on SVC morphology and dynamics in healthy subjects. This influence would become less in the patients with SVCS, suggesting that SVC Doppler spectra could reflect the severity of SVCS.

7. References

Behar DM., Reisner SA., Ben-Ami H (2001). Superior vena cava syndrome diagnosed by transesophageal echocardiography. *Isr Med Assoc J*, Vol 3, No.6, pp. 457–460.

De Crespigny AJ., Howard D., D'Arceuil H., et al (1999). Dynamic contrast-enhanced MRI of Implanted VX2 tumors in rabbit muscle: comparison of Gd-DTPA and NMS60. *Magn Reson Imaging,*Vol. 17, No. 9, pp. 1297-1305.

Goldberg SN., Walovitch RC., Straub JA., et al (1999). Radio-frequency-induced coagulation necrosis in rabbits: immediate detection at US with a synthetic microsphere contrast agent. *Radiology, Vol.* 213, No. 2, pp. 438-444.

Ishida H., Murata N., Yamada H., et al (2000). Pneumoperitoneum with carbon dioxide enhances liver metastases of cancer cells implanted into the portal vein in rabbits. *Surg Endosc*, Vol 14, No. 3, pp. 239-242.

Jellinek H., Krenn H., Oczenski W, et al (2000). Influence of positive airway pressure on the pressure gradient for venous return in humans. *J Appl Physiol,* Vol 88, No.3, pp. 926–932.

Kim TK., Choi BI., Park SW., et al (2000). Gadolinium mesoporphyrin as an MR imaging contrast agent in the evaluation of tumors: an experimental model of VX2 carcinoma in rabbits. *Am J Roentgenol,* Vol 175, No. 1, pp. 227-234.

Liu JB., Goldberg BB., Merton DA., et al (2001). The role of contrast-enhanced sonography for radiofrequency ablation of liver tumors. *J Ultrasound Med,* Vol 20, No. 5, pp. 517-523.

Tighe DA., Paul JJ., Huhta JC (2000). Superior vena caval syndrome: color flow Doppler detection of collateral venous channels. *J Am Soc Echocardiogr*, Vol 13, No. 8, pp. 780–784.

Vieillard Baron A., Augarde R., Prin S., et al (2001). Influence of superior vena caval zone condition on cyclic changes in right ventricular outflow during respiratory support. *Anesthesiology*, Vol 95, No. 5, pp. 1083–1088.

Yano S., Shimada K (1997). Changes in superior vena cava pulsed Doppler flow patterns: Possible indicator of improvement of superior vena cava syndrome due to lung cancer. *Ultrasound Med*, Vol 16, No. 10, pp. 707–710.

2

The use of Tricuspid Annular Plane Systolic Excursion and Tissue Doppler Imaging Velocities for the Estimation of Pulmonary Hypertension and Right Ventricular Function in Mechanically Ventilated Patients

Vasilios Papaioannou and Ioannis Pneumatikos
Democritus University of Thrace, Alexandroupolis Hospital, Intensive Care Unit
Greece

1. Introduction

Right ventricular (RV) function can be seriously compromised due to either left ventricular (LV) failure or severe pulmonary hypertension (PH) and pulmonary vascular dysfunction of extra-cardiac origin, especially in critically ill patients, and can be associated with worse prognosis. Echocardiography in the Intensive Care Unit (ICU) can provide significant information to the caregivers, when confronted with a patient with unexplained hemodynamic instability. However, right ventricular echocardiographic assessment can be a challenge in day-to-day clinical practice in the ICU, mostly because of complex interactions between mechanical ventilation, fluid balance and critical illness *per se,* whereas right-to-left interdependence can lead to significant hemodynamic collapse in patients with severe respiratory diseases, septic cardiomyopathy or pulmonary embolism. Finally, the complex geometry of the chamber in association with lack of optimal visualization may limit the accuracy of conventional variables, which have bee proven to be reliable in other clinical settings. For the above reasons, novel indices have been adopted for easier, highly reproducible and less variable evaluation of RV function, such as the tricuspid annular plane systolic excursion (TAPSE) and the Tissue Doppler Imaging (TDI) velocities of tricuspid valve. Their accuracy has already been tested in patients with cardiovascular diseases. Nevertheless, their adoption as monitoring tools in critically ill patients under mechanical ventilation remains to be established. In this chapter we will review the different areas of application of TAPSE and TDI velocities and try to discuss their possible potential as accurate and reproducible diagnostic and prognostic techniques in adult critical care.

2. Conventional hemodynamic measurements in ICU

The pulmonary circulation is a high-flow and low-resistance system. Contrary to the left ventricle (LV) the thin-walled right ventricle (RV) cannot easily tolerate acute increase in afterload, leading to acute distention, paradoxic intra-ventricular septal movement and consequently, reduced LV filling and cardiac output (CO) (Pinsky, 2002, 2007; Sibbald & Driedger, 1983). Due to ventricular interdependence superficial myocardial fibers enrich both LV and RV. As a result, the two ventricles share the septum and are contained within the same pericardial cavity, explaining the decrease in LV output during positive pressure ventilation and application of different levels of positive end-expiratory pressure (PEEP) (Taylor et al., 1967; Fellahi et al., 1998).

Right ventricular dysfunction is common in critically ill patients. Any cause of RV pressure overload such as pulmonary hypertension (PH) or reduced RV contractility, such as RV infarction, sepsis, cardiomyopathy, myocarditis and pericardial disease may lead to RV failure in patients during their stay in Intensive Care Unit (Bunnell & Parrillo, 1996; Parker et al., 1990). Furthermore, pulmonary vascular dysfunction is associated with many disease processes in the ICU setting, whereas pulmonary embolism (PE) and acute respiratory distress syndrome (ARDS) are considered the two main causes of acute *cor pulmonale* (ACP) in adults (Jardin et al., 1985; Vieillard-Barron et al., 2002). The elevation in pulmonary vascular resistance (PVR) can increase the transpulmonary gradient and lead to RV failure. For these reasons, adequate assessment of RV function is very important, especially in hemodynamic unstable patients, since the presence of RV dysfunction may alter treatment and has severe impact upon final outcome (Beaulieu & Marik, 2005).

Pulmonary hypertension is defined at right heart catheterization with resting pulmonary artery systolic pressure (PASP) exceeding 35 mmHg, whereas absence of echocardiographic evidence of increased left atrial pressure or pulmonary artery occlusion pressure (PAOP) < 15 mmHg, obtained through a pulmonary artery catheter (PAC), describes PH associated with primary pulmonary disease (Rubin, 1997; Berger et al., 1985). The gold standard for the diagnosis of pulmonary hypertension and RV dysfunction in ICU is considered to be the pulmonary artery catheterization (Price et al., 2010). However, different studies have shown that assessment of PASP, LV and RV with PAC seems to be inaccurate in patients under mechanical ventilatory support, whereas overall outcomes are not improved when the PAC is used in general in critically ill patients (Vieillard-Barron et al., 2002; Price et al., 2010; Hadian & Pinsky, 2006).

For the above reasons, the role of both transthoracic and transesophageal echocardiography is increasingly recognized in assessing both RV and LV function in critically ill patients, providing significant information regarding RV geometry in different clinical scenarios. Normally, RV systolic function can be quantified using the right ventricular function area change (RVFAC) and ejection fraction (RVEF), whereas RV dilatation can be estimated by measuring RV end-diastolic area (RVEDA) in the long axis, from an apical four-chamber view. The ratio between RVEDA and LVEDA is one of the best ways to assess RV distention and quantify pressure and volume overload. A ratio ≥ 0.6 corresponds to moderate dilatation whereas a ratio ≥ 1 reflects a severe RV dysfunction (Jurcut et al., 2010). Moreover, in cases of severe RV overload, the septum becomes flat (in diastole indicating volume overload and in systole when there is pressure overload) and the LV takes the 'D' shape, limiting LV preload. In addition, the pulmonary pressures can be calculated using the modified Bernoulli equation by estimating the systolic-pressure gradient across the tricuspid valve and after measuring right atrial pressure (RAP) (Jurcut et al., 2010; Kaul et al., 1984).

2.1 Common limitations of traditional echo-derived measurements in ICU

However, the presence of tricuspid regurgitation (TR) varies among studies, based on different levels of severity of pulmonary hypertension. Furthermore, narrow acoustic windows due to lung hyperinflation or marked respiratory variations in intrathoracic pressure, particularly in patients with severe lung disease, may limit the ability to detect an adequate TR jet (Berger et al., 1985; Arcasoy et al., 2003). In a cohort study of 374 lung transplant candidates with a prevalence of pulmonary hypertension around 25%, it was found that estimation of pulmonary artery systolic pressure by echocardiography was frequently inaccurate, compared with data derived from right heart catheterization, leading to considerable overdiagnosis of pulmonary hypertension (Arcasoy et al., 2003).

Another possible limitation for PASP estimation with pulse wave (PW) Doppler is associated with the method used for RAP assessment. Right atrial pressure depends not only on RV preload but also on pleural pressures transmitted to the right atrium, leading to differences between intravascular and transmural pressures under mechanical ventilation. Only a few studies have evaluated different echo-derived measures for the assessment of RAP in mechanically ventilated patients (Lichtenstein & Jardin, 1994; Yock & Popp, 1984). Different techniques for calculating inferior vena cava (IVC) diameter have been proposed to impact on accuracy of RAP estimation (Bendjelid et al., 2003). The method that seems more accurate was developed by Lichtenstein, and calculates IVC diameter longitudinally at end-expiration and end-diastole and during the R wave on electrocardiogram (ECG), 2 cm before the right atrium and with the M-mode on short axis view (Lichtenstein & Jardin, 1994). The estimation of RAP using IVC diameter and its respiratory collapse has been shown to correlate better with central venous pressure (CVP) in patients with RV dysfunction and PH (Mintz et al., 1981). It seems that since the normal respiratory augmentation in venous return is limited by RV enlargement, normal IVC diameter variations are reduced, increasing diagnostic accuracy of this technique. Furthermore, measurement of distensibility index of IVC has been proposed for RAP calculation in mechanically ventilated patients (Barbier et al., 2004). Finally, traditional echocardiographic indices, such as RVFAC, are time-consuming and not always easy to perform because of difficulties to well delineate the RV endocardial border.

3. Estimation of TAPSE and RV TDI velocities in different clinical studies

For the above reasons, different methods have been suggested for echo-Doppler derived diagnosis of pulmonary hypertension and assessment of RV function in patients under mechanical ventilatory support, such as Tricuspid Annular Plane Systolic Excursion (TAPSE) calculation (Kaul et al., 1984; Hammarstrom et al., 1991) and recently, the ratio of peak tricuspid regurgitant velocity (TRV, ms) to the right ventricular outflow tract time-velocity integral (TVI_{RVOT}, cm) that seems to accurately determines pulmonary vascular resistance (Abbas et al., 2003).

Moreover, tissue Doppler imaging (TDI) techniques that measure velocities of cardiac tissue have been studied for the assessment of left ventricular diastolic function in the ICU (Combes et al., 2004; Vignon et al., 2008), whereas only a limited number of researchers have investigated their diagnostic accuracy on right ventricular (RV) dysfunction, in different clinical settings (Meluzin et al., 2001; Sundereswaran et al., 1998; Moustapha et al., 2001).

Finally, an increased ratio of RV diameter to tissue Doppler velocity of tricuspid annular motion has been suggested by others as useful predictor of pulmonary hypertension (McLean et al., 2007)

3.1 Calculation of TAPSE in cardiovascular patients

Since RV muscle fiber orientation results in a contraction that occurs predominantly along the longitudinal plane, systolic displacement of the tricuspid annulus toward the RV apex closely correlates with right ventricular fractional area change. TAPSE as a measure of RV base-to-apex shortening during systole is recorded on M-mode using the 2D four-chamber view. The cursor is placed to the junction of tricuspid valve plan with the free wall of the RV, whereas data are averaged over five beats (Figures 1 & 2). Normal values for TAPSE are 15-20 mm (Price et al., 2010; Meluzin et al., 2001; Lang et al., 2005).

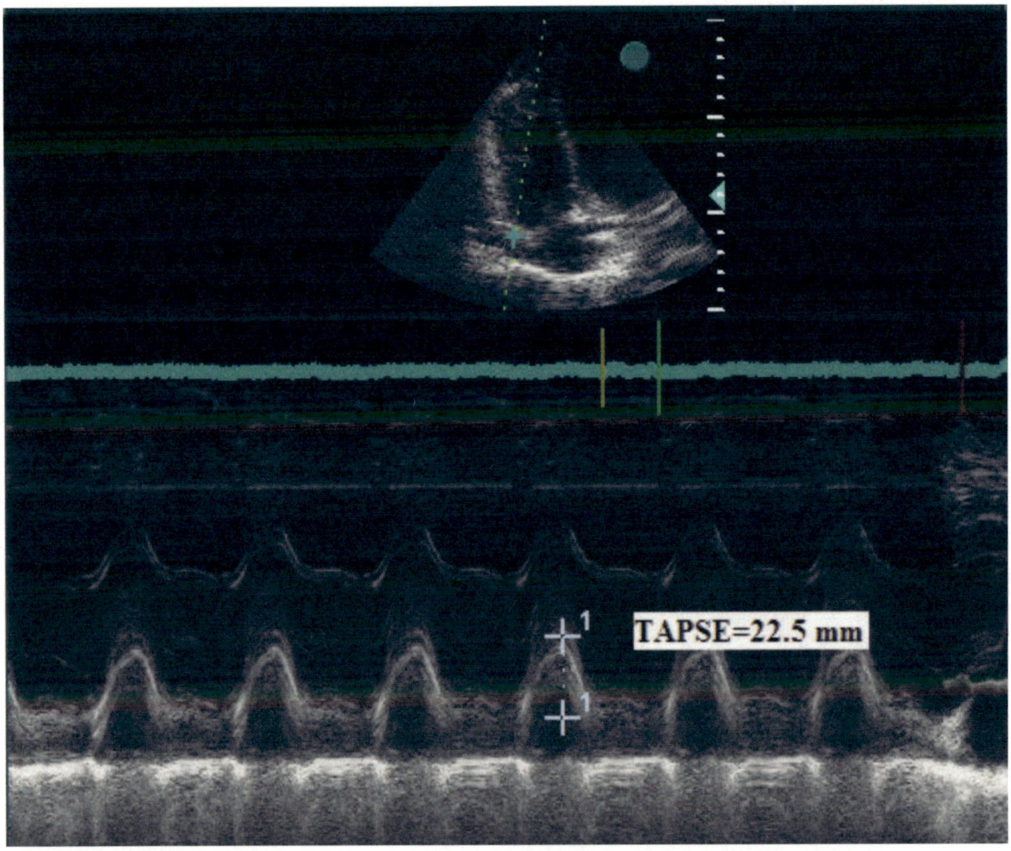

Fig. 1. Measurement of tricuspid annular plane systolic excursion (TAPSE)

TAPSE calculation in a patient under spontaneous respiration by M-mode, using the 2D four-chamber view. The cursor was placed to the junction of tricuspid valve (TV) plan with the free wall of the right ventricle (RV), whereas data were averaged over five beats. In this case, TAPSE value is normal (22.5 mm).

Samad assessed TAPSE in patients after a first myocardial infarction and showed that values ≤ 15 mm were associated with increased mortality (45% at 2 years) compared with patients having TAPSE > 20 mm (4%) (Samad et al., 2002). Kaul and coworkers found that TAPSE was more closely related with the RV area change during systole compared with radionuclide estimation of RV ejection fraction (Kaul et al., 1984). Both of these studies have shown that TAPSE is decreased in patients with depressed right ventricular function (RVFAC< 25%), whereas low TAPSE values have been found to predict a poor outcome in patients with dilated cardiomyopathy and pulmonary hypertension (Ghio et al., 2000; Forfia et al., 2006). In 63 patients with PH, Forfia and colleagues found that a TAPSE ≤ 18 mm was associated with greater RV systolic dysfunction (RVFAC 24 vs 33%), right heart remodeling and RV-LV disproportion (RVEDA / LVEDA: 1.7 vs 1.2). In addition, for every 1-mm decrease in TAPSE, the unadjusted risk of death increased by 17%, which persisted after adjusting for other hemodynamic and echocardiographic measurements and treatment regimens. Finally, one year survival in patients with TAPSE of 18 mm or greater was 94% versus 60% in subjects with TAPSE less than 18 mm, respectively.

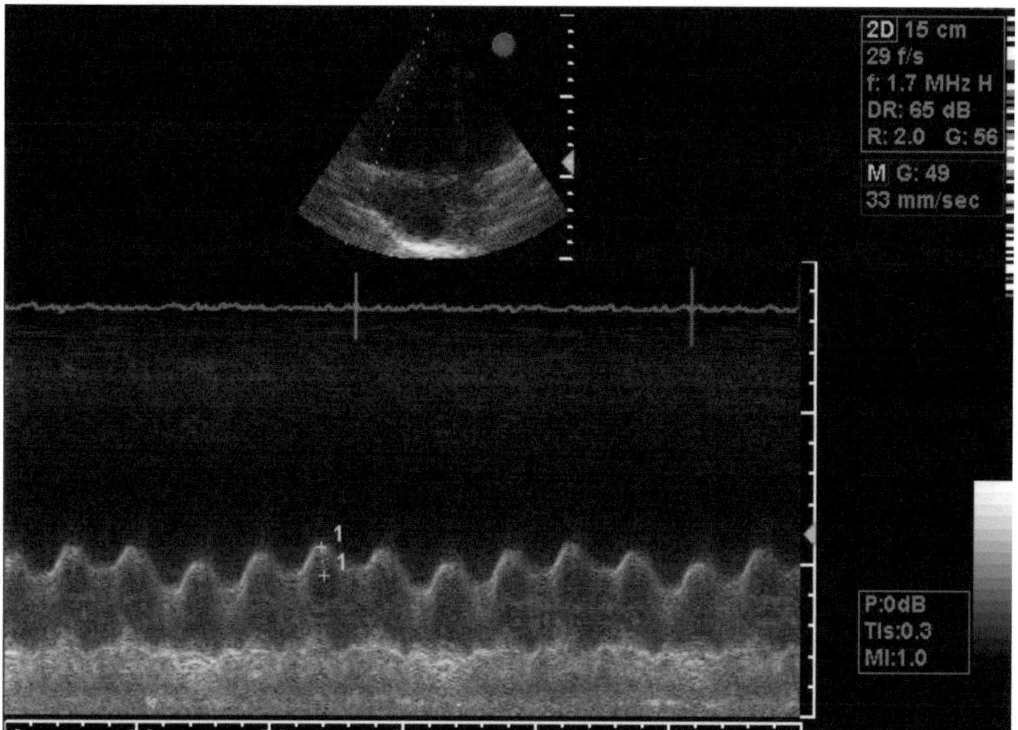

Fig. 2. TAPSE calculation. in a mechanically ventilated patient with severe pulmonary hypertension and RV failure due to acute respiratory distress syndrome (ARDS). TAPSE values were 9.8 mm

In conclusion, patients with normal LV function and depressed TAPSE have increased pulmonary vascular resistance, reflecting afterload at the level of proximal pulmonary arteries. The increase in RV filling pressure and a trend toward a reduction in TAPSE can also be signs of right ventricular function deterioration in cases of preload increase and a reduction in contractility. We have observed a decrease in TAPSE during a trial of separation from mechanical ventilation (weaning trial) in a cohort of medical critically ill patients with different diagnoses of admission, associated with increase in RV preload that was estimated with RVEDA, probably due to augmented venous return during spontaneous negative pressure ventilation (unpublished data).

3.2 Use of Tricuspid annular tissue Doppler imaging in cardiovascular patients

Tissue Doppler is superior to blood flow Doppler as it reflects directly myocardial function and is less subject to preload changes. TDI imaging has been used for differentiating different levels of PASP and for assessing left and right ventricular systolic and diastolic functions (Isaaz, 2000, 2002). Low values of systolic (Sm) and diastolic [Em (early) & Am (late atrial)] velocities have been proposed to reflect systolic and diastolic RV dysfunction, respectively (Waggoner & Bierig, 2001). Figures 3 & 4 demonstrate TDI measurements at the level of tricuspid valve in two patients with normal PASP and RV function and pulmonary hypertension with RV failure, respectively.

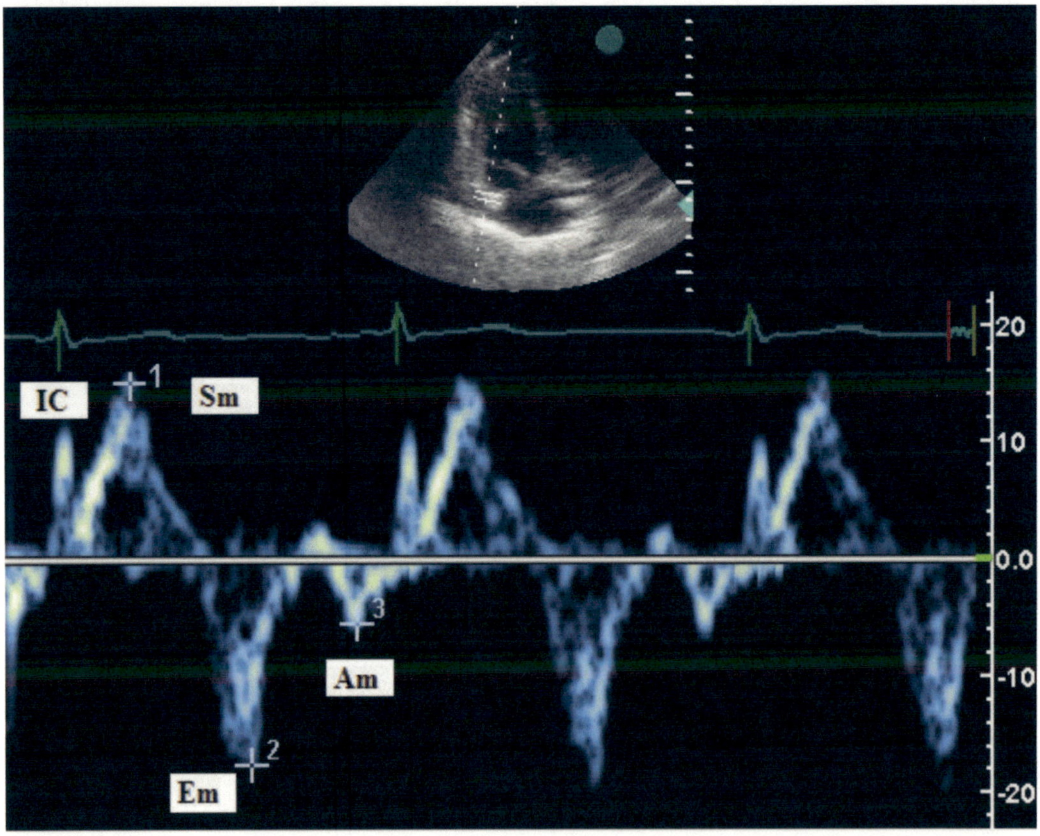

Fig. 3. Tissue Doppler Imaging (TDI) velocities of tricuspid valve.
After placing the cursor at the junction of the RV free wall and the anterior leaflet of the tricuspid valve, using the 2D four-chamber view. The systolic phase consists of two waves: 1. the first peak represents isovolumic contraction (IC) and 2. the second peak represents systole (Sm). Sm (1): Peak systolic velocity at the anterior leaflet of TV (15 cm/sec), Em (2): peak early diastolic velocity at the anterior leaflet of TV (18 cm/sec), Am (3): peak late diastolic (atrial) velocity at the anterior leaflet of tricuspid valve (6 cm/sec)

Meluzin J has shown that RV TDI systolic annular velocity correlated with RVFAC, assessed using radionuclide angiography and with prognosis, in 44 patients with LV heart failure (Meluzin, 2001, 2005). Moreover, a systolic annular velocity of less than 11.5 cm/sec predicted right ventricular dysfunction (RVEF < 45%) with a sensitivity of 90% and specificity of 85%. Dokainish has found that RV TDI systolic annular velocity detected mild degrees of RV dysfunction not yet apparent from visual assessment and concluded that Sm was an independent predictor of cardiac death or rehospitalization (Dokainish et al., 2007). Saxena demonstrated that the peak systolic tricuspid annular velocity (Sm) obtained from TDI measurements was able to determine RV systolic function, regardless of pulmonary artery pressures and was strongly correlated with both RVFAC and TAPSE, in 52 patients with varying degrees of pulmonary hypertension (Saxena et al., 2006). Similar results were found in a cohort of 22 heart transplant recipients, supporting that both Sm and TAPSE might be clinically useful for RV function determination (Doutreleau et al., 2007).

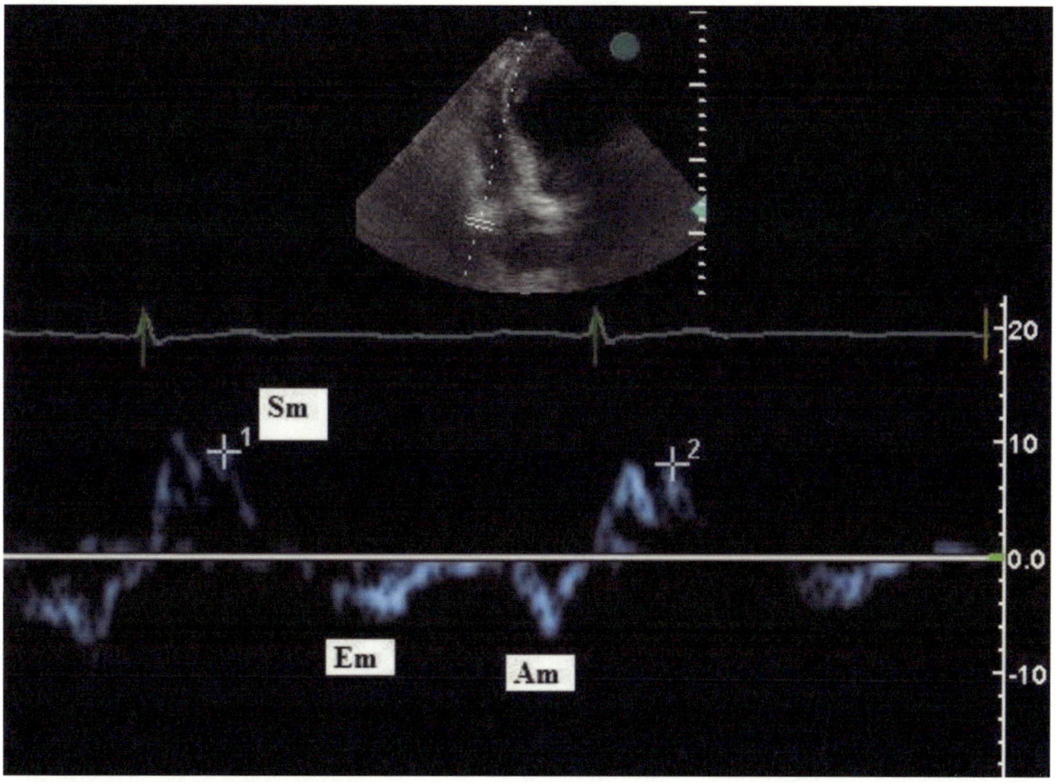

Fig. 4. Pulsed-wave tissue Doppler imaging (TDI) velocities of tricuspid valve in a patient with pulmonary hypertension and severe RV failure.
In this case, there is significant decrease in both systolic [Sm (1,2): 8-9 cm/sec] and diastolic velocities (Em, Am), indicating severe systolic and diastolic right ventricular dysfunction

3.3 Use of TAPSE and Tricuspid annular tissue Doppler imaging in the ICU

Recently, Sade showed that in ICU patients (35% under mechanical ventilation) the E (from the trans-tricuspid flow) /Em ratio was strongly correlated with right atrial pressure (Sade et al., 2007), whereas Denault proposed an algorithm for the diagnosis and classification of RV diastolic function during weaning from cardio-pulmonary bypass, based on a combination of indices derived from pulsed-wave Doppler of the tricuspid valve, hepatic vein flow and tricuspid annulus TDI velocities(Denault et al., 2005).

In a recent study we demonstrated that TAPSE and RV TDI velocities obtained by 2D echocardiography were significantly correlated with E/e' (transmitral early wave and mitral annulus motion ratio at its lateral aspect), left ventricular ejection fraction (LVEF), RVFAC, PASP and length of ventilatory support in a cohort of 32 mechanically ventilated patients with acute pulmonary edema (Papaioannou et al., 2010). Furthermore, these indices were proven to discriminate successfully patients with different duration of weaning. Liberation from mechanical ventilation can impose a significant load upon the cardiovascular system, especially in patients with heart disease. The shift from positive to negative intrathoracic pressure can augment venous return and central blood volume, increasing left ventricular preload and afterload. Moreover, high levels of catecholamines may reduce supply of oxygen to the heart due to tachycardia and decrease cardiac output due to increased pulmonary and vascular resistance (Lemaire et al., 1988).

Different studies in mechanically ventilated patients have confirmed that increased pulmonary artery systolic and occlusion pressures during weaning trials are associated with weaning failure (Schmidt et al., 1997 & Delooz, 1976) whereas only one study using echocardiography investigated the relation between the echo-derived index E/e' and PAOP during liberation from the ventilator, in patients without pre-existing heart diseases (Lamia et al., 2009). However, baseline filling pressures have not been proven to successfully predict weaning outcome (Lemaire et al., 1988 & Jubran et al., 1998), whereas early assessment of weaning readiness with echocardiography during the course of mechanical ventilation had not been studied previously. The direct correlations that were found in our study between low TAPSE and RV TDI velocities with LVEF reflect systolic ventricular interdependence, while the inverse correlations between the RV function parameters and E/e' indicate that LV filling pressures comprise an important part of RV afterload in the context of acute pulmonary edema.

In a similar study, Lamia and colleagues tested the hypothesis that TAPSE is related to RV function at baseline and increases in parallel with RVFAC following positive inotropic therapy, in 86 mechanically ventilated patients with varying diagnoses. Contrary to these initial hypotheses, they found that TAPSE was either weakly related or totally unrelated to RV systolic function, whereas a more significant correlation was found between TAPSE and left ventricular ejection fraction in comparison with RVFAC, especially after performing a set of dynamic maneuvers, such as fluid challenge, passive leg raising and dobutamine infusion (Lamia et al., 2007).

Although simple to use, highly reproducible and fast, especially in the ICU setting where it can be performed by less experienced practitioners, TAPSE has some inherent limitations as a measure of RV function. It may be difficult to obtain a clear visualization of the tricuspid annulus, particularly in obese patients and in those suffering from chronic obstructive pulmonary disease (COPD). LV failure may induces changes in TAPSE independently of RV dysfunction, whereas Lamia's finding of a cut-off value of 22 mm that identified patients with LVEF < 45% with 85% sensitivity and 62% specificity, makes this measure unsuitable for the assessment of LV function, at least in heterogeneous populations of critically ill patients (Lamia et al., 2007). In addition, RV assessment is restricted to the longitudinal movement of the RV free wall and does not measure the contribution of the intraventricular septum and RV outflow tract (RVOT) (Lopez-Candales et al., 2006). Finally, apical akinesis may preserve normal TAPSE values with impairment of RV function whereas severe tricuspid regurgitation can also underestimate RV dysfunction and correlation with RV ejection fraction (Lopez-Candales et al., 2006 & Hsiao et al., 2006).

4. Conclusions

The echocardiographic assessment of left ventricle in the ICU has gained increased interest in the last years. However, the estimation of both systolic and diastolic right ventricular function is much more difficult to perform in mechanically ventilated patients and is mainly based on hemodynamic data derived from right heart catheterization. Heterogeneous pathologic processes that may lead to pulmonary hypertension and ARDS, application of different levels of PEEP and models of mechanical ventilation and a continuous dynamic change in fluid balance may have profound implications in heart-lung interactions and finally, the estimation of cardiac output. Severe sepsis and septic shock can also impair both the left and right ventricle, through changes in contractility, venous return and dramatic decrease in systemic vascular resistance. Finally, the development of ARDS due to either pulmonary or extra-pulmonary causes (i.e., severe sepsis) can be associated with acute cor pulmonale, pulmonary hypertension, RV and subsequently LV failure and hemodynamic collapse.

For these reasons early and accurate assessment of cardiac function is urgently recommended in the ICU setting. Different Intensive Care Medicine Societies have already published guidelines concerning theoretical and practical education of intensivists in performing daily echocardiography (Cholley et al., 2006). The development of novel indices for the estimation of RV, such as TAPSE and TDI velocities seems very promising, since they are easily obtained at the bedside, they need less computational load and optimal visualization in comparison with conventional indices, such as RVFAC or RVEF and finally, can be performed by less experienced personnel, especially in the acute care setting (Salem et al., 2008). Moreover, intra- and inter-observer variability seems to be limited with the adoption of these techniques (Forfia et al., 2006).

Their value in the ICU needs to be further investigated for their future use as basic echocardiographic assessment tools, since there are only two studies in the literature exploring significance of TAPSE and RV TDI velocities, as diagnostic or prognostic methods in mechanically ventilated patients with different diagnoses of admission. Although their application for LV assessment seems scientifically ground, evaluation of RV function and primary PH using these tools can be biased by the presence of LV failure, excluding their possible adoption in patients with biventricular dysfunction. However, in cases with normal LV, TAPSE and RV TDI velocities could be of significant value for continuous and indirect evaluation of pulmonary hypertension and RV function, in patients with severe respiratory failure. New studies must be undertaken for assessing their accuracy for predicting successful or failed liberation from the ventilator and for evaluation of possible impact of high levels of PEEP upon RV contractility during ARDS. Finally, daily and sequential estimations can be adopted as an alternative method for therapeutic monitoring of positive inotropic treatment upon cardiac performance, during shock states of different origin.

5. References

Abbas, AE., Fortuin, FD., Schiller, NB., Appleton, CP., Moreno, CA., & Lester, SJ. (2003). A simple method for noninvasive estimation of pulmonary vascular resistance. *J Am Coll Cardiol*, 41, 1021-1027, ISSN : 0735-1097.

Arcasoy, SM., Christie, JD., Ferrari, VA., Sutton, M., Zisman, DA., Blumenthal, NP., Pochettino, A., & Kotloff, RM. (2003). Echocardiographic assessment of pulmonary hypertension in patients with advanced lung disease. *Am J Respir Crit Care Med,* 167, 735-740, ISSN: 1535-4970 (electronic).

Barbier, C., Loubieres, Y., Schmit, C., Hayon, J., Ricom, JL., Jardin, F., & Vieillard-Barron, A. (2004). Respiratory changes in inferior vena cava diameter are helpful in predicting fluid responsiveness in ventilated septic patients. *Intensive Care Med*, 30, 1740-1746, ISSN : 0342-4642.

Beaulieu, Y., & Marik, PE. (2005). Bedside ultrasonography in the ICU. Part I. *Chest,* 128, 881-895, ISSN: 0012-3692.

Bendjelid, K., Romand, JA., Walder, B., Suter, PM., & Fournier, G. (2003). Correlation between inferior vena cava diameter and right atrial pressure depends on the echocardiographic method used in patients who are mechanically ventilated. *J Am Soc Echocardiogr,* 15, 944-949, ISSN : 0894-7317.

Berger, M., Haimowitz, A., Van Tosh, A., Berdoff, RL., & Golderg, E. (1985). Quantitative assessment of pulmonary hypertension in patients with tricuspid regurgitation using continuous wave Doppler ultrasound. *J Am Coll Cardiol*, 6, 359-365, ISSN: 0735-1097.

Bunnell, E., & Parrillo, JE. (1996). Cardiac dysfunction during septic shock. *Clin Chest Med,* 17, 237-248, ISSN: 0272-5231.

Cholley, BP., Vieillard-Baron, A., & Mebazaa, A. (2006). Echocardiography in ICU: time for widespread use! *Intensive Care Med,* 32, 9-10, ISSN : 0342-4642.

Combes, A., Arnoult, F., & Trouillet, JL. (2004). Tissue Doppler imaging estimation of pulmonary artery occlusion pressure in ICU patients. *Intensive Care Med*, 30, 75-81, ISSN: 0342-4642.

Delooz, HH. (1976). Factors influencing successful discontinuance of mechanical ventilation after open heart surgery: a clinical study of 41 patients. *Crit Care Med,* 4, 265-270, ISSN: 0090-3493.

Denault, AY., Coutoure, P., Buithieu, J., Haddad, F., Carrier, M., Babin, D., Levesque, S., & Tardif, JC. (2006). Left and right ventricular diastolic dysfunction as predictors of difficult separation from cardiopulmonary bypass. *Can J Anaesth,* 53, 1020-1029, ISSN: 1496-8975 (electronic).

Dokainish, H., Sengupta, R., Patel, R., & Lakkis, N. (2007). Usefulness of right ventricular tissue Doppler imaging to predict outcome in left ventricular heart failure independent of left ventricular diastolic function. *Am J Cardiol,* 99, 961-965, ISSN: 0002-9149.

Doutreleau, S., Talba, S., Di Marco, P., Lebourg, F., Rouyer, O., & Geny, B. (2007). Does tricuspid annular plane systolic excursion (TAPSE) or systolic velocity (Sm) allow an easier determination of right ventricular function after heart transplantation? *J Heart Lung Transplant*, 26 (3), 302-303, ISSN: 1053-2498.

Fellahi, JL., Valtier, B., Beauchet, A., Bourdarias, JP., & Jardin, F. (1998). Does positive end-expiratory pressure ventilation improve left ventricular function? A comparative study of transesophageal echocardiography in cardiac and noncardiac patients. *Chest*, 114, 556-562, ISSN: 0012-3692.

Forfia, PR., Fisher, MR., Mathai, SC., Housten-Harris, T., Hemmes, AR., Borlaug, BA., Chamera, E., Corretti, MC., Champion, HC., Abraham, TP., Girgis, RE., & Hassoun, PM. (2006). Tricuspid annular displacement predicts survival in pulmonary hypertension. *Am J Respir Crit Care Med*, 174, 1034-1041, ISSN: 1535-4970 (electronic).

Ghio, S., Recusani, F., Klersy, C., Sebastiani, R., Laudisa, ML., Campana, C., Gavazzi, A., & Tavazzi, L. (2000). Prognostic usefulness of the tricuspid annular plane systolic excursion in patients with congestive heart failure secondary to idiopathic or ischemic dilated cardiomyopathy. *Am J Cardiol*, 85, 837-842, ISSN: 0002-9149.

Hadian, M., & Pinsky, MR. (2006). Evidence-based review of the use of pulmonary artery catheter impact data and complications. *Crit Care*, 10, Suppl 3 , S8, ISSN: 1364-8535.

Hammarstrom, E., Wranne, B., Pinto, FJ., Puryear, J., & Popp, RL. (1991). Tricuspid annular motion. *J Am Soc Echocardiogr*, 4, 131-139, ISSN : 0894-7317.

Hsiao, SH., Lin, SK., Wang, WC., Yang, SH., Gin, PL., & Liu, CP. (2006). Severe tricuspid regurgitation shows significant impact in the relationship among peak systolic tricuspid annular velocity, tricuspid annular plane systolic excursion and right ventricular ejection fraction. *J Am Soc Echocardiogr*, 19, 902-910, ISSN : 0894-7317.

Isaaz, K. (2000). What are we actually measuring by Doppler tissue imaging? *J Am Coll Cardiol*, 36(3), 897-899, ISSN: 0735-1097.

Issaz, K. (2002). Tissue Doppler imaging for the assessment of left ventricular systolic and diastolic functions. *Curr Opin Cardiol*, 17, 431-442, ISSN: 0268-4705.

Jardin, F., Gueret, P., Dubourg, O., Farcot, JC., Margairaz, A., & Bourdarias, JP. (1985). Two-dimensional echocardiographic evaluation of right ventricular size and contractility in acute respiratory failure. *Crit Care Med*, 13, 952-956, ISSN: 0090-3493.

Jubran, A., Marthu, M., Dries, D., & Tobin, MJ. (1998). Continuous recording of mixed venous oxygen saturation during weaning from mechanical ventilation and the ramifications thereof. *Am J Respir Crit Care Med*, 158, 1763-1769, ISSN: 1535-4970 (electronic).

Jurcut, R., Giusca, S., La Gerche, A., Vasile, S., Ginghina, C., & Voigt, J-U. (2010). The echocardiographic assessment of the right ventricle: what to do in 2010? *Eur J Echocardiogr*, 11, 81-96, ISSN; 1525-2167.

Kaul, S., Tei, C., Hopkins, JM., & Shah, PM. (1984). Assessment of right ventricular function using two-dimensional echocardiography. *Am Heart J*, 107, 526-531, ISSN: 0002-8703.

Lamia, B., Teboul, JL., Monnet, X., Richard, C., & Chemla, D. (2007). Relationship between the tricuspid annular systolic excursion and right and left ventricular function in critically ill patients. *Intensive Care Med*, 33, 2143-2149, ISSN: 0342-4642.

Lamia, B., Maizel, J., Ochagavia, A., Chemla, D., Osman, D., Richard, C., & Teboul, JL. (2009). Echocardiographic diagnosis of pulmonary artery occlusion pressure elevation during weaning from mechanical ventilation. *Crit Care Med*, 37, 1696-1701, ISSN: 0090-3493

Lang, RM., Bierig, M., Devereux, RB., Flachskampf, FA., Foster, E., Pellikka, PA., Picard, MH., Roman, MJ., Seward, J., Shanewise, JS., Solomon, SD., Spencer, KT., Sutton, MS., & Stewart, WJ. (2005). Recommendations for chamber quantification: a report from the American Society of Echocardiography's Guidelines and Standards Committee and the Chamber Quantification Writing Group, developed in conjunction with the European Association of Echocardiography, a branch of the European Society of Cardiology. *J Am Soc Echocardiogr*, 18, 1440-1463, ISSN: 0894-7317.

Lemaire, F., Teboul, JL., Cinotti, L., Giotto, G., Abrouk, F., Steg, G., Macquin-Mavier, I., & Zapol, WM. (1988). Acute left ventricular dysfunction during unsuccessful weaning from mechanical ventilation. *Anesthesiology*, 69, 171-179, ISSN: 0003-3022.

Lichtenstein, D., & Jardin, F. (1994). Appréciation non invasive de la pression veineuse centrale par la mesure échographique du calibre da la veine cave inférieure en réanimation. *Rean Urg*, 3, 79-82.

Lopez-Candales, A., Rajagopolan, N., Saxena, N., Gulyasy, B., Edelman, K., & Bazaz, R. (2006). Right ventricular systolic function is not the sole determinant of tricuspid annular motion. *Am J Cardiol*, 98, 973-977, ISSN : 0002-9149.

McLean, AS., Ting, I., Huang, SJ., & Wesley, S. (2007). The use of the right ventricular diameter and tricuspid annular tissue Doppler velocity parameter to predict the presence of pulmonary hypertension. *Eur J Echocardiography*, 8, 128-136, ISSN: 1525-2167.

Meluzin, J., Spinarova, L., Bakala, J., Toman, J., Krejci, J., Hude, P., Kara, T., & Soucek, M. (2001). Pulsed Doppler tissue imaging of the velocity of tricuspid annular systolic motion. A new, rapid and non-invasive method of evaluating right ventricular systolic function. *Eur Heart J*, 22, 340-348, ISSN : 1522-9645 (electronic).

Meluzin, J., Spiranova, L., Hude, P., Krejci, J., Kincl, V., Panovsky, R., & Dusek, L. (2005). Prognostic importance of various echocardiographic right ventricular functional parameters in patients with symptomatic heart failure. *J Am Soc Echocardiogr*, 18, 435-444, ISSN: 0894-7317.

Mintz, GS., Kotler, MN., Parry, WR., Iskandrian, AS., & Kane, SA. (1981). Real-time inferior vena caval ultrasonography: Normal and abnormal findings and its use in assessing right heart function. *Circulation*, 64, 1018-1025, ISSN : 0009-7322.

Moustapha, A., Lim, M., Saikia, S., Kaushik, V., Kang, SH., & Barasch, E. (2001). Interrogation of the tricuspid annulus by Doppler tissue imaging in patients with chronic pulmonary hypertension: implication for the assessment of right ventricular systolic and diastolic function. *Cardiology*, 95, 101-104, ISSN: 0008-6312.

Papaioannou, V., Stakos, D., Dragoumanis, C., & Pneumatikos, I. (2010). Relation of tricuspid annular displacement and tissue Doppler imaging velocities with duration of weaning in mechanically ventilated patients with acute pulmonary edema. *BMC Cardiovasc Disord*, 10 (1), 20, ISSN: 1471-2261 (electronic).

Parker, MM., McCarthy, KE., Ognibene, FP., & Parrillo JE. (1990). Right ventricular dysfunction and dilatation, similar to left ventricular changes, characterize the cardiac depression of septic shock in humans. *Chest,* 97, 126-131, ISSN: 0012-3692.

Pinsky, MR. (2002). Recent advances in the clinical application of heart-lung interactions. *Curr Opin Crit Care,* 8, 26-31, ISSN: 1070-5295.

Pinsky, MR. (2007). Heart-lung interactions. *Curr Opin Crit Care,* 13, 528-531, ISSN: 1070-5295.

Price, LC., Wort, SJ., Finney, SJ., Marino, PS., & Bret, SJ. (2010). Pulmonary vascular and right ventricular dysfunction in adult critical care: current and emerging options for management: a systematic literature review. *Crit Care,* 14, R169, ISSN: 1364-8535.

Rubin, LJ. (1997). Primary pulmonary hypertension. *N Engl J Med,* 336, 111-117, ISSN: 0028-4793.

Sade, LE., Gulmez, O., Eroglu, S., Sezgin, A., & Muderrisoglu, H. (2007). Noninvasive estimation of right ventricular filling pressure by ratio of early tricuspid inflow to annular diastolic velocity in patients with and without recent cardiac surgery. *J Am Soc Echocardiogr,* 20, 982-988, ISSN: 0894-7317.

Salem, R., Vallee, F., Rusca, M., & Mebazaa, A. (2008). Hemodynamic monitoring by echocardiography in ICU: the role of the new echo techniques. *Curr Opin Crit Care,* 14, 561-568, ISSN: 1070-5295.

Samad, BA., Alam, M., & Jensen-Urstad, K. (2002). Prognostic impact of right ventricular involvement as assessed by tricuspid annular motion in patients with acute myocardial infarction. *Am J Cardiol* , 90, 778-781, ISSN: 0002-9149.

Saxena, N., Rajagopalan, N., Edelman, K., & Lopez-Candales, A (2006). Tricuspid annular systolic velocity: a useful measurement in determining right ventricular systolic function regardless of pulmonary artery pressures. *Echocardiography,* 23 (9), 750-755, ISSN: 0742-2822.

Schmidt, H., Rohr, D., Bauer, H., Bohrer, H., Motsch, J., & Martin, E. (1997). Changes in intrathoracic fluid volumes during weaning from mechanical ventilation in patients after coronary artery bypass grafting. *J Crit Care,* 12, 22-27, ISSN: 0883-9441.

Sibbald, WJ., & Driedger, AA. (1983). Right ventricular function in acute disease states: pathophysiologic considerations. *Crit Care Med,* 11, 339-345, ISSN: 0090-3493.

Sundereswaran, L., Nagueh, SF., Vardan, S., Middleton, KJ., Zoghbi, WA., Quinones, MA., & Torre-Amione, G. (1998). Estimation of left and right ventricular filling pressures after heart transplantation by tissue Doppler imaging. *Am J Cardiol,* 82, 352-357, ISSN : 0002-9149.

Taylor, RR., Covell, JW., Sonnenblick, EH., & Ross, J. (1967). Dependence of ventricular distensibility on filling of the opposite ventricle. *Am J Physiol,* 213, 711-718, ISSN: 0363-6135.

Vieillard-Barron, A., Prin, S., Chergoui, K., Dubourg, O., & Jardin, F. (2002). Echo-Doppler demonstration of acute cor pulmonale at the bedside in the medical intensive care unit. *Am J Respir Crit Care Med,* 166, 1310-1319, ISSN: 1535-4970 (electronic).

Vignon, P., AitHssain, A., François, B., Preux, PM., Pichon, N., Clavel, M., Frat, JP, & Gastinne, H. (2008). Echo-cardiographic assessment of pulmonary artery occlusion pressure in ventilated patients: a transoesophageal study. *Crit Care,* 12, R18, ISSN : 1364-8535.

Waggoner, AD., & Bierig, SM. (2001). Tissue Doppler imaging: a useful echocardiographic method for the cardiac sonographer to assess systolic and diastolic ventricular function. *J Am Soc Echocardiogr*, 14(12), 1143-1152, ISSN: 0894-7317.

Yock, PG., & Popp, RL. (1984). Noninvasive estimation of right ventricular systolic pressure by Doppler ultrasound in patients with tricuspid regurgitation. *Circulation*, 70, 657-662, ISSN : 0009-7322.

3

Endomyocardial Biopsy Guided by Echocardiography

Alfredo Inácio Fiorelli, Wilson Mathias Junior
and Noedir Antonio Groppo Stolf
Heart Institute of Sao Paulo University
Brazil

1. Introduction

In the recent year, transcatheter endomyocardial biopsy is a procedure relatively simple that has been increasingly utilized in cardiomyopathy diagnosis. It is estimated that over 50,000 biopsies are performed annually in the United States in general to control rejection episodes after heart transplantation.

Endomyocardial biopsy plays important role in the diagnosis and treatment of adult and pediatric cardiovascular disease due to many specific myocardial disorders the etiology is seldom discovery by noninvasive testing. The indication this procedure may be especially challenging for many nonspecialists because the method is invasive and always must weigh the risks and benefits. The percutaneous transvenous endomyocardial biopsy has become the procedure safe and more convenient for rejection control after heart transplantation, histopathological diagnosis of cardiomyopathies or tumors[1,2,3]. The endomyocardial biopsy technique is safe in experienced hands however the method may lead to several complications, the most serious them is the right ventricle perforation with cardiac tamponade[4,5].

Heart biopsy already experimented investigation with different methods such as: open thoracotomy[6]; partial extrapleural thoracotomy with resection of a rib to facilitate the exposition[7]; percutaneous introduction of Vim-Silverman and Menghini needle[8,9,10]; introduction of a modified Ross transseptal needle through the superior vena cava or carotid artery[11]; and the use of cutting blades introduced through a catheter for endomyocardial biopsy[12]. Unfortunately, the heart biopsy history was marked by severe complications, which included pericardial tamponade, cardiac perforation, pneumothorax and hemothorax, and eventually death. Since 1980, the technique has become routinely used.

Weinberg et al., in 1958, reported their experience with five patients who were undergone pericardial and myocardial biopsy[13]. The procedure was performed percutaneously under local anesthesia and the thorax was opened by resection of the fourth cartilage on the left. This invasive method did not gain ample acceptance due to high risk. The cardiac biopsy with needle through a limited thoracotomy was associated with pulmonary injuries, cardiac tamponade, coronary vessels laceration, arrhythmia, and sometimes with death. Despite these risks, direct needle biopsy was carried out in some centers.

In 1960, Sutton and Sutton reported the use of the myocardial biopsy in 150 patients whose specimens was obtained with needle introduced percutaneously at the left ventricular apex[14]. The guidance was done by fluoroscopy or electrocardiography but surgical risk maintained high. Ventricular premature beats or pulsation felt through needle indicated contact with left ventricle surface. This technique was repeated experimentally with few variations by Timmis et al., in 1972, using either Vim-Silverman or Menghini needle[15]. An electrocardiogram electrode extension was attached at needle to help in recognition of the epicardium through the lesion current; however without risk significative reduction.

In 1962, Sakakibara and Konno became responsible for the introduction of the endomyocardial biopsy modern era with use of a flexible bioptome with sharpened cusps through transvascular approach to obtain endomyocardial tissue by a bite as opposed to cutting technique[16]. A long catheter was introduced into a peripheral vein or artery by dissection technique and advances to the right or left ventricle and small movable cutting jaws obtaining pieces of myocardial about 3 mm in diameter.

In 1965, Bulloch et al. improved the safety of cardiac biopsy proposing the use of vascular access through the right external or internal jugular vein by introduction of a capable needle of withdrawing specimens from the right interventricular septum[17].

In 1972, Caves et al. at Stanford University developed another bioptome model that is in use until today for assessment of cardiac allograft rejection. The bioptome contains a moving jaw so that the longer and thinner is used for left ventricular biopsy and the shorter and thicker for right ventricular biopsy[18]. In the same year, Shirey et al., presented experience with left ventricle biopsy[19].

In 1973, Ali et al., publishing experience with the technique of Sakakibara and Konno for right ventricular endomyocardial biopsy by transvenous access employed in 28 patients with a variety of myocardial diseases of known and unknown etiology[20].

In 1974, Richardson reported another transvascular technique that gained wide acceptance with use of a modified Olympus bronchoscope biopsy forceps, called the King's College endomyocardial bioptome, introduced through a long sheath for either left or right ventricular biopsy[21].

In 1980, Kawai proposed the use of a new flexible model catheter to able of monitoring simultaneously the intraventricular electrocardiogram[22].

Table 1 shows the main diagnostic finding in endomyocardial biopsy and the main indications to endomyocardial biopsy at Heart Institute of Sao Paulo University include:

1. Assessment and management of graft rejection after heart transplantation;
2. Remission control of Chagas' disease reactivation after specific therapy administration, in general after heart transplantation;
3. Evaluation and diagnosis of the cardiomyopathies with unknown etiology;
4. Diagnostic and orientation of the infectious myocarditis, inflammatory, drug induced, and others;
5. Evaluation and management of malignant ventricular arrhythmias with unknown etiology;
6. Evaluation and orientation of restrictive cardiomyopathies with unknown etiology;
7. Etiologic diagnosis of the intracardiac tumor mass;
8. Cardiomyopathy evaluation after use of immunosuppressive therapy;
9. Controlled research protocols approved by the ethics committee and research of the institution.

Inflammatory or Immunology	Infiltrative
• Heart allograft rejection	• Amyloidosis
• Chagas 'disease reactivation	• Hemochromatosis
• Myocarditis	• Glycogen deposit disease
• Cytomegalovirus infection	• Fabry' disease
• Toxoplasmosis	• Gaucher' disease
• Sarcoidosis	**Degenerative**
• Rheumatic myocarditis	• Idiopathic cardiomyopathy
• Eosinophilic myocarditis	• Drug-induced cardiomyopathy
• Kawasaki' disease	• Actinic cardiomyopathy
• Differentiation between restrictive cardiomyopathy and pericarditis	
Ischemic	**Tumor**
• Acute or chronic ischemic cardiomyopathy	• Primary cardiac neoplasm
• Shönlen-Henoch purpura	• Metastatic cardiac neoplasm

Table 1. Principal findings of the endomyocardial biopsy

2. Technique of the endomyocardial biopsy

2.1 Special care

All biopsies must be performed with cardiac rhythm control, blood pressure, and continuous oxygen saturation. Patients with coagulopathies, thrombocytopenia, or under use of anticoagulant agents or antiplatelet should be well analyzed before biopsy to avoid hematoma formation and bleeding. The patients must be informed about all procedure stages and that during the withdrawal of myocardial fragment they may have a temporary pulling painful sensation.

No premeditation is given for routine biopsy either child as adult patient. To adult patient is not necessary the venous access temporary maintenance or sedation and the biopsies are usually performed with local anesthesia. Eventually in adolescent patients may be necessary a small sedation to comfort.

To patients with venipuncture fear may be utilized anesthetic cream existing market and which contains lidocaine and prilocaine under the trade name EMLA cream™ (*an abbreviation for Eutectic Mixture of Local Anesthetics*). To be effective EMLA cream™ must be applied topically in puncture site two hours before to reduce the procedure discomfort.

Patient is encouraged usually to have a regular meal and if possible increase oral fluid amount up to 6 or 8 hours prior to biopsy. This maneuver is not mandatory but may facilitate the puncture. To infants and children this fasting period is minor and they should receive parenteral hydration by dehydration possibility and hypoglycemia.

However, in children or pediatric patients require sedation and general anesthesia which must be accomplished with all cares that cover this procedure. In these cases the patient oxygenation must be ensured by mechanical ventilation through endotracheal intubation or laryngeal mask airway. The pediatric patients with low ejection fraction have an increased surgical risk and care must be redoubled.

It is recommended that the endomyocardial biopsy should not be performed without a prior echocardiographic analysis, especially in pediatric patients or in diagnostic investigation of dilated cardiomyopathies. Echocardiography that will be utilized as guide at endomyocardial biopsy cannot be the first echocardiographic exam accomplished in the patient because it is very important to procedure planning the prior knowledge of anatomy and heart function.

It should be taken great care with the air inadvertent entry through sheath to the right heart chambers by air embolization possibility to pulmonary trunk with consequent decrease of the cardiac output, or to systemic circulation in cases with intracardiac shunts.

Endomyocardial biopsies can be performed through the following venous access or arterial: subclavian, jugular or femoral however these two last approaches are more frequently utilized. Subclavian access rarely is employed because the possibility of severe vascular injuries is greater. The procedure is more frequently performed at cardiac catheterization laboratory and uses the fluoroscopic to guide endomyocardial biopsy. But 2 two-dimensional echocardiography almost always offers additional resource, either alone or combined with fluoroscopy.

In patients with multiples previous biopsies the passage of dilators with caliber gradually increased will facilitate the placement of the sheath. Venacavography realized prior in patients with antecedents of the venous thrombosis, presence of intravenous catheters or venous puncture attempts without success should be seen before biopsy to avoid accidents (Figure 1).

All the recommendations above are strongly emphasized mainly to critical patients with decompensated heart failure or pediatric patients. The cares must also be extended to the place where the biopsy will be performed as well as necessary material and equipment (Table 2). This procedure is only a diagnostic exam easily executable; however it is an invasive method of risk. Nevertheless, once when the preconized classic principles are rigorously respected, the endomyocardial biopsy evolves low values of morbidity and mortality.

Emergence Material and Cardiovascular Control
• Cardiac rhythm control, noninvasive blood pressure and O_2 Saturation. • Portable Cardiac Defibrillator. • Fluoroscopy or Disposable Two-dimensional Echocardiography. • Temporary Pacemaker Generator and Electrode. • Material to Pericardiocentesis and Pericardial Drainage. • Drugs and Equipments to Cardiovascular Reanimation.
Material to Endomyocardial Biopsy Realization
• Sterile Surgical Drapes and Gowns. • Antiseptic, Lidocaine 2% without vasoconstrictor, Saline Solution, and Heparin. • 10mL and 20mL Syringes, Gauze, Bandages and Hypodermic Needles. • Material to Vascular Puncture: Surgical knife, Needle punctures 5Fr, 7Fr, 8Fr or 9Fr, Guidewire, Dilator, Sheath and Bioptome. • Surgical instruments: Anatomical forceps, Scissors, Needle holder, Forceps type Halstead and Backaus.

Table 2. Material and Equipment utilized during Endomyocardial Biopsy

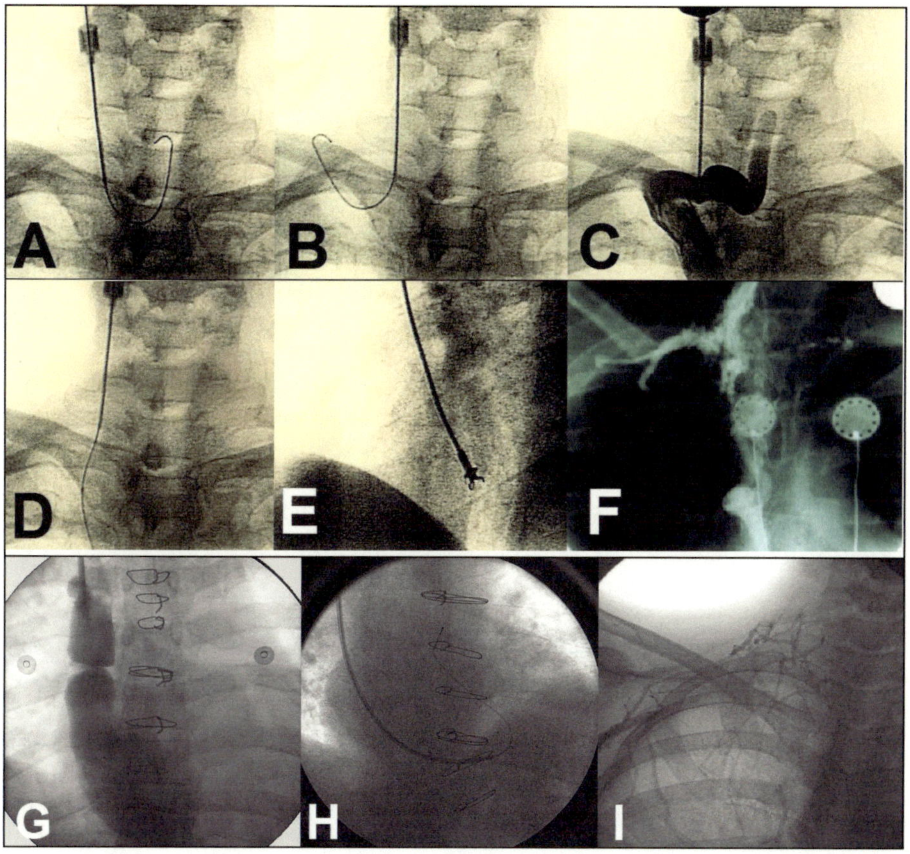

Fig. 1. A - Attempted passage of guidewire through the right internal jugular vein. B- Guidewire deviated to the right subclavian vein. C - Contrast injection showing the venous anatomy. D - Passing of the guidewire after needle to be gently sloping. E - Introduction of the bioptome with two jaw. F - Superior vena cava with obstruction. G - Superior vena cava anastomosis with stenosis after cardiac transplantation by bicaval technique. H - Sheath positioned into right ventricle with the aid of the guidewire. I - Upper venous system with obstruction

2.2 Bioptomes

Currently, there are disposable bioptomes and sheaths available for percutaneous insertions and biopsy either left ventricle as right. Over the years the development of modern devices became the cardiac biopsy of a high risk technique to an insurance procedure and simple.

Two basic types of bioptomes are available concerning the format with pre-shaped distal end (*stiff shape – Konno, and Caves-Shultz bioptome*) and unshaped maintained straight (*floppy shaft – King, Cordis, Cook bioptome*). The pre-shaped bioptome does not require long sheath or pre-shaped it can be short and straight because the bioptome curvature allows easily the entry into intraventricular chamber. Pre-shaped bioptomes have greater stiffness and offer better control to operator during biopsy. The forceps curvature angle can be modified to facilitate the passage of the instrument across tricuspid valve guiding

the forceps against interventricular septum. Table 3 shows main bioptomes commercially available.
On the other hand, the straight bioptome necessitates pre-shaped long sheath to locate the forceps tip against interventricular septum. The pre-shaped long sheath can be located in intraventricular cavity by long guidewire or fluid filled catheter with or without balloon-tipped. The sheath maintenance into ventricular cavity has as advantage main the quick positioning of the forceps; however this attitude may facilitates the development of arrhythmias and the ventricular perforation. In general the pre-shaped bioptomes are used in jugular approach or subclavian and straight bioptomes in femoral approach.
It is possible to find in the market either disposable bioptome as reusable to be utilized for any conventional access approach and ventricular chambers being that the femoral vein requires a long sheath. Right ventricular endomyocardial biopsy can be performed percutaneously from one of the following approaches: internal jugular, subclavian or femoral veins. Left ventricular endomyocardial biopsy is normally performed retrograde access from one of the femoral veins.
Both fluoroscopy as echocardiography can be used to guidance during endomyocardial biopsy for any approach differing only bioptome kind and sheath. The bioptome can have one or two articulated jaws (Figure 2).

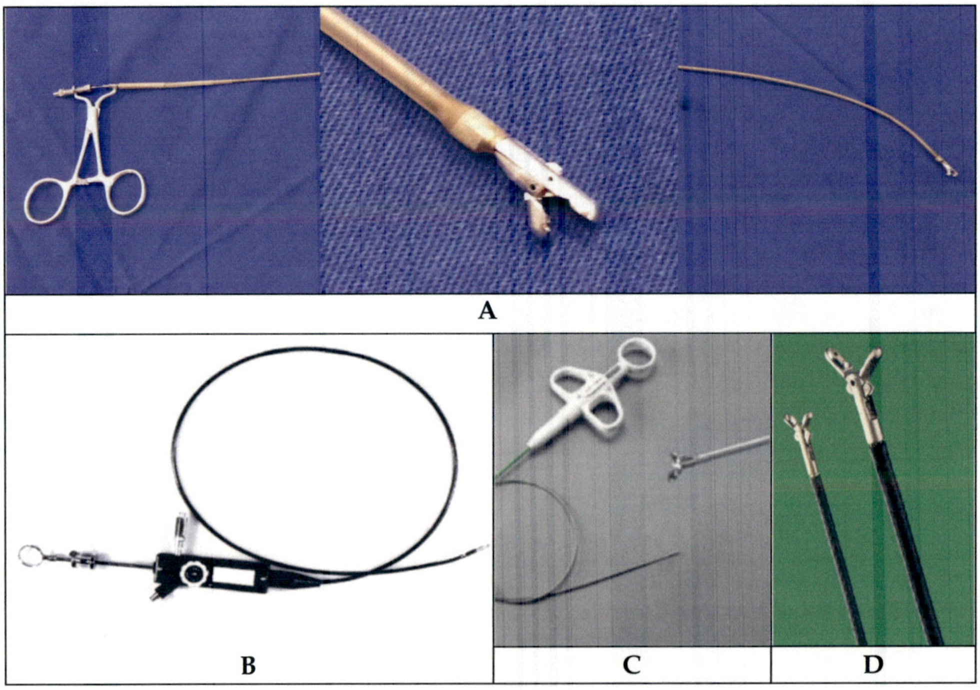

Fig. 2. A - Caves-Shultz bioptome is pre-shaped and has only one articulated jaw while the other is fixed and the introduction into cardiac chamber is done through a sheath. Jaw open. B - Kawai-model® flexible bioptome is straight and has a stainless steel shaft. It has two articulated jaws and need of a long sheath-guiding catheter introduced into ventricular chamber. C - Cook® straight bioptome. D - Straight bioptome with two articulated jaw requires a pre-shaped sheath. Jaws open

Model	Jaw		Flexible Shaft Length (cm)	Reusable
	size (Fr)	Articulated		
Scholten Bioptome®	5.0, 6.5, 8.0 and 9.0	1	50 and 100	yes
Novatome™	6.0, 7.0, 8.0 and 9.0	1	50 and 100	no
Cordis®	5.4, 7.0 and 7.5	2	50 and 104	no
SparrowHawk®	6.0	2	50	no
Cook®	3.0 and 5.2	2	60 and 120	no

Table 3. Characteristics of some bioptomes commercially available

2.3 Internal jugular vein approach

The right internal jugular vein is the most common percutaneous access site for right ventricular endomyocardial biopsy. Patient is placed on supine position with the neck extended and the head should be turned to the left about 45 degree to facilitate venous puncture site. The skin of the surgical region receives conventional asepsis and surgical drapes are positioned comfortably.

It is very important careful identification of the triangle formed by the medial heads and lateral of the sternocleidomastoid muscle and the clavicle because the puncture is performed at upper vertex this triangle in direction to the ipsilateral nipple. During the needle introduction is performed anesthesia with lidocaine and the intermittent aspiration confirms vein localization. Excessive use of the lidocaine may infiltrate the recurrent nervous or the carotid sheath and lead transitorily to vocal cords paralysis or Horner's syndrome respectively.

Use of ultrasound should be considered if there is any difficulty in locating the vein or artery because it facilitates the location of the blood vessel and demonstrates adjacent structures (Figure 3). Although ultrasonography is not absolutely necessary for the procedure it is a very valuable tool, mainly for patients undergo the procedure repeatedly. Valsalva maneuver or elevation of the legs may be very useful because it help to dilate the vessel and makes it more evident. Sometimes if the vein is collapsed or scarred, the use of the great gauge needle may compress the vein and make cannulation difficult and the use of thin gauge needle help to locate the vessel.

The guidewire is inserted into right internal jugular vein by standard Seldinger technique as usually is performed in all punctures to introduce intravascular catheters[23]. Either fluoroscopy (Figure 4E) or two-dimensional echocardiography (Figure 5) can be used to confirm appropriate wire-guide position before sheath introduction, because occasionally the wire-guide is deflected toward the arm instead of advancing toward the right atrium.

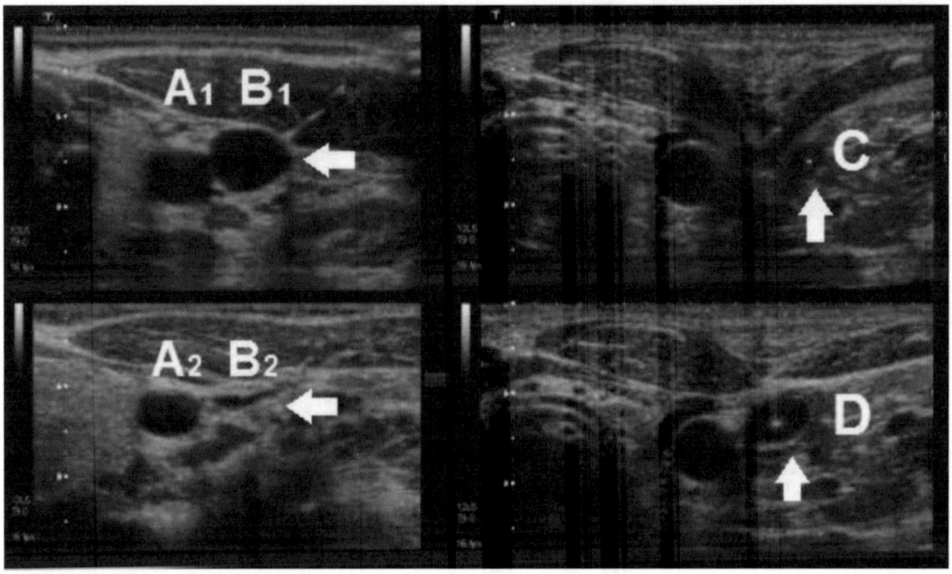

Fig. 3. The ultrasonography is a powerful resource to help the vascular puncture in difficult situations. The images above were obtained by ultrasound of the right cervical region and show the anatomical relationship between the carotid artery (A) and internal jugular vein (B) and can be observed that the vein is much more compressible. The images to left side show venous distention with (A1B1) and without (A2B2) use of the Valsalva maneuver, respectively. C – During percutaneous venous puncture the image echogenic represents the correct position of the needle into internal jugular vein (arrow)

Saline solution injection through sheath produces diluted microbubbles that serve as a contrast-enhanced and facilitates intracardiac anatomy identification and the wire-guide by echocardiography. Microbubbles have a high degree of echogenicity which are able of reflect the ultrasound waves and help to differentiate the anatomical structures. Wire-guide is a metallic object and has higher echogenicity in relation to other cardiac structures being easily identified.

In Figure 4A is represented the main cervical anatomical structures for orientation of the right intern jugular vein. The triangle vertex formed by sternal head muscles bundles and clavicular of the sternocleidomastoid muscle serve as orientation anatomic point to internal jugular vein puncture (Figure 4A). The needle should be oriented in direction to ipsilateral nipple forming an angle of the 45 degree with skin (Figure 4B).

An 18-gauge needle is located into right internal jugular vein through of a small incision in the skin is made with a scalpel to facilitate subsequent passage of the dilator and sheath. The needle must not be inserted in same plane of the carotid artery on the contrary should be move away from it as much as possible. If occur an inadvertent arterial puncture, the needle must be removed and an external compression is applied for 8 to 10 minutes to avoid bleeding and hematoma formation with serious consequences. Other arterial complication reported refers to carotid artery dissection or occlusion, and stroke related to emboli from thrombus or atheroma secondary to inadvertent carotid puncture.

The sheath gauge should be chosen adequately to each bioptome, for example Caves-Schultz bioptome requires a 9F or 8.5F sheath. The sheath only should be introduced into vein after confirm by fluoroscopy or echocardiography that the guidewire is adequately into vein. Once finished biopsy, the sheath is removed and should be apply an external compression on the puncture site for half to one hour or more because the venous orifice left by puncture is big.

We prefer the right jugular approach to pediatric patient or infants with pre-shaped 5Fr-bioptome.

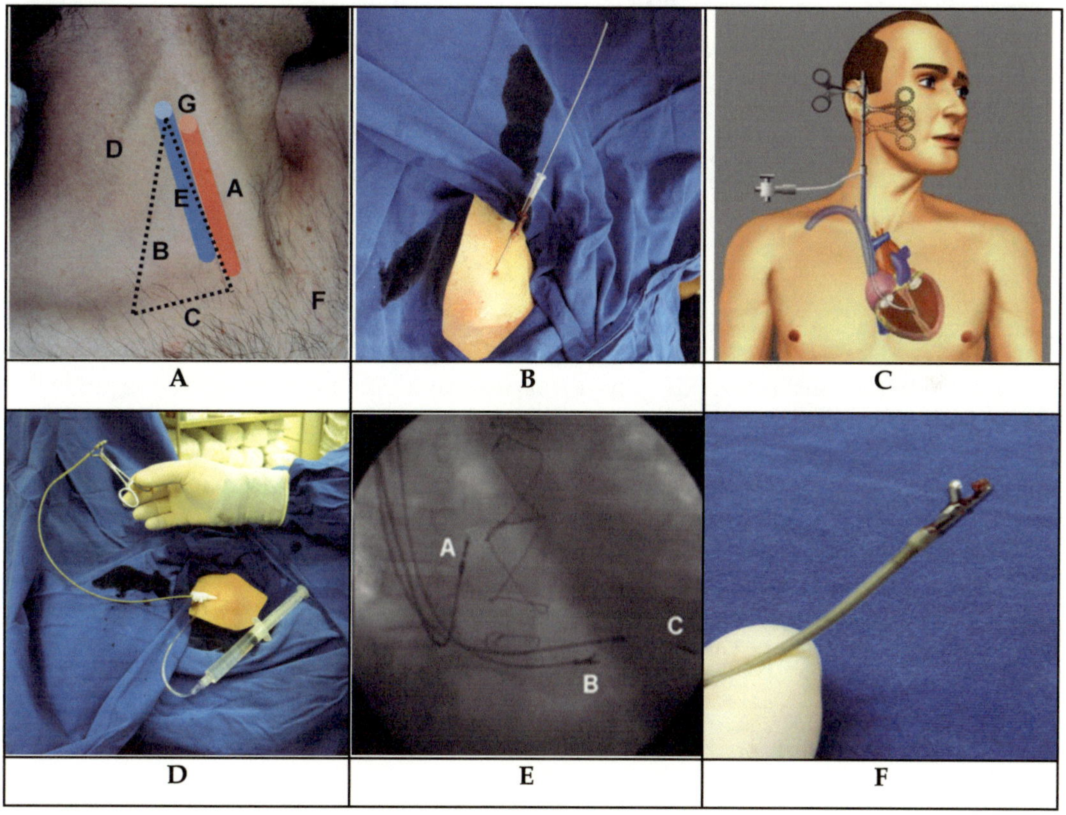

Fig. 4. Endomyocardial biopsy performed through right internal jugular vein. A - Depiction of the main cervical anatomical structures that serves to help in the right venous puncture. (A) Sternal head lateral border of the sternocleidomastoid muscle; (B) Clavicular head medial border of the sternocleidomastoid muscle; (C) Clavicule; (D) Right external jugular vein; (E) Right internal jugular vein; (F) Manubrium; and (G) Right carotid artery. B – Right internal jugular vein punctured com needle and guidewire. C - Schematic diagram showing bioptome position during withdrawal of myocardial fragment. D – Pre-shaped bioptome passing through the sheath. E - Routine endomyocardial biopsy to monitoring of acute rejection after heart transplantation guided by fluoroscopy on patient with dual chamber pacemaker. (A) – Atrial electrode; (B) – Bioptome; and (C) – Ventricular electrode. F – Myocardial fragment at pre-shaped bioptome

The left internal jugular vein approach is similar to above description done to the right with mirror image. Despite these considerations, the left internal jugular vein approach offers more difficulties because the trajectory since puncture site until right ventricle is more sinuous with critical angles in relation to right approach. Left jugular puncture allows also the deviation of the guidewire to left through subclavian vein because this latter vein receives that first perpendicularly.

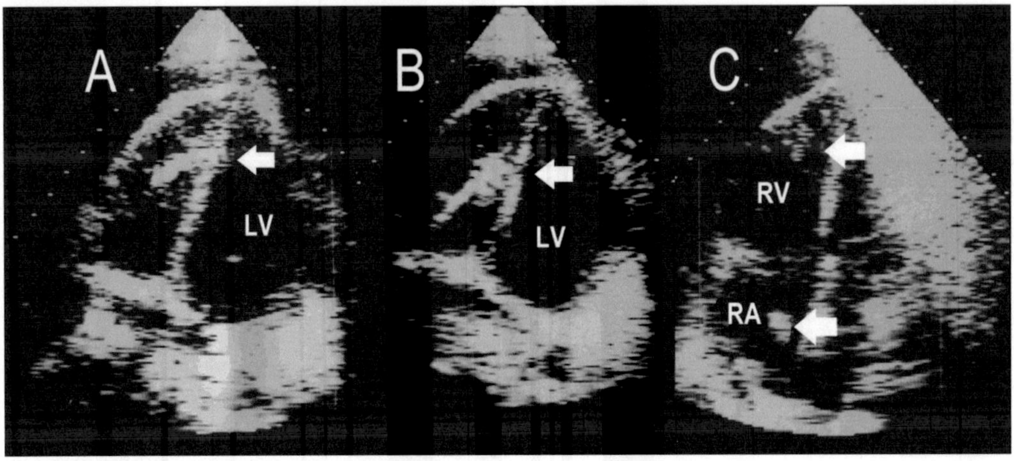

Fig. 5. Two-dimensional echocardiography images in apical four chambers used to guide the bioptome during endomyocardial biopsy. Transient echogenic image created from of saline solution infusion through sheath lateral access that facilitates the anatomical structures identification. The bioptome is adequately positioned with the tip directed to interventricular septum only in situations A and B. A - Tip of the bioptome is removing a fragment of the interventricular septum apical portion (arrow). B - Forceps open at middle portion of the interventricular septum (arrow). C - Image showing the bioptome tip in direction to right ventricle free wall (arrow). This position is not adequate for perforation risk high and in same plane can be seen also the bioptome inside the right atrium (arrow). LV – Left ventricle; RV – Right ventricle; and RA – Right atrium

2.4 Subclavian vein approach

Subclavian vein approach is not preferential access to perform the endomyocardial biopsy and should be used in special situations. Eventually, the internal jugular vein approach must be prevented for venous obstruction, infection, hematoma or for any other reason. So, the subclavian vein may be an alternative access to accomplish the endomyocardial biopsy. Either the left subclavian vein as right may be utilized as access approach to biopsy. The left subclavian vein generally offers less resistance to bioptome advance when compared to right due to path curvature to have major radius and without acute angle.

The subclavian vein puncture site should be more lateral than that utilized usually in venous catheters insertions to increase the puncture angle. If the right subclavian vein entry angle into superior vena cava was very acute, it may difficult the bioptome progression and with venous perforation possibility.

Before venous insertion of the dilator and sheath should be confirmed the guidewire correct position to avoid vascular injuries or put the catheter at inadequate place. The guidewire is easily detected by dimensional echocardiography as an echogenic image into superior vena cava toward right atrium. As in any vascular puncture the insertion elements must glide smoothly without offer endurance.

In local puncture should be maintained compression for an hour or more after the sheath removal to prevent bleeding and hematoma, however this period must be further if the patient has coagulation disturbance or the puncture was difficult and complicated.

2.5 Femoral vein approach

Femoral vein puncture offers less technical difficulty compared to other venous access to endomyocardial biopsy (Figure 6). This approach is extremely disseminated among interventional cardiologists and it represents the preferred access them. The femoral vein approach has as main advantages the lower risk hematoma and arterial injuries[24]. If occur an inadvertent arterial puncture, the external compression is more efficient and less uncomfortable. Many patients prefer femoral access for aesthetic reasons because multiples prior biopsies can lead to keloid formation that is visible at cervical region.

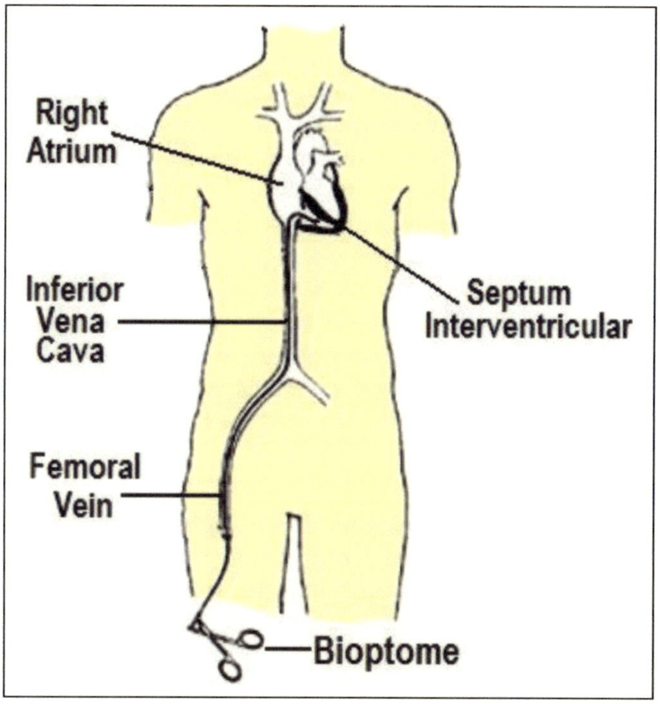

Fig. 6. Endomyocardial biopsy performed through left femoral vein. The bioptome advances by inside of the long sheath that runs along the inferior vena cava, passes through the tricuspid valve until the right side of the interventricular septum

It should be emphasized that inguinal region is potentially contaminated and this way the care with asepsis must be redoubled. Inguinal region should be widely shaved and washed with antiseptic solution before the usual surgical preparation. This considerations have more relevance to patients underwent to heart transplantation for increased susceptibility to infections.

As disadvantage the femoral access should be noted the need for a pre-shaped long sheath with curvature angle of 135-degree or catheter guidance to facilitate the direction of bioptome across the tricuspid valve. This approach may offer more difficulty to withdraw of myocardial specimens of an appropriate region of septum as well as fragments of larger size because the device is thinner. Moreover this long sheath increases the risk of lead to clots and deep venous thrombosis.

The operator may have the sensibility reduced by femoral approach because the trajectory of bioptome is long and may increase the ventricular perforation risk. Therefore, it is very important that the patients remain supine for approximately 2 to 4 hours after sheath removal to prevent bleeding.

In 2008, Holzmann et al., reported experience with 3048 biopsy only for femoral approach and had the following complications: pericardial tamponade with pericardiocentesis in 0.08%; permanent complete AV block with permanent pacemaker required in 0.04%; AV block III temporary requiring atropine and temporary pacemaker in 1.47%; small pericardial effusions in 0.74%; and persistent atrial fibrillation with cardioversion in 0.18%[25].

2.6 Femoral arterial approach

The left ventricular biopsy is indicated only in specials situations because the right ventricular biopsy is sufficient to study of most cardiomyopathies. Left ventricle biopsy has more importance in the diagnosis of intracardiac masses than in cardiomyopathies assessment.

The guidewire used is long and advances through abdominal aorta retrogradely until into left ventricular cavity. After, this guide helps a pigtail catheter or pre-shaped sheath to be positioned into ventricular cavity too. In left ventricular biopsy is sufficient guide the bioptome away from mitral valvular apparatus because all walls are equally thick.

It must be dispensed much attention to inadvertent entry of air into the system for arterial embolism risk. During the procedure the sheath is washed continuously with heparin diluted into saline solution to avoid thrombus formations and embolism.

2.7 Heterotopic heart approach

For heterotopic heart transplantation, the donor right atrium is located into right hemithorax. Heterotopic heart approach requires a special strategy to achieve the donor right ventricle. The connection of the hearts may be performed between the anastomosis combinations of flowing donor-recipient structures vena cava and right atria. Metallic clips are put above and below that anastomosis to identification the bioptome entry site into donor heart. Right internal jugular vein remains the preferential route of approach. The other venous access may be used with the following order of increasing difficulty: left subclavian, left internal jugular, right subclavian, and finally femoral vein with much more difficulty.

Two-dimensional echocardiography offers good guidance in expert hands however with the fluoroscopy seems be easier. Figure 7 shows different stages in endomyocardial biopsy performing on heterotopic heart transplantation.

3. Guidance for endomyocardial biopsy

Endomyocardial biopsy usually is performed safely under fluoroscopic guidance because it provides information to the operator about the course of the bioptome and site of biopsy. Fluoroscopy presents several advantages because is widely known; easy handling, safe method, allows complete visualization of the procedure, and does not require an additional operator to biopsy achievement. It is the most accepted method and universally widespread.

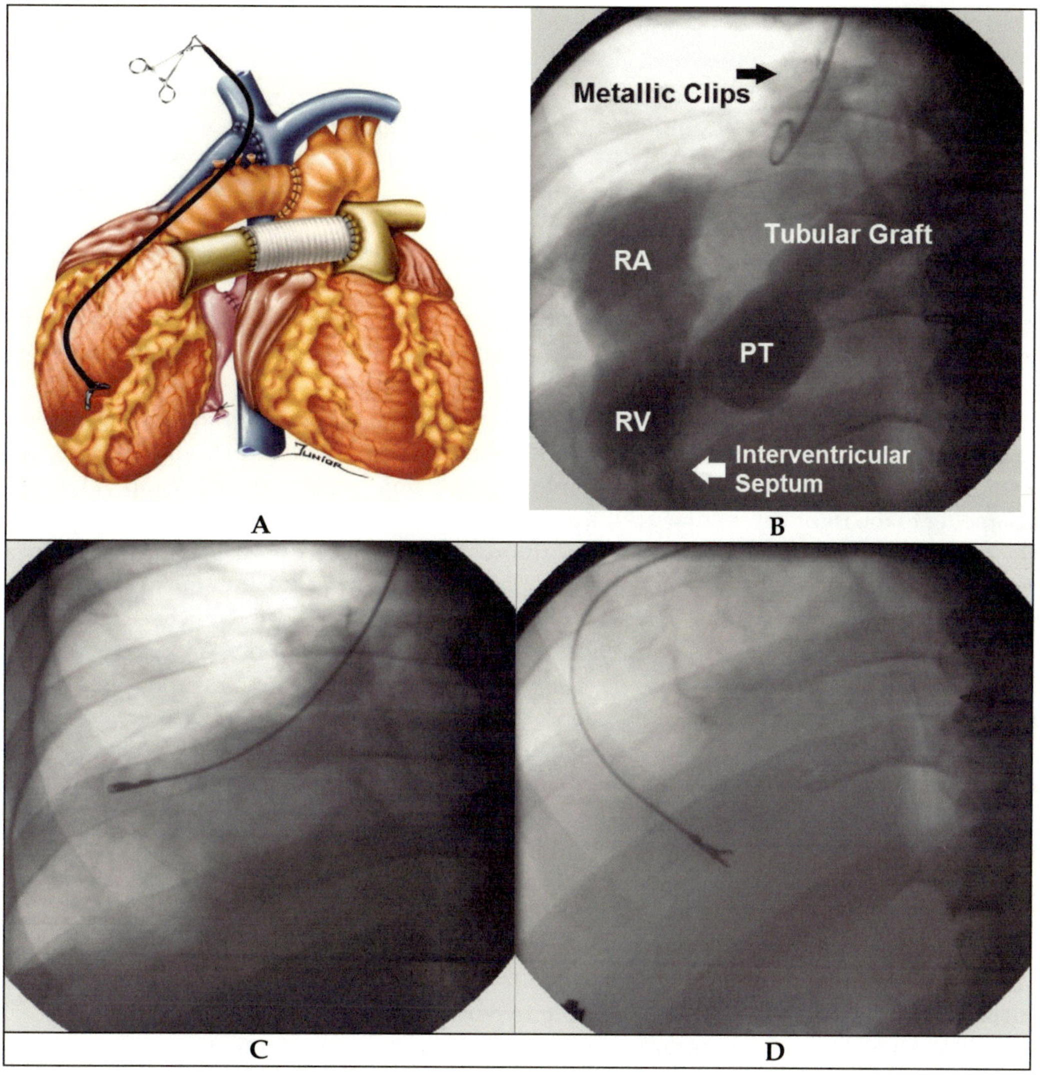

Fig. 7. A - Illustration showing bioptome trajectory during the performing of the endomyocardial biopsy on heterotopic heart transplantation. B - Contrast injection into graft superior vena cava. In superior vena cava anastomosis was placed metallic clips for easy identification of the bioptome entry site into cardiac graft. C – Inside the right atrium the bioptome tip tends to move away from the tricuspid valve. D – After rotating 180 degree the bioptome reaches the interventricular septum. Sometimes the forceps opening may offer resistance by trajectory tortuosity of bioptome

Other noninvasive methods may offer additional information about anatomic aspects and improved guidance of the bioptome[26]. For example, computed tomography may be used to assess the angle of the intraventricular septum relative to the superior vena cava or inferior vena cava, and cardiac magnetic resonance imaging may be of value to detection of a focal disease process may identify the area of the left or right ventricle that would be most likely to demonstrate the underlying pathological process. These methods have more application to guide biopsy with needle on investigation of the extracardiac thoracic mass.

3.1 Endomyocardial biopsy guidance by echocardiography

In this chapter we give more emphasis to two-dimensional echocardiography as guidance method for endomyocardial biopsy realization as well as hybrid method i.e. association of both methods for special situations.

In 1983, Hanley et al., published the use of echocardiography to guide endomyocardial biopsy in diagnosis of the left ventricle melanoma[27].

In 1984, Piérard et al. reported the use of two-dimensional echocardiography as bioptome guidance method during the endomyocardial biopsy[28]. In the same year, Copeland et al., extended this procedure to investigation of intracardiac mass[29].

In 1985 Williams et al., described the use of the two-echocardiography as guide to endomyocardial biopsy with successful in 83 patients being that in 96% of the cases was possible visualize the bioptome entering into right atrium, crossing the tricuspid valve, and advancing to the right ventricular apex and free wall[30].

The echocardiographic technique without fluoroscopy has been used primarily to critical patients that cannot go to catheterization room, present contraindication for radiation or to biopsy intracardiac masses. In contrast to fluoroscopy and angiography, echocardiography is able to provide direct assessment of soft tissues and heart anatomy, and can assess the relationship between catheters or devices and adjacent structures.

Some operators use fluoroscopy and echocardiography in combination, also called hybrid method, to enhance entry into the right ventricle and direction of the bioptome. Three-dimensional echocardiography may enhance visualization and reduce the reliance on radiographic imaging in the future.

Endomyocardial biopsy technique employs routinely the fluoroscopy to guide the bioptome very easily and with few adverse effects. In most cases, when there is high risk to transfer the patient at catheterization room or contraindication to use of fluoroscopy as in the pregnancy the echocardiography is very practical. Sometimes the transthoracic or transesophageal echocardiography are useful to confirm the position of intracardiac tumors but also to guide the bioptome for providing two or three-dimensional images.

Two-dimensional echocardiography advantages over other imaging modalities are equipment mobility, X-ray elimination, and offer in real time image during all procedure. It can be recorded at the bedside, into cardiac catheterization laboratory, cardiovascular intensive care unit, emergency room-indeed, any place that can accommodate a wheeled cart. It provide in real time images with adequate spatial orientation and anatomic definition. It is helpful in the cardiomyopathy diagnosis, intracardiac masses visualization, intracardiac catheters detection, and in the catheter placement and localization mainly in a pediatric population. However, it has as main disadvantage the necessity of a specialist operator becoming the process more expensive.

The most advantage with use of the two-dimensional echocardiography to guide endomyocardial biopsy is the possibility of realize the procedure to bedside and perhaps to may reduce the risk of perforation by a better anatomic definition of the myocardial sampling site. It permits sampling from different ventricular sites giving preference to the septum. Table 4 resumes advantages and disadvantages of endomyocardial biopsy guided by two-dimensional echocardiography.

Advantages
• It does not require the use of hemodynamic laboratory.
• Both patient and operator are not exposed to radiation.
• As two-dimensional echocardiography apparatus is portable the exam can be realized in intensive care unit, surgical room or even in the hemodynamic laboratory.
• It allows the realization of hybrid exam.
• Biopsy samples can be obtained from different site such as upper interventricular septum or middle, apex, and free wall, which increase the diagnostic yield.
• More accuracy to achieve the bioptome on intracavitary tumor mass.
Disadvantages
• It requires an operator specialized in echocardiography.
• Lack of window for viewing.

Table 4. Advantages and disadvantages two-dimensional echocardiography to guide endomyocardial biopsy

In our institution endomyocardial biopsy and Gallium-scintigraphy are the main methods to rejection control and Chagas' disease reactivation after heart transplantation, and research too[31-39]. The two-dimensional echocardiography has been used in last 25 years to guide endomyocardial biopsy examination with emphasis in critical patients with cardiomyopathy or after heart transplantation; to help in the visualization of the intracardiac tumors' position and in patients that cannot go at catheterization room[40,41].

The patient is putting in supine position and the transducer is placed at the point of maximal impulse of the heart this way is possible obtain cardiac image in four chamber. This position offers the best view to follow the bioptome into cardiac chambers until interventricular septum. The transducer may be then moved medially in the same plane until it lay over the right ventricular apex.

After the heart global echocardiographic evaluation with propose of studied cardiac chambers and ejection fraction, the transducer was placed at the subcostal area apex and kept the image with apical four-chamber view. This position provides better image to guidance and accompaniment of the exam, and allows observing very well the movements of the bioptome extremity inside of the heart. It is possible identify the passage of bioptome within the superior vena cava, right atrium, crossing the tricuspid valve to reach the interventricular septum right side.

An echocardiographic-dense image identifies the bioptome and the forceps removing the fragments of the interventricular septum. Contrast saline solution injection into venous system by jugular vein improves the cardiac chambers identification.
Once contact with the endocardium is confirmed by two-dimensional echocardiography, the bioptome is withdrawn 1 to 2 cm and its jaws were opened. After, the bioptome is advanced slowly to engage the endocardium. Gentle forward pressure is maintained while the jaws are closed.
In each exam was removing between 5 to 7 myocardial specimens for histopathological analysis. The bioptome containing the specimen is removed by gentle traction on the shaft.
Recently, we published our experience with the use of two-dimensional echocardiography as a guidance method to performance of endomyocardial biopsies. We avoided the withdrawal from myocardial samples of right ventricle free wall by higher risk of perforation[40,41]. The preferred route of access for bioptome percutaneous introduction was the right internal jugular vein with 8.5 Fr introducer in 62(81.6%) biopsies, left internal jugular in 11(14.5%) and femoral vein in 3(3.9%). The guide catheter was useful in lots of situations mainly when femoral vein was the access route.

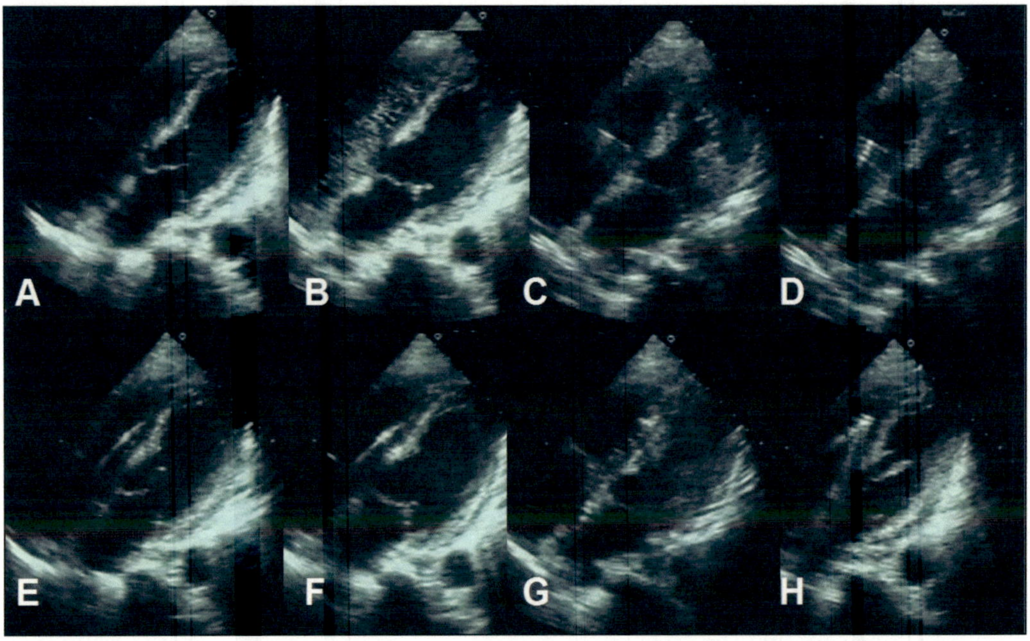

Fig. 8. Sequential images of the endomyocardial biopsy guided by two-dimensional echocardiography. A - Apical four-chamber view. B - Contrasted image obtained by saline solution injection. C - Bioptome tip on the tricuspid valve. D - Bioptome passing across tricuspid valve. E - Bioptome advancing against middle of the interventricular septum. F - Bioptome withdrawing myocardial fragment. G - Bioptome withdrawing myocardial fragment at apex. H - Bioptome coming out the right ventricle

In patients who needed of the continuous invasive cardiac monitoring the Swan-Ganz catheter is easily installed after biopsy by echocardiography too. Hybrid guidance with fluoroscopy and two-dimensional echocardiography was very useful to carry out the bioptome with more safety during the learning period and in patients with cardiac tumor.

Heart transplantation operative technique, biatrial or bicaval, was not impeditive factor to realize the endomyocardial biopsy two-dimensional echocardiography guidance; however may have difficulty if the vena cava anastomosis had stenosis. The Figure 7 shows details of an endomyocardial biopsy image guided by two-dimensional echocardiographic in patient after heart transplantation by bicaval technique.

Two-dimensional echocardiography advantages over other imaging modalities are equipment mobility, X-ray elimination, and offer in real time image during all procedure. It can be recorded at the bedside, into cardiac catheterization laboratory, cardiovascular intensive care unit, emergency room-indeed, any place that can accommodate a wheeled cart. It provides in real time images with adequate spatial orientation and anatomic definition. It is helpful in the cardiomyopathy diagnosis, intracardiac masses visualization, intracardiac catheters detection, and in the catheter placement and localization mainly in a pediatric population. However, it has as main disadvantage the necessity of a specialist operator becoming the process more expensive.

In 2004, Bedanova et al. reported experience with 1,262 biopsies collected under echocardiography guidance in 156 patients and only in 11 patients there was conversion to X-ray guidance and no case of significant tricuspid regurgitation was related due to biopsy[42].

After our learning period, the procedure duration time with echocardiographic guidance was comparable with fluoroscopy, between 10 and 15 minutes. The percutaneous right jugular vein approach was more employed due to its facility in offer few curves during the bioptome advance and both models can be used with guide catheter or sheath. In patients with artificial cardiac pacing the puncture was performed on an opposite side.

In our series, the surgical technique of the heart transplantation did not offer additional difficulties to endomyocardial biopsy by two-dimensional echocardiography guidance agreement with other investigations. Difficulties to progression of the bioptome occur frequently when there is severe stenosis at the site of the superior vena cava anastomosis.

Recently the use of real-time transthoracic three-dimensional echocardiography in endomyocardial right ventricular biopsies has been investigated both in children as in adults with easiness and safe perhaps until with more benefits[43].

In experienced hands to accomplish endomyocardial biopsy by fluoroscopy the learning will be easier with two-dimensional echocardiography as orientation guide. The view by fluoroscopy is in the frontal plane (or coronal plane) being possible following the bioptome advance until there occurs transition of superior or inferior vena cava to right atrium, and the entry into right ventricle across tricuspid valve. The view by two-dimensional echocardiographic is in the transverse plane and the transducer is then located in the subcostal position, and a short-axis plane is visualized, showing the junction between the inferior vena cava and the right atrium. If the femoral vein approach is used, the bioptome can be seen entering the right atrium from the inferior vena cava.

When the forceps enters the right atrium, the transducer is rotated to obtain at frontal plane the subcostal four-chamber view that is the more appropriate (Figure 1). The tricuspid leaflets are easily visible by two-dimensional echocardiography and helps the operator pass the bioptome across valve with minimal trauma. The bioptome advances under echocardiographic control and is seen crossing the tricuspid valve and entering the right ventricular cavity.

Into the right atrium, an anterior counterclockwise rotation helps guide the bioptome overcome the tricuspid valve. This maneuver must be performed delicately by atrium perforation risk or injuries on valvar apparatus. Generally, the primary positioning is not satisfactory, and the catheter must be manipulated using two-dimensional echocardiography to position the tip optimally, in front of the interventricular septum. Further counterclockwise rotations straighten the curve and orient the bioptome to central ventricular septum.

Under two-echocardiography is possible withdraw myocardial fragments of all septum region and avoiding the ventricle free wall.

The most appalling during the endomyocardial biopsy accomplishment is the perforation of the right or left ventricle with cardiac tamponade by its high morbidity with death risk, especially if an inexperienced team does the manipulation. Sometimes it has been observed by fluoroscopy dislocation of the tip of the bioptome until the cardiac apex and is very difficult differentiating between apical portion septum and the free wall. These are the situations of more risk of the ventricular perforation mainly in dilated cardiomyopathies.

It is probably that the endomyocardial biopsy guidance by two-dimensional echocardiographic may reduce the complications incidence by providing a better anatomic view of the adequate site where the specimens must to be withdrawn, from the septum and not from the right ventricular free wall.

On the other hand, by two-dimensional echocardiography is possible adequately distinguishes the septum from the right ventricular free wall. It also permits patient follow-up after the procedure and immediate detection of complications such as pericardial effusion or the appearance of thrombus. Sometimes it is possible to identify the opening and closing of the bioptome jaw (Figure 5).

The local pain, hematoma and other minor complications may be more frequents and are related with the puncture difficulties.

3.2 Risks of the endomyocardial biopsy

The most potential complications due to endomyocardial biopsy occur during the procedure and the diagnosis or the suspect diagnostic is done also during the intervention period. Occasionally, the injuries due to endomyocardial biopsy have clinical manifestations late and during the intervention there was not any lesion suspect.

Main complications are ventricular perforation and tamponade cardiac; pneumothorax, hemothorax or both; cervical hematoma or mediastinal; ventricular arrhythmias or supraventricular; transitory cardiac block; carotid puncture or femoral; transitory phrenic nerve paralysis; pain; and unsuccessful puncture or guidewire progression. Except ventricular perforation the others may be more frequent however are considered benign complications and rarely put the patient in life risk.

Endomyocardial biopsy is a simple procedure but non-free of risk and the ventricular perforation followed of tamponade is the most terrible of them because the mortality is related with this severe complication. Patients with coagulopathies, increased right ventricular systolic pressures, recent receipt of heparin, or right ventricular enlargement seem to be at higher risk.

Every center that performs endomyocardial biopsy must have available echocardiography because is useful to confirm pericardial effusion and should be performed whenever the operator suspects of ventricle perforation even before the patient leaves the catheterization room. This terrible complication may manifest initially with lightweight chest discomfort and without cardiovascular shock evident and that is getting worse due to the injury degree and the pericardial effusion intensity.

Immediate pericardiocentesis and the capability to surgically evacuate the pericardial space should be available at centers that perform endomyocardial biopsy. The right ventricle is more susceptible because the wall has about of 1 to 2 mm thickness. In patient with dilated cardiomyopathy this complication is more severe because right ventricular wall is thinner.

To reduce the chance of perforation, the operator must always open the bioptome jaws before touching the ventricle wall to increase contact area and after few seconds close the forceps slowly. This maneuver allows the bioptome accommodate among the trabecular and withdraw a myocardial fragment gently. The procedure must be repeated to removal of 5 to 7 fragments.

The bleeding risk after perforation increases in patients with pulmonary hypertension or coagulopathies. Small perforations may have spontaneous resolution because right ventricle pressure is low.

The contact of the bioptome with ventricular wall or during withdraw myocardial fragment may generate temporary ventricular arrhythmias. Malign arrhythmias rarely occur and are related with cardiomyopathy gravity. In our experience with more of 10,000 biopsies there is only related one case which needed of the cardiac defibrillation for ventricular fibrillation as primary event. Same in cardiomyopathies severe risk of malignant arrhythmias sustained is very rare.

The risks of endomyocardial biopsy are related with clinical picture of the patient and the operator experience. Patients with cardiogenic collapse or unstable ventricular arrhythmias require most care and carry to catheterization room is not recommendable. In these cases endomyocardial biopsy guidance by echocardiography is highly suitable.

Major complications	Minor complications
Haemopericardium / Tamponade	Chest pain (transient)
Mediastinitis	Nerve palsy
Pneumothorax / Air embolism	Rupture of chordae tendineae (small)
Pericardial fibrosis/thickening	Deep vein thrombosis
Thromboembolism	Haematoma
Myocardial infarction	Hypotension
Infectious transmission (hepatitis B/C)	Vascular fistulae
Tricuspid or mitral valve damage with possible severe regurgitation	Electrocardiographic abnormalities (transient)

Table 5. Complications of endomyocardial biopsies

Complications average rate is variable in different centers due to service experience and of adopted criteria in the database construction. Rate complications will be greater the more extensive and detailed is the database. Complications incidence varies since values inferior to 1% until 7%, being that the more severe injuries as well as the mortality do not exceed to 0.5%. Table 6 shows the main complications at experience for different authors.

Author	**Olsen**	**Fowles and Mason**	**Deckers**	**Han**	**Fiorelli**	**Fiorelli**
Year		**1982**	**1992**	**2006***	**2010**	**2011***
Biopsy number	**3097**	**n>4000**	**546**	**90**	**1228****	**76**
Possible ventricular perforation (pain)			0.7%		0.0%	0.0%
Tamponade		0.14%	0.5%***	3.3%	0.8%	0.0%
Hemo/Pneumothorax		3 cases			1.1%	0.0%
Atrial fibrillation		3 cases			0.1%	0.0%
Ventricular arrhythmia		1 case	1.1%	1.1%	0.5%	0.8%
AV block permanent					0.0%	0.0%
Neurological complications		1 case			0.0%	0.0%
Vasovagal reaction			0.4%	2.2%	0.0%	0.0%
Prolonged venous oozing after sheath removal			0.2%		0.0%	0.0%
Local pain				6.7%	8.3%	5.6%
Puncture failure					5.8%	6.6%
Tricuspid injury					0.8%	0.0%
Arterial puncture during local anesthesia			2.0%		3.1%	2.8%
Local hematoma					3.7%	5.3%
Arteriovenous fistula					0.1%	0.0%
Superior vena cava injuries					0.1%	0.0%
Mortality			**0.4%**	**0.0%**	**0.0%**	**0.0%**
Total of complications	**1.55%**	**<1%**	**6.0%**	**5.6%**	**9.2%**	**4.5%**

* - only guided by echocardiography; ** - only patients with heart transplantation, *** - 2 deaths.

Table 6. Complications after endomyocardial biopsy for different authors

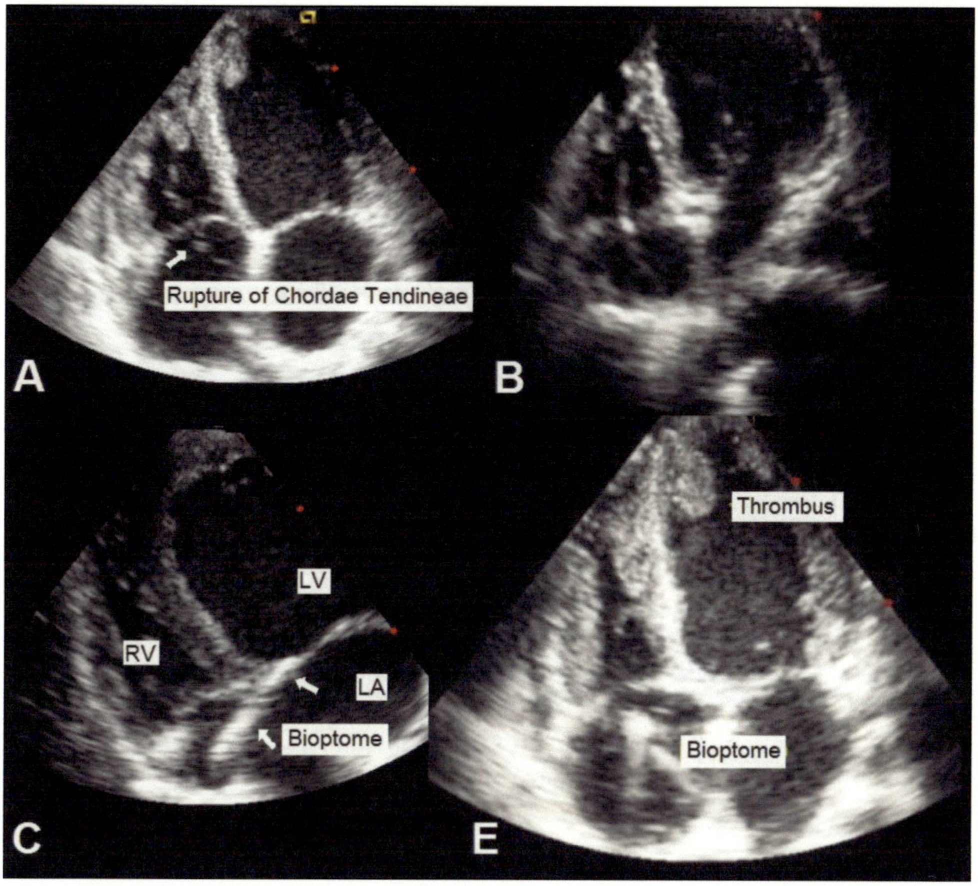

Fig. 9. A - Rupture of chordae tendineae due endomyocardial biopsy. B - Bioptome in normal position toward the interventricular septum. C - Bioptome inside coronary sinus. D - Bioptome in normal position inside right atrium and left intraventricular thrombus finding echocardiographic
Courtesy of Dr. Arnaldo Rabischoffsky

3.3 Conclusion

Although there have been numerous studies comparing non-invasive imaging techniques to endomyocardial biopsy for the diagnosis of graft rejection, infiltrative disorders, and even intracardiac masses, there are still considerable limitations to these techniques. The endomyocardial biopsy remains the gold standard to assess and diagnose myocardial disease in the living patient.

The endomyocardial biopsy procedure is a safe, simple, and effective interventional procedure with a very low rate of morbidity and mortality. Fluoroscopy is the guide method to endomyocardial biopsy more used and safe; however in many times presents serious restrictions or same it cannot be utilized. Critical patients and pregnancy are good examples these situations.

Two-echocardiography is a fantastic recourse by information reliability, practicality and portable. Two-dimensional echocardiography is a special feature to guidance endomyocardial biopsies mainly in critically ill patients because it can be realized to bedside and without offers additional risk, and presents still advantages on the fluoroscopy. In special situations, the hybrid combination can be very useful mainly in intra-cardiac tumor cases.

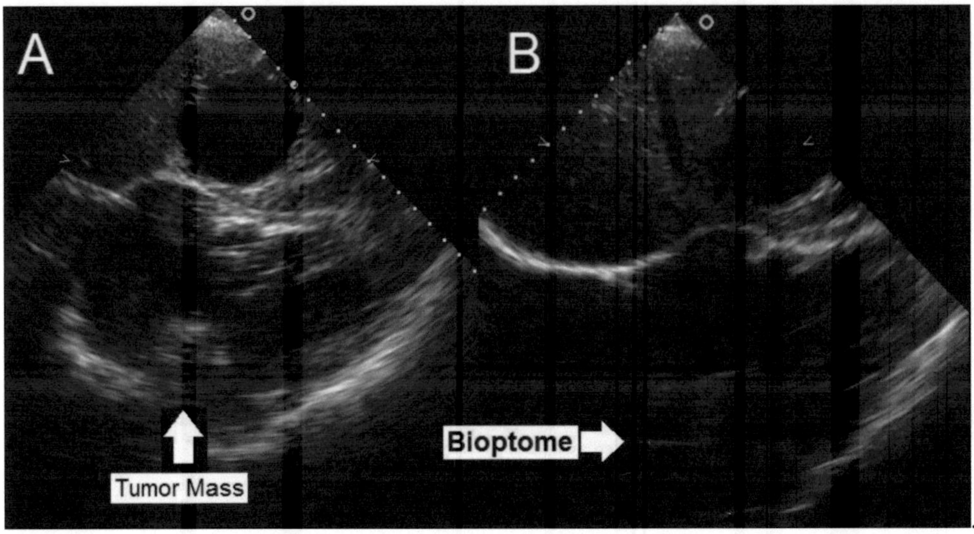

Fig. 10. A - Patient with tumor into right atrium confirmed by two-echocardiography. B – Bioptome withdrawing myocardial fragment and anatomic pathological exam confirmed the presence of angiosarcoma

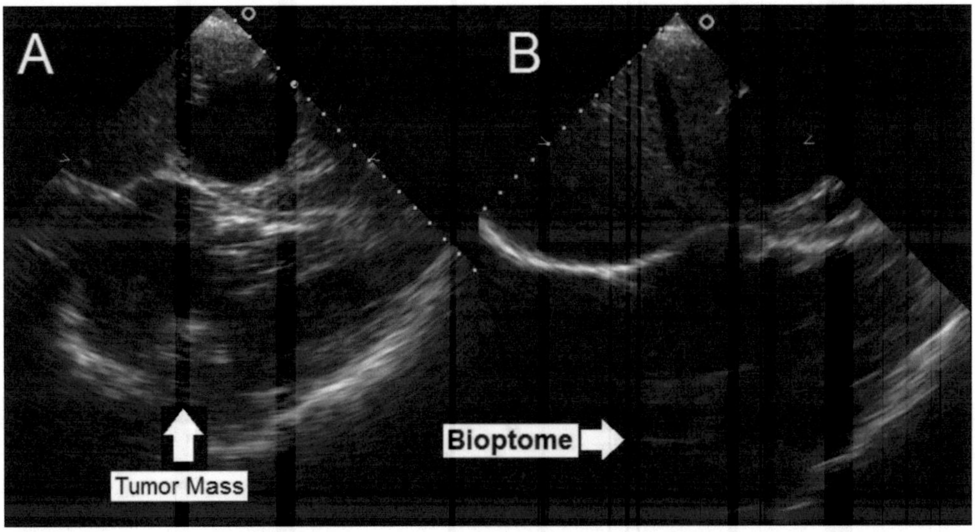

Fig. 11. A - Patient with tumor into right atrium confirmed by two-echocardiography. B – Bioptome withdrawing myocardial fragment and the anatomic pathological exam confirmed the angiosarcoma diagnosis

4. Acknowledgements

We thank to
To all members of the Echocardiography Department of Heart Institute of Sao Paulo University/Brazil for excellent care to patients and by working together that we have developed over the years which resulted in this publication.
To Dr. Arnaldo Rabischoffsky - Director of the Echocardiography Unit of the Pro-Cardiac Hospital, Rio de Janeiro / Brazil - for gently in provides images of his personal collection.
To Marcelo Fiorelli Alexandrino da Silva – Medical student of Sao Paulo University – for data collection.

5. References

[1] Elliott P, Arbustini E. The role of endomyocardial biopsy in the management of cardiovascular disease: a commentary on joint AHA/ACC/ESC guidelines. *Heart.* 2009;95:759-60.
[2] Pytlewski G, Georgeson S, Burke J et al. Endomyocardial biopsy under transesophageal echocardiographic guidance can be safely performed in the critically ill cardiac transplant recipient. *Am J Cardiol* 1994;73:1019-20.
[3] Cooper LT, Baughman KL, Feldman AM, Frustaci A, Jessup M, Kuhl U, Levine GN, Narula J, Starling RC, Towbin J, Virmani R. The role of endomyocardial biopsy in the management of cardiovascular disease: a scientific statement from the American Heart Association, the American College of Cardiology, and the European Society of Cardiology. Endorsed by the Heart Failure Society of America and the Heart Failure Association of the European Society of Cardiology. *European Heart Journal* 2007;28,3076–3093.
[4] Jackson CE, Gardner RS, Connelly DT. A novel approach for a novel combination: a trans-septal biopsy of left atrial mass in recurrent phyllodes tumour. *Eur J Echocardiogr* 2009;10:171-2.
[5] Abramowitz Y, Hiller N, Perlman G et al. - The diagnosis of primary cardiac lymphoma by right heart catheterization and biopsy using fluoroscopic and transthoracic echocardiographic guidance. *Int J Cardiol* 2007;118:e39-40.
[6] Raffensperger J, Driscoll J, Sutton G, et al: Myocardial biopsy. *Arch Surg* (Chicago) 1964;89:1021.
[7] Weinberg M, Egbert HF, Lydield J: Diagnostic biopsy of the pericardium and myocardium. *Arch Surg* (Chicago) 1958;76:825.
[8] Price KC, Weiss JM, Hata JM, et al: Experimental needle biopsy of myocardium of dogs with particular reference to histological study by electron microscopy. *J Exper Med* 1955;101:687.
[9] Bercu B, Heinz J, Chaudhry AS, et al: Myocardial biopsy -A new technique utilizing the ventricular septum. *Am J Cardiol* 1964;14:675.
[10] Timmis CG, Gordon S, Baron RH, et al: Percutaneous myocardial biopsy. *Am Heart J* 1965;70: 499.
[11] Leighton RF, Hamlin RL, Scarpelli DG, et al: Drill biopsy of the canine interventricular septum: A new cardiac catheterization technique. *Am J Cardiol* 1967;19:365.
[12] Bulloch RT, Murphy LM, Pearce BM: Intracardiac needle biopsy of the ventricular septum. *Am J Cardiol* 1965;16:227,.

[13. Weinberg M, Fell Eh, Lynfield J. Diagnostic biopsy of the pericardium and myocardium. *AMA Arch Surg*. 1958;76:825-9.
[14] Sutton Dc, Sutton Gc. Needle biopsy of the human ventricular myocardium: review of 54 consecutive cases. *Am Heart J*. 1960;60:364-70.
[15] Timmis GC, Gordon S, Baron RH, Brough AJ. Percutaneous myocardial biopsy. *Am Heart J*. 1965;70:499-504.
[16] Sakakibara S, Konno S. Endomyocardial biopsy. *Jpn Heart J*. 1962;3:537-43.
[17] Bulloch Rt, Murphy Ml, Pearce Mb. Intracardiac needle biopsy of the ventricular septum. *Am J Cardiol*. 1965;16:227-33.
[18] Caves PK, Stinson EB, Graham AF, Billingham ME, Grehl TM, Shumway NE. Percutaneous transvenous endomyocardial biopsy. *JAMA*. 1973;225:288-91.
[19] Shirey EK, Hawk WA, Mukerji D, Effler DB. Percutaneous myocardial biopsy of the left ventricle. Experience in 198 patients. *Circulation*. 1972;46:112-22.
[20] Ali N, Ferrans VI, Roberts WC, Maswmi RA. Clinical evaluation of transvenous catheter technique for endomyocardial biopsy. *Chest* 1973;63;399-402.
[21] Richardson PJ. King's endomyocardial bioptome. *Lancet*. 1974;7859:660-1.
[22] Kawai C, Matsumori A, Kawamura K. Myocardial biopsy. *Annu Rev Med*. 1980;31:139-57.
[23] Seldinger SI. Catheter replacement of the needle in percutaneous artenography: a new technique. *Acta Radiol* (Stockh) 1953; 36: 368-76.
[24] Anderson JL, Marshall HW. The femoral venous approach to endomyocardial biopsy: comparison with internal jugular and transarterial approaches.*Am J Cardiol*. 1984;53:833-7.
[25] Holzmann M, Nicko A, Kühl U, Noutsias M, Poller W, Hoffmann W, Morguet A, Witzenbichler B, Tschöpe C, Schultheiss HP, Pauschinger M. Complication rate of right ventricular endomyocardial biopsy via the femoral approach: a retrospective and prospective study analyzing 3048 diagnostic procedures over an 11-year period. *Circulation*. 2008;118:1722-8.
[26] Borchert B, Lawrenz T, Bartelsmeier M, Röthemeyer S, Kuhn H, Stellbrink C. Utility of endomyocardial biopsy guided by delayed enhancement areas on magnetic resonance imaging in the diagnosis of cardiac sarcoidosis. *Clin Res Cardiol*. 2007;96:759-62.
[27] Hanley PC, Shub C, SeWard JB, Wold LE. Intracavitary cardiac melanoma diagnosed by endomyocardial left ventricular biopsy. *Chest* 1983; 54:195-8
[28] Piérard L, El Allaf D, D'Orio V, Demoulin JC, Carlier J. Two-dimensional echocardiographic guiding of endomyocardial biopsy. *Chest*. 1984 Jun;85(6):759-62.
[29] Copeland JG, Valdes-Cruz L, Sahn DJ. Endomyocardial biopsy with fluoroscopic and two-dimensional echocardiographic guidance: case report of a patient suspected of having multiple cardiac tumors. *Clin Cardiol*. 1984;7:449-52.
[30] Williams GA, Kaintz RP, Habermehl KK, Nelson JG, Kennedy HL. Clinical experience with two-dimensional echocardiography to guide endomyocardial biopsy. *Clin Cardiol*. 1985;8:137-40.
[31] Higuchi ML, de Assis RV, Sambiase NV, Reis MM, Kalil J, Bocchi E, Fiorelli A, Stolf N, Bellotti G, Pileggi F, et al. Usefulness of T-cell phenotype characterization in endomyocardial biopsy fragments from human cardiac allografts. *J Heart Lung Transplant*. 1991;10:235-42.

[32] Coelho V, Moliterno R, Higuchi ML, Guilherme L, Cunha-Neto E, Fiorelli AI, Kalil J. Gamma delta T cells play no major role in human heart allograft rejection. *Transplantation*. 1995;60:980-4.

[33] Bacal F, Veiga VC, Fiorelli AI, Bellotti G, Bocchi EA, Stolf NA, Ramires JA. Treatment of persistent rejection with methotrexate in stable patients submitted to heart transplantation. *Arq Bras Cardiol*. 2000;74:141-8.

[34] Benvenuti LA, Roggério A, Sambiase NV, Fiorelli A, Higuchi Mde L. Polymerase chain reaction in endomyocardial biopsies for monitoring reactivation of Chagas' disease in heart transplantation: a case report and review of the literature. *Cardiovasc Pathol.* 2005;14:265-8.

[35] Benvenuti LA, Roggério A, Freitas HF, Mansur AJ, Fiorelli A, Higuchi ML. Chronic American trypanosomiasis: parasite persistence in endomyocardial biopsies is associated with high-grade myocarditis. *Ann Trop Med Parasitol*. 2008;102:481-7.

[36] Fiorelli AI, Coelho GH, Lima JL, Lourenço DD, Gutierres P, Bacal F, Bocchi E, Dias RR, Stolf NA. Massive degeneration and atrophy of the native heart after heterotopic transplantation: a case report. *Transplant Proc*. 2009;41:965-6.

[37] Bacal F, de Freitas AF Jr, Moreira LF, F orelli AI, Mangini S, Abuhab A, de Lima Oliveira J Jr, Santos RH, Stolf NA, Bocchi EA. Validation of a cutoff value on echo Doppler analysis to replace right heart catheterization during pulmonary hypertension evaluation in heart transplant candidates. *Transplant Proc.* 2010;42:535-8.

[38] Benvenuti LA, Roggério A, Coelho G, Fiorelli AI. Usefulness of qualitative polymerase chain reaction for Trypanosoma cruzi DNA in endomyocardial biopsy specimens of chagasic heart transplant patients. *J Heart Lung Transplant*. 2011; [Epub ahead of print].

[39] Fiorelli AI, Santos RH, Oliveira JL Jr, Lourenço-Filho DD, Dias RR, Oliveira AS, da Silva MF, Ayoub FL, Bacal F, Souza GE, Bocchi EA, Stolf NA. Heart transplantation in 107 cases of Chagas' disease. *Transplant Proc*. 2011;43:220-4.

[40] Fiorelli AI, Coelho GH, Oliveira JL Jr, Aiello VD, Benvenuti LA, Santos A, Chi A, Tallans A, Igushi ML, Bacal F, Bocchi EA, Stolf NA. Endomyocardial biopsy as risk factor in the development of tricuspid insufficiency after heart transplantation. *Transplant Proc*. 2009;41:935-7.

[41] Fiorelli AI, Coelho GB, Santos RH, Oliveira JL Jr, Aielo V, Benvenuti L, Oliveira AS, Da Silva MA, Chizzola PR, Costa R, Mathias W Jr, Bacal F, Bocchi EA, Stolf NA. Successful endomyocardial biopsy guided by transthoracic two-dimensional echocardiography. *Transplant Proc*. 2011;43:225-8.

[42] Bedanova H, Necas J, Petrikovits E, Pokorny P, Kovalova S, Malik P, Ondrasek J, Cerny J. Echo-guided endomyocardial biopsy in heart transplant recipients. *Transpl Int.* 2004;17:622-5.

[43] Platts D, Brown M, Javorsky G, West C, Kelly N, Burstow D. Comparison of fluoroscopic versus real-time three-dimensional transthoracic echocardiographic guidance of endomyocardial biopsies. *Eur J Echocardiogr*. 2010;11:637-43.

[44] Olsen EG. The value of endomyocardial biopsies in myocarditis and dilated cardiomyopathy. *Eur Heart J*. 1991;12 Suppl D:10-2.

[45] Rabischoffsky A. Echo-guided endomyocardial biopsy. *Rev Bras Ecocardiogr* 2008;21:27-30.

[46] Han J, Park Y, Lee H, Kang H, Kim H, Yang DH, Park HS, Cho Y, Chae SC, Jun JE, Park WH. Complications of 2-D echocardiography guided transfemoral right ventricular endomyocardial biopsy. *J Korean Med Sci*. 2006;21:989-94.

[47] Fowles RE, Mason JW. Myocardial biopsy. *Mayo Clin Proc*. 1982;57:459-61.

[48] Deckers JW, Hare JM, Baughman KL. Complications of transvenous right ventricular endomyocardial biopsy in adult patients with cardiomyopathy: a seven-year survey of 546 consecutive diagnostic procedures in a tertiary referral center. *J Am Coll Cardiol*. 1992;19:43-7.

[49] Han J, Park Y, Lee H, Kang H, Kim H, Yang DH, Park HS, Cho Y, Chae SC, Jun JE, Park WH. Complications of 2-D echocardiography guided transfemoral right ventricular endomyocardial biopsy. . *J Korean Med Sci*. 2006;21:989-94.

Part 2

Pulmonary Factors Influencing Doppler

4

Doppler Echocardiographic Changes in Respiratory Diseases

Mohammed Al-Biltagi[1] and Adel Salah Bediwy[2]
[1]*Pediatric Department, Cardiology Unit, Faculty of Medicine, Tanta University,*
[2]*Chest Department, Faculty of Medicine, Tanta University*
Egypt

1. Introduction

The heart is one of the most important organs which can be affected by several systems including respiratory system. The in common function of both heart and lung is to provide tissues with oxygen and to get rid of the Carbon dioxide. So; they work in harmony and interact in a proper way with each other. This interaction may be neural, mechanical and/or humeral. The neural effects are either central through the brain stem centres in medulla oblongata or peripheral through baro-reflexes or lung-stretch reflexes. Being together inside the thoracic cavity; the heart can be affected by lung inflation and deflation. This is called mechanical heart–lung interactions (Figure 1).

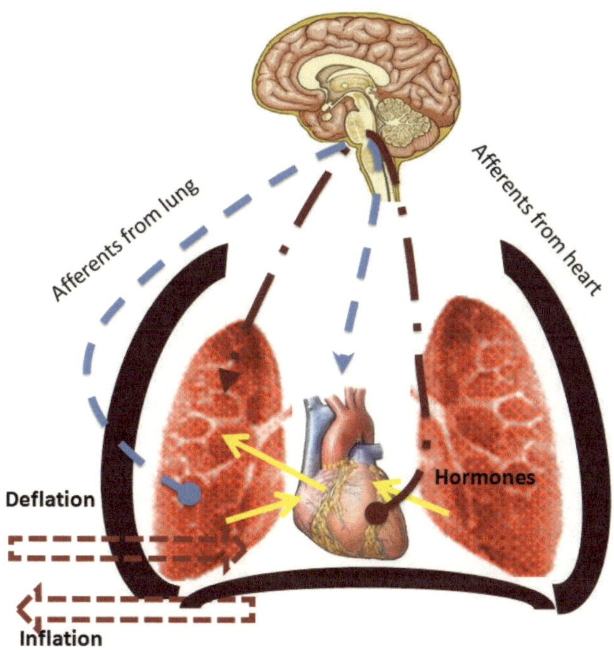

Fig. 1. The heart-lung interaction; neural, mechanical and humoral

The lung may act as an endocrine gland secreting certain hormones or substances that can affect heart functions forming what is known as humoral heart–lung interaction. The lung helps in deactivation of 5-hydroxytryptmine, acetylcholine, norepinephrine, bradykinin and prostaglandins E1, E2 and F2. It produces angiotensin converting enzyme that helps in activation of angiotensin I to angiotensin II and helps in synthesis of prostaglandins E1, E2. All these humoral products can affect the heart in a way or another. Atrial natriuretic peptide (ANP) and brain natriuretic peptide (BNP) are two polypeptide hormones secreted by the atrial cardiocytes. The ANP is well known to have a bronchodilating effect more prominent in the larger central airways than in the peripheral airways. The lung also supplies the cardiac muscle with the needed oxygen and the heart supplies the respiratory muscles with oxygenated blood. So; respiratory pump failure may occur if the heart cannot supply the needed requirement. These heart-lung interactions occur all the time with every breath and every cardiac cycle. However; their effects are subtle under normal circumstances but become significant in certain pathological situations *(Said 2001).*

2. Respiration induced changes in echocardiography

Respiration can bring on physiological changes of cardiovascular haemodynamics. These changes are mostly related to changes in intra-thoracic and intra-abdominal pressure which can affect both systemic and pulmonary venous return. Respiration can also affect the intra-pericardial pressure which in turn affects the filling of the four cardiac chambers. Respiration can affect all the modalities of the echocardiographic examination. It can affect the image quality as well as the measurements in Two-Dimensional echocardiography, M-mode and Doppler studies.

2.1 The image quality

The respiration may affect the image quality of the echocardiographic study especially when visualizing the posterior wall of the left ventricle (LV). Even normal respiration may have undulating, distorting, and blocking effect during echocardiographic examination of the heart; particularly the posterior wall of LV to the extent that the patient may need to hold his breath in order to obtain clear echoes (*Fenichel et al 1976*).

These effects are due to both physiological and anatomical changes that occur with respiration. The physiological changes are due to pressure variations (intra-thoracic, intrapericardial and intra-abdominal), changes in systemic and pulmonary venous return, diminished LV filling pressure during inspiration, pericardial constraint, ventricular interdependence and variation in the angle of incidence of the transducer beam. The anatomical changes are due to the diaphragmatic movements, lung inflation and with interference and dropping out of the lateral shadows together with longitudinal rotation and posterior motion of heart. Inspiration increases the antero-posterior diameter of the chest, and the lungs expand particularly anteriorly, and fill the space previously occupied by the heart. However; sub-costal view is an exception where the heart images become clearer with inspiration. However with deep inspiration; the abdomen becomes too tense to allow the transducer to be placed under the sternum. So; half a breath is preferred during sucostal examination of the heart. Lung deflation by expiration (particularly in steep left lateral position with left arm up to spread the ribs) can improve the image quality especially with the parasternal and often apical view of the heart. Left lateral rotation of the patient will deflate the left lung and avoid the pulmonary interference and improve the clarity of echocardiograms. Improving the quality of image can be done by using device-driven systems, which can acquire signal averaging of echocardiographic frames over multiple cardiac cycles (*Ginghina et al 2009, Lang 2005, Klingler 1989*)

2.2 Two-D and M-mode measurements

The respiration does not only affect the image quality but also can alter the measurement taken during 2-D and M-mode study. There is an inspiratory decrease in LV end diastolic dimensions as measured by M-mode due to reduction of the LV filling during inspiration. Respiration also can change the position of the heart relative to the location of the echo transducer which can cause measurement error due to anatomical translation and rotation of the heart, which may change with respiratory phases. There may be a significant inspiratory decrease of LV diastolic dimension while the inspiratory decrease of LV mean systolic dimension is usually insignificant. The echocardiography-derived inspiratory decrease in stroke volume is about 16% (*Brenner et al 1978*). This reduction in the LV dimensions during inspiration may be due actual reduction of LV stroke volume as a result of decrease preload due to decrease diastolic filling, increased after load (due to increased impedance to LV emptying) or due to the anatomical medial rotation of the short axis of the heart during inspiration. There is an existed consistent relation between the respiratory excursion and the resultant displacement of the recorded echoes (*Fenichel et al 1976*).

	Findings in deep Inspiration
Anterior echoes	Increased especially with deep inspiration
Posterior echoes	Displaced posteriorly (about 2 cm). The echogenicity may decreased or even eliminated.
Septum	Can be seen displaced posteriorly just before and after the appearance of dense mass tissue
Posterior wall of LV	There is blunting of its systolic anterior motion and decreased its pulsation but still can be identified.
RV end-diastolic volume	Increased
LV end-diastolic volume	Decreased
Total end-diastolic heart volume	Unchanged
Mitral leaflets	Echos are displaced posteriorly but the opening and closing slopes remain the same
Aortic root and semilunar valves	Posterior deviation up to 1 cm
Posterior wall of the left atrium	Posterior deviation parallel to the aortic root.
Tricuspid valve	Displaced posteriorly

Table 1. The changes in M-mode and 2-D measurements observed during deep inspiration

In a Study done in 1992, the effects of the quiet respiration and body position on RV size and function using 2-D and M-mode echocardiography were observed in 15 healthy children. All the end-diastolic and end-systolic echocardiographic dimensions, areas, and volumes increased slightly but significantly with inspiration. RV ejection fractions were found to be significantly higher during inspiration, as were stroke volume indices. The study also found that RV dimensions increased from supine to left lateral decubitus position (*Norgård and Vik-*

Mo 1992). On the other hand a previous study done in 1979 found that the changes observed in RV and LV diemensions during respiration were opposite in direction and approximately equal in magnitude, so that total internal diastolic cardiac dimension remained essentially constant (*Lendrum et al 1979*).

These respiration-related changes in the cardiac measurements should be considered while doing serial follow up measurements of LV functions during various hemodynamic interventions. These changes should also be considered in doing any correlation between echocardiographic dimensions and other methods of assessing LV function. To obtain more accurate measurement during two-dimensional quantitation; the American Society of Echocardiography recommended to obtain the image during quiet or suspended respiration (at end-expiration). However, many patients may not be able to follow even careful instructions. If the images are to be obtained during held end-expiration; the patient is advised to avoid Valsalva manoeuvre, as it can degrade image quality and produces undesired physiologic changes that disrupt the basic measurements. Table 1 showed the 2-D and M-mode findings observed in deep inspiration

2.3 Doppler measurements

During inspiration; the blood flow increases in the right side of the heart and decreases in the left side because of the decreased flow out of the pulmonary veins into the left atrium and left ventricle. The reverse occurs during expiration. These respiratory-induced changes in the intra-cardiac blood flow were reflected in the Doppler estimated trans-mitral and trans-tricuspid blood inflow as well as the trans-pulmonary and trans-aortic blood outflow.

Respiration does not only affect the intracardiac blood inflow and outflow; but also affecting the intracardiac pressures. The right atrial pressure which is needed to estimate the systolic right ventricular, pulmonary artery pressures and left atrial pressure; can be expected by the changes in the diameter of the IVC during inspiration. Respiratory variation in SVC systolic forward flow may be a useful Doppler flow index for expecting the systolic pulmonary pressure and to assess the severity of pulmonary hypertension. During inspiration the E/A ratio of transmitral flow may be reduced but of no significance in healthy subjects. However this effect may become significant in certain cardiac diseases as in coronary artery diseases and abnormal LV relaxation pattern (*Ginghina et al 2009*).

2.3.1 Mitral and tricuspid inflow

The normal changes in the intra-thoracic pressure occurring during normal breathing have insignificant effects on the trans-mitral and trans-tricuspid flow. However these changes become significant with strained breathing. *Uiterwaal et al 1989* found that the maximum velocity during early diastole of right ventricle (VmaxE) and during atrial contraction (VmaxA) were significantly higher during inspiration than during expiration. They found the reverse on the mitral side; as the VmaxE and VmaxA were significantly lower during inspiration than during expiration. *Tsai et al* 1998 found that early diastolic peak flow velocity and flow velocity integral, the ratio of early/late diastolic peak flow velocity, and the ratio of early/late diastolic flow velocity integral at end-inspiration were significantly lower than those at end-expiration. The mitral peak E velocity decreased by 4-9% while the A wave remains unchanged. On the other hand the Tricuspid peak E velocity increased 15% while the A wave increased by 10% which maintain E/A ratio to be unchanged.

Riggs and Snider 1989 found reduction of early diastolic LV filling parameters in normal children (decreased E wave by 8 %) while active atrial emptying (peak A velocity and

A/total area ratio) may remain unchanged with respiration. This led to marked reduction of transmitral E/A ratio (by 14%). The effect was marked on the right side of the heart. The tricuspid peak E increased by 26% while peak A velocities increased by 18%. The E/A ratio remained unchanged. *Yuan et al 2004* quantitatively investigated the effect of the different intra-thoracic pressure on the blood flow velocities across the four cardiac valves. They found significant difference from the transvalvular velocities recorded during spontaneous respiration with the velocities recorded during various intrathoracic pressures. They concluded that the respiratory intrathoracic pressure changes may cause change in the velocity across the valves. However *Riggs et al 1989* showed that the inspiratory changes in Tricuspid valve Doppler indexes had less marked changes in neonates. This could be due to the faster heart and respiratory rates plus the reduced right ventricular compliance. To minimize the effect of respiration on the trans-mitral and trans-tricuspid flow velocities, the patient is advised to hold breathing in shallow end-expiration.

2.3.2 Aortic and pulmonary outflow

Ferreira T et al 1990 found significant higher peak early velocity in the inflow tract and in the maximal velocity in the outflow tract of the LV during expiration. There were also no significant changes in the time intervals observed in their study. *Buda et al 1979* studied the effects of Valsalva and Müller manoeuvres on LV functions. They observed that the negative intra-thoracic pressure may affect LV functions by increasing LV transmural pressures and consequently after load. The same observation was documented by *Buda et al 1981* who showed that deep inspiration decreased the LV outflow tract (LVOT) gradient and decreased the LV ejection time in patients with muscular subaortic stenosis. They linked this decrease in the pressure gradient across LVOT to the increasing LV afterload through an increase in LV transmural pressure as a result of the negative intra-thoracic pressure caused by the deep inspiration. *Weyrnan et a1 1973* studied the specific effects of respiratory movements on the recorded echocardiogram. They found an influence of respiratory changes on the pulmonary arterial pressure and its pulmonary valvular echoes.

2.3.3 Inferior vena cava and hepatic veins

The inferior vena cava and the hepatic veins flows are best recorded from the subcostal sagittal view; where the forward flow is away from the transducer (below the baseline) and the retrograde flow is towards the transducer. This flow is continuous with one large peak in systole (S wave) which coincides with relaxation of the right atrium and the descent of tricuspid annulus during RV systole. There is another large peak during diastole (D wave) which occurs during the rapid filling phase of ventricular diastole. A third wave (A wave) occurs in some normal subjects due to reversed flow secondary to right atrial contraction. There is a fourth wave in the hepatic flow called V wave which is due to reverse flow in late systole (*Reynolds et al 1991; Lee et al 2007*). The respiration induces marked changes in Doppler velocity curves of hepatic veins. During inspiration there is a significant increase in both normal forward systolic (S) and diastolic (D) flow velocities as well as retrograde A velocity (*Ginghina et al 2009*). During expiration, there is decreased diastolic flow and increased reversals. The RA pressure can be determined by the respiratory variation in inferior vena cava diameter observed through the subcostal window; where the diameter of the IVC decreases in response to inspiration with minimal size observed at end inspiration (*Kircher et al 1990*). However, the position of the patient must be considered, as the largest diameter is measured in the right lateral position, becomes intermediate in the supine position, and the smallest diameter is measured in the left lateral position. For an adult; the normal IVC diameter is less than 1.7 cm and there is a 50% decrease in the diameter when the RA pressure is normal (0–5 mm Hg). When the IVC diameter is dilated (>1.7 cm) with normal inspiratory collapse (>50%), the RA pressure is suggestive to be mildly elevated (6–10 mm Hg). However when the inspiratory collapse is less than 50%, the RA pressure is usually between 10 and 15 mm Hg. If the IVC is dilated without any collapse; this suggests markedly elevation of RA pressure (greater than 15 mm Hg). With intravascular volume depletion, the IVC is small (usually < 1.2 cm) with spontaneous collapse (*Ginghina et al 2009*).

2.3.4 Superior vena cava

The superior vena cava flow can be best recorded from the suprasternal notch or subcostal view. The flow has the same wave like the IVC flow. It lacks the A wave of hepatic flow. However; the effect of respiration on SVC flow waves is less marked than in the hepatic flow; perhaps because of the pressure differences in the abdominal and thoracic cavities with respiration (*Reynolds et al 1991, Lee et al 2007*). Respiration makes appropriate fixed pulsed wave Doppler trace sampling to be difficult due the continuous movement of pulsed Doppler sample volume as a result of the change in heart position and diaphragmatic movement. Errors due to respiratory movement during Doppler estimation must be considered and manoeuvres that minimize the effect of respiration should be tried (*Kircher et al 1990*). The following measures may help to minimize the effect of respiration on Doppler studies:

1. Holding breathing at end expiration. Even patients with heart failure can do multiple holding of their breathing for 6 seconds.
2. Avoidance of angle of incidence by parallel positioning.
3. Taking the average velocities during multiple consecutive 3-5 quality tracing.

3. Respiratory maneuvers that may help in diagnosis of cardiac diseases

3.1 Valsalva maneuver

It is performed by attempting forceful expiration against a closed airway when the mouth is closed and the nose is pinched. There are 4 phases occurring during this maneuver. In the first phase; there is rise of the blood pressure coincide with onset of straining and increase the intra-thoracic pressure. The second phase coincides with the decrease in venous return and consequent reduction of stroke volume and pulse pressure and increase in heart rate. In the third phase, there is a release of straining; allowing re-expansion of the pulmonary vessels and the aorta causing increase of the pulmonary blood flow and cardiac output starts to increase. The last phase; there is marked increase of venous return which increase the cardiac output and leads to blood pressure overshoot (in normal heart) and return of the heart rate to the baseline. Performing Valsalva maneuver during echocardiography can help in diagnosis and evaluation of certain cardiac disorders e.g. aortic and pulmonic stenosis as well as tricuspid regurgitation *(Stoddard et al 1993)*. It is also helpful in diagnosis of hypertrophic cardiomyopathy, and mitral valve prolapse (MVP). In patients with obstructive hypertrophic cardiomyopathy and mild or dynamic LV outflow tract obstruction; Valsalva maneuver can unmask latent gradients/to increase LVOT gradient specially during the straining phase of Valsalva maneuver. During this phase, the preload, end-diastolic LV volume and after load decreased. So the systolic anterior motion (SAM) occurs earlier in systole, and mitral-septal contact lasts longer and LV outflow tract gradient increases (*Ginghina et al 2009*).

Valsalva maneuver helps also to augment the diagnosis of mitral valve prolapse, as it increases the intensity of mitral regurgitation associated with MVP and it makes regurgitation to start earlier in systole due to reduction of left ventricular volume. Patent foramen ovale is another cardiac disease in which Valsalva maneuver can help diagnosis. It can be reliably detected with contrast echocardiography or by using agitated saline through either trans-thoracic or trans-esophageal echocardiography. During Valsalva maneuver, the atrial shunting from right to left will be enhanced and begin during the third (release) phase. However, *Stoddard et al 1993* found that cough test is superior to the Valsalva maneuver in delineating a patent foramen ovale during contrast trans-esophageal echocardiography. Valsalva maneuver can be used for better assessment of the cardiac functions. The transmitral Doppler flow can be used to assess the diastolic functions of LV. There are small changes (<15%) in transmitral peak flow velocities that occur with spontaneous respiration. Valsalva maneuver was found to be effectively unloading the heart and unmask an impaired relaxation pattern and high filling pressures in patients with a baseline pseudonormal flow pattern (*Yuan et al 2007*).

3.2 Mûller maneuver

The Mûller maneuver is used to augment tricuspid regurgitation and is rarely used during echocardiographic examination. It is performed by holding the breathing in inspiration while the nose is closed and the mouth is sealed for 10 seconds. This exaggerated inspiratory effort, will increase the negative pressure in the chest and lungs is made very subatmospheric. This will augment the right-sided filling and hence augment the tricuspid regurgitation (*Buda et al 1981*).

4. Echocardiography in various respiratory conditions

Table 2 summarizes the indications of echocardiography in respiratory diseases.

a. **Congenital diseases:**
1. Choanal atresia
2. Congenital mal-development of the lung: Agenesis, hypoplasia, and dysplasia of lung
3. Congenital hiatus hernia or diaphragmatic hernia
4. Chest wall deformity as in Pectus excavatum; Pectus carinatum; Kyphoscoliotic heart disease
5. Situs inversus e.g. kartagener syndrome
6. Total anomalous pulmonary venous connection
7. Partial anomalous pulmonary venous connection

b. **Acquired:**
1. Traumatic chest conditions: Pulmonary insufficiency following trauma and surgery; Unspecified injury of heart with open wound into thorax; Contusion of heart with open wound into thorax; other trauma).
2. Obstructive sleep apnea (adult) (pediatric)
3. Reactive airway diseases (Asthma & COPD)
4. Pulmonary Vascular disorders (Aneurysm of pulmonary artery; arteriovenous fistula of pulmonary vessels (Contrast Echocardiography)).

5. Pulmonary embolism
6. Primary pulmonary hypertension, follow-up of pulmonary artery pressures in patients with pulmonary hypertension to evaluate response to treatment,
7. Swelling, mass, or lump in chest, malignancy.
8. Patients being considered for lung transplantation or other surgical procedure for advanced lung disease to exclude possible cardiac disease.
9. Acute respiratory infections: pneumonia especially if associated with empyema or septic shock
10. Chronic pulmonary infection: tuberculosis, fungal disease
11. ICU patient: Respiratory failure, mechanically ventilated patient, exacerbated reactive airway disease; Acute cor pulmonale and for routine re-evaluation of right ventricular function in patients with cor pulmonale, Iatrogenic pulmonary embolism and infarction, acute pulmonary edema; and chest pain: if associated with: hemodynamic instability, unexplained hypotension in Intensive Care or emergency settings;

Table 2. The indications of Echocardiography in respiratory conditions

4.1 Congenital respiratory diseases

4.1.1 Choanal atresia

Choanal atresia results from the persistence of the bucconasal membrane, which separates the nasal cavity and the nasopharynx in the early embryological development period. It may be unilateral or bilateral. Unilateral cases are often diagnosed later in life with unilateral nasal obstruction and discharge, while bilateral atresia almost always present with respiratory emergency. It may be found as isolated anomaly or associated with other defects as seen in CHARGE association. The most common cardiac lesions associated with choanal atresia are PDA and/or VSD, singly or in combination. Over half of the patients with choanal atresia may have multiple cardiac anomalies e.g. Endocardial cushion defect, conotruncal anomalies, or fallot's tetralogy. (*Zagnoev et al 1981*)

4.1.2 Congenital mal-development of the lung

Lung agenesis is defined as complete absence of lung tissue, carina, main bronchus and pulmonary vasculature while in lung aplasia there are a carina and main bronchus without lung tissue. In pulmonary hypoplasia there is bronchial underdevelopment associated with reduced amount of lung tissue. About 50% of patients with lung agenesis have other congenital anomalies especially cardiac anomalies. The incidence is being greater in those with right-sided agenesis. The congenital heart anomalies that may be associated with lung agenesis have a broad range, from simple isolated congeital cardiac defects like atrial septal defcts to extreme dextroversion and displacement of the heart. Tricuspid atresia; pulmonary artery sling; and total anomalous pulmonary venous drainage are among the recorded congnital heart diseases associated with lung agenesis. Some cardiac malformations (eg, tetralogy of Fallot, and scimitar syndrome) may lead to pulmonary hypoplasia. Echocardiography alone may be not enough for detailed diagnosis. Cross-sectional imaging modalities such as magnetic resonance imaging (MRI) and computed tomography (CT) and pulmonary angiography may be needed for accurate determination of anomalous vasculature, particularly in the presence of coexisting lung agenesis (*rzykowski et al 2007*).

Bridging bronchus is a malformation in which an aberrant bronchus arising from the left main stem bronchus to supply the right middle and /or lower lung lobes. Bridging bronchus may be associated with many malformations like cardiovascular (a sling-like left pulmonary artery and left-sided obstructive lesions including coarctation of the aorta), skeletal, genitourinary and abdominal malformations.

4.1.3 Congenital hiatus hernia or diaphragmatic hernia

Congenital diaphragmatic hernia (CDH) is protrusion of the abdominal viscera into the thoracic cavity due to absence of the diaphragm, or through a hole in it. This can occur on the left or right side, but is most common on the left. Hiatus hernia occurs when part of the stomach is present the thoracic cavity through the esophageal hiatus of the diaphragm. Cardiovascular malformations are common in cases with congenital diaphragmatic hernia (25-50%). Ventricular septal defect (VSD), atrial septal defect (ASD), conotruncal defects such as tetralogy of Fallot, transposition of great vessels, or aortic coarctation are among the cardiac anomalies seen in such cases. Hypoplastic left heart syndrome, is sometimes seen in cases with left-sided CDH. Dextroposition of the heart (e.g., the heart is shifted into the right chest) is also seen in left-sided CDH. Pulmonary hypertension and pulmonary hypoplasia are common complications of CDH. (*Tonks et al 2008*)

Echocardiography is needed immediately after diagnosis of CDH. It is helpful to exclude any associated congenital heart defect. It also helps in assessing cardiac functions and determining any reduction of the LV mass. Increased pulmonary vascular resistance is an almost universal finding in CDH. Determination of pulmonary artery pressures is essential as many surgeons prefer to operate when echocardiography has shown normal pulmonary artery pressures which are maintained for at least 24 to 48 hours (*Bosenberg et al 2008*). Echocardiographic findings of increased pulmonary artery pressure are flattening of the intraventricular septum, presence of tricuspid regurgitation, and/or right-to-left or bidirectional shunting at the ductal level. Estimation of RV pressure can be done by estimation of tricuspid regurgitation jet. Patency of the ductus allows RV to decompress and prevents right heart failure when the pressure becomes suprasystemic (*Bohn 2000*).

4.1.4 Chest wall deformity

There is a wide range of congenital chest wall deformities. The most frequent ones are pectus excavatum (more than 90% of congenital chest wall deformities), pectus carinatum and kyphoscoliosis. Pectus excavatum (Funnel chest) is caused by an abnormality of connective tissue, which results in depression of the sternum. It is sometimes associated with Marfan and Ehlers Danlos syndromes. Pectus carinatum (Pigeon chest) is thought to be associated with rickets, severe childhood asthma; congenital heart diseases as in ventricular septal defect (VSD) or with scoliosis. Kyphoscoliosis may be due to neuromuscular, congenital vertebral deformity or may be idiopathic. The usual cardiac manifestations presented in chest wall deformity are pain, dyspnea, and palpitation. ECG may show incomplete right bundle block, right anterior fascicular block, right axis deviation, or LV hypertrophy (*Kara et al 2009*).

Echocardiography may be indicated in patients with chest wall deformity to evaluate cardiac compression and to exclude associated cardiac abnormalities. In pectus excavatum, the sternum depressed the right atrium and right ventricle, interfering with diastolic filling of these structures. Mitral valve prolapse is a common finding and usually presented with chest pain and palpitations. Evaluation of the aortic root is specially needed if there is suspicion of Marfan syndrome as aortic root dilatation is a common finding. Evaluation of the cardiac function particularly in the sitting, or upright, position is of utmost importance.

No significant impairment to cardiac function could be observed when the patient with pectus excavatum is lying flat especially in mild to moderate cases (*Colombani 2009*). However, unless the patient is symptomatic, echocardiography is not mandatory in the workup of patients with pectus excavatum.

Echocardiography may be considered if congenital heart disease is suspected in cases with pectus carinatum. In a study performed by *Iakovlev et al 1990, it was found* that 97% out of 70 children with pectus carinatum had echocardiographically documented MVP. Some of those patients had hemodynamic and cardiodynamic changes as well as decreased myocardial contractility. These abnormalities were more frequently observed in the patients with pigeon chest.

In Kyphoscoliosis, there is increased incidence of dilatation of the ascending aorta, dilatation of the pulmonary artery, bicuspid aortic valve, subaortic septal hypertrophy, and MVP with or without mitral regurgitation. Kyphoscoliosis complicated with chronic hypoxemia, may induce both functional and anatomic changes in the pulmonary vascular bed. Chronic hypoxemia and reduction in the pulmonary vascular bed due to small lungs in kyphoscoliotic patient may cause cor pulmonale as an end result. Myocardial noncompaction of the ventricular myocardium which is a rare congenital cardiomyopathy characterized by excessively protrusive trabeculae and deep trabecular recesses in one or more segments of the ventricle was observed in some cases. Echocardiography shows trabeculations and deep intratrabecular recesses along the ventricular cavity in the apical and lateral segments of LV. Colour Doppler imaging shows blood flow in these recesses. Dilatation of LV and LA may be noted with LV global hypokinesia. Eustachian valve may be thikened in some cases which may appear as mass in RA and need transesophageal echocardiography for better evaluation. There is an increased incidence of MVP in patients with skeletal abnormalities (*Velibey et al 2010*).

4.1.5 Situs inversus e.g. kartagener syndrome

Kartagener's syndrome is a very rare congenital malformation due to abnormal ciliary motility or immotile cilia with impaired mucociliary transport. So; the ciliated epithelium situated in the airways, brain ventricles, oviducts, and vasa efferentia of the testes all may be affected. The classic syndrome is a triad of situs inversus, bronchiectasis, and sinusitis which was first described by Kartagener 1904 (*Leigh et al 2009*). Situs inversus is present only in 47.7% of cases so some authors prefer to name this syndrome as *the immotile cilia syndrome or the dyskinetic cilia syndrome.* Heterotaxy (situs ambiguous) is present in about 6% of cases with Kartagener syndrome. However, the prevalence of CHD with heterotaxy was noted to be 200-fold higher in primary ciliary dyskinesia than in the general population.

Diagnosis is usually confirmed by studies of ciliary function and ultrastructure, and by immunohistochemistry of cilia and by measurements of nasal nitric oxide. Isolated dextrocardia is almost always associated with other cardiac anomalies, which are often serious. When accompanied by situs inversus, serious cardiac malformations are less common, but described. Echocardiography allows identification of the cardiac malformations that may be associated with Kartagner syndrome. Among these cardiac malformations are: tetralogy of Fallot, L-transposition of the great arteries, aortic coarctation, subpulmonic stenosis, right or left atrial isomerism, atrial septal defect, common atrium, atrioventricular septal defect; ventricular septal defect, double outlet right ventricle, left ventricular outflow tract obstruction, bilateral superior vena cava, inferior vena cava drainage via azygous or via hemiazygous. (*Kennedy et al 2007*)

4.2 Acquired respiratory diseases

4.2.1 Traumatic chest conditions

Pulmonary insufficiency may occur following cardiac trauma and surgery. Unspecified injury of heart may occur with open wound into thorax. Contusion of heart may present with open thoracic wound. Though traumatic myocardial contusion or traumatic pericardial lesions are usually well tolerated and the clinical findings are transient; the sequelae of the cardiac trauma may be serious and difficult to be recognized. Blunt chest trauma might lead to cardiac injury ranging from simple arrhythmias to lethal conditions such as cardiac rupture. Therefore, a careful evaluation of every traumatized individual for cardiovascular injury is essential so that the more serious complications will be recognized and treated effectively. *Parmley et al 1958*; found that the most commonly encountered cardiac lesion at necropsy was myocardial rupture of a septum or a chamber wall. *Bjørnstad et al 2009* described a case with coronary artery dissection and acute myocardial infarction following blunt chest trauma.

Blunt trauma is uncommonly followed by intracardiac valve injuries but it does occur specially with car accidents. The valve most commonly affected is the tricuspid. *Hasdemir et al 2010* described occurrence of severe tricuspid regurgitation and second-degree Mobitz II atrioventricular block in a 68 years old woman due to blunt cardiac trauma secondary to car accident. Echocardiography could demonstrate rupture of tricuspid chordae tendinae or papillary muscles with prolapse of the valve cusps into the right atrium during systole and remarkable tricuspid regurgitation. Close follow-up may suffice in some patients with stable hemodynamic conditions, and regression of tricuspid regurgitation can be expected during follow-up. Mutilating mitral valve lesion secondary to cardiac trauma can induce mitral incompetence. The most common site of lesion is the papillary muscles (PM), followed by the chordae and then the mitral valve leaflets. The clinical course can be indolent or devastating, and most often requires urgent or delayed surgical treatment, either with mitral valve repair or replacement (*Pasquier et al 2010*). When the aortic valve is traumatically injured, it usually has a tear or avulsion on the cusp or on a commissure as well. The injury is often combined with trauma to the ascending aorta (*Kan & Yang 2005*).

4.2.2 Obstructive sleep apnea (adult & pediatric)

Obstructive sleep apnea (OSA) is a common but under-diagnosed condition that increases the risk of cardiovascular morbidity and mortality. Repetitive episodes of upper airway narrowing and/or occlusion; characteristic of OSA may lead to significant hypoxemia and cyclical alterations of arterial oxygen saturation. These episodes cause oxygen desaturation in response to apnoea, followed by the resumption of oxygen saturation during hyperventilation leading to a phenomenon called hypoxia/reoxygenation injury due to alteration of the oxidative balance through the induction of excess oxygen-free radicals, quite like in the sequelae of ischemia/reperfusion injury. These acute cardiovascular (CV) stressors together with swings in intrathoracic pressure, and central nervous system (CNS) arousals are potentially forming the basis for heightened CV risk in individuals with OSA (*Marrone et al 1998*). The development of pulmonary hypertension (PHT) and right heart dysfunction are well-known complications of OSA. Hypoxemia and hypercarbia-induced respiratory acidosis, which results from the apnoea episodes, are potent mediators of pulmonary vasoconstriction that can lead to reversible and irreversible chronic changes in the pulmonary vasculature. It is likely that production of various neurohumoral factors in response to hypoxemia and respiratory distress may further promote PHT, right ventricular (RV) dysfunction and consequent impairment of systemic cardiac output (*Blum & McGowan 2004*).

Adenotonsillar hypertrophy is being the most common cause for upper airway obstruction and sleep apnoea in paediatric patients. Many studies showed the cardiac changes in children with OSA. *Kirk et al 2010* showed that all the Caucasian children with OSA included in their study had nocturnal systolic systemic hypertension and half of them had diurnal systolic systemic hypertension as well. However, they found no echocardiographic findings of LVH and/or RV hypertrophy. On the other hand; *Weber et al 2007* found dilatation of the RV systolic and diastolic diameters with significant reduction of RV functions in children with OSA. They also found reduction of the LV functions but without significance. The same finding was also documented by *Biltagi et al 2008* who found that there was significant reduction of both systolic and diastolic function of both RV and LV in the children with OSA and higher clinical score than in control children and children with OSA and lower clinical score. There was also a positive correlation between the echocardiographic finding of impairment of the cardiac functions with the level of the inflammatory breath markers and also with the clinical score of OSA. They also found that the Tissue Doppler is more sensitive to discover the impairment of the cardiac function than the conventional Doppler. The pulmonary pressure in the children with OSA and higher clinical score was significantly more than the control and children with OSA and lower clinical score. These findings were also confirmed by *Attia et al 2010* who found that the Tissue Doppler imaging can detect the subtle, subclinical changes in cardiac performance that occur in OSA due to adenotonsillar hypertrophy. They also found that these changes were reversible after surgical treatment.

Cardiac affection is well documented in adults with OSA. Atherosclerosis, secondary hypertension, atrial fibrillation, conduction disorders, coronary artery disease, congestive heart failure (CHF), pulmonary hypertension, stroke, and cardiac death; all are documented to occur in adults with OSA. *Romero-Corral et al 2007* found that echocardiographic examination documented impaired RV and LV functions and increased left atrial volume in cases with moderate to severe OSA. *Koshino et al 2010* explain these cardiac changes by the occurrence of negative intrathoracic pressure during apnea. They found that RV and LV longitudinal deformation was significantly reduced during the Müller maneuver. *Cioffi et al 2010* also documented occurrence of high prevalence of concentric LV hypertrophy in Moderate to severe OSA. They related these changes to the increase in myocardial end-systolic stress, venous return and sympathetic activity. Early recognition of RV dysfunction before development of pulmonary arterial (PA) hypertension is important for preventing further progression to heart failure and even death. *Shanoudy et al 1998* found by contrast transesophgeal echocardiography; an increased prevalence of PFO in adults with OSA which indicates that the pathophysiology of OSA may predispose to the maintenance of patency of a foramen ovale.

4.2.3 Bronchial asthma & COPD

Bronchial asthma (BA) is a common chronic inflammatory condition affecting the airways. Bronchial asthma does not affect only the lung but affects other organs including the heart. Even with mild cases, subclinical cardiac dysfunction can be documented and the severity of cardiac affection is parallel to the severity of the disease. Diastolic dysfunction of the RV was the earliest hemodynamic change in BA. RV hypertrophy and dilation and LV diastolic dysfunction were observed in severe BA. Echocardiography detected RV systolic and diastolic dysfunction in a considerable percent of asthmatic children even with mild cases. Left ventricular dysfunction is usually detected in severe asthmatic cases. Tissue Doppler Echocardiography was found to be more sensitive in detecting cardiac dysfunction than conventional Doppler. However, these cardiac dysfunctions may be reversible especially in acute cases (*Peng et al 2006, Zeybek et al 2007*). The occurrence of supraventricular tachycardia in BA is related to presence of interventricular septal hypertrophy, LV dysfunction, and increased PAP (*Chicherina et al 2007*). Asthmatic medications can also affect the echocardiographic findings. Chronic administration of theophylline may cause a slight increase in percent fractional shortening, outflow peak velocity and atrial contribution to ventricular filling in the asthmatic children as compared to normal though these findings were found to be insignificant (*Aoki et al 1994*).

The cardiac manifestations of chronic obstructive pulmonary disease (COPD) are numerous. RV dysfunction and pulmonary vascular disease are well known to complicate the clinical course of COPD and correlate inversely with survival. Although RV dysfunction and PH are common in COPD; the increase in mean pulmonary artery pressures tends to be mild to moderate. The manifestations of pulmonary hypertension in patients with COPD are usually subtle and are often obscured by the manifestations of the lung disease. However, there is a dramatic increase in pulmonary pressure observed during exercise, nocturnal desaturations and acute exacerbations. Despite that the cardiac catheterization remains the "gold standard" for the measurement of pulmonary arterial pressures, but recent studies showed that continuous wave Doppler echocardiography is able to detect the increase in pulmonary pressure and is sufficiently sensitive to detect changes in pulmonary arterial pressure. Presence of progressive worsening of diastolic and systolic function of the LV is an additional factor aggravating hemodynamic compromise in patients with COPD which should be kept in mind when choosing the appropriate therapy (*Falk et al 2008, Higham et al 2001, Fisher et al 2009, Strutynskiĭ et al 2010*).

4.2.4 Pulmonary vascular disorders

Pulmonary artery (PA) aneurysm is a rare clinical condition, either congenital or acquired. It is defined as PA dilation greater than 4 cm. Large PA aneurysm can cause airway obstruction and compromise. Two-D echocardiography appears to be a useful non-invasive technique in the recognition of PA aneurysms. It can localize the site; the type; single or multiple; and the size of PA aneurysm. The fusiform aneurysms may reach a huge size, which may make it impossible to be imaged completely by a single 2-D sector plane and can cause displacement of the left atrium (*Bhandari & Nanda 1984*).

However; accurate diagnosis and evaluation of PA aneurysms may be difficult without angiography, computed tomography (CT) and MRIs. Associated cardiac lesions may be detected by echocardiography. Pulmonary hypertension is rarely found in some patients with aneurysm of the main pulmonary artery. However, severe pulmonary hypertension may be the cause of the aneurysm. Thrombus may be found inside the aneurysm with its characteristic echocardiographic features of having a laminated appearance, variably increased echodensity compared with surrounding tissues, stagnation caused by low blood flow state in the aneurysm and lack of obvious tumor features, such as narrow stalk and origin from PA wall. Echocardiography may detect associated lesions like atrial septal defects, mitral stenosis, aortic coarctation etc (*Güler et al 2003*).

Pulmonary arterio-venous fistula (PAVF) is a rare vascular anomaly. In PAVF, there is a direct communication between the PA branches and the pulmonary vein, without intervening pulmonary capillary bed. PAVFs are found in approximately 15–20% of patients with Rendu-Osler-Weber (ROW) disease. The M- mode and Two-D echocardiography may be normal and show normal intracardiac anatomy with no evidence of atrial or ventricular septal defect. However, if PAVF is suspected a contrast echocardiography showed be performed. After the injection of the contrast rapidly into the right antecubital vein; the right atrium and ventricle will be opacified but the left heart chambers will remain free of contrast until three cardiac cycles (3 s) after that the contrast will be seen in the left heart side. These findings are compatible with a right-to-left shunt at the pulmonary vasculature level and not intracardiac. (*Roolvink 2004*)

4.2.5 Pulmonary embolism

Pulmonary embolism (PE) is a common and serious disease. The prognosis depends on the speed of diagnosis and initiation of therapy. Since 1990; a large number of diagnostic tests and strategies have been evaluated for PE. Echocardiography has certain criteria to improve the diagnosis of acute PE. Presence of RV hypokinesis and dilation (without RV wall hypertrophy, and RV diameter becomes equal to or larger than the diameter of LV), tricuspid regurgitation velocity >2.7 m/sec without inspiratory collapse of the inferior vena cava, paradoxical septal movements and widening of pulmonary artery diameter together with the clinical suspicion of PE will increase the sensitivity of echocardiography to diagnose PE. Transesophageal echocardiography can show the central pulmonary arteries and may show a thrombus in the dilated segment of pulmonary artery. However, the echocardiography may fail to diagnose PE in about half of the cases. Despite that, echocardiography is one of the preferred first diagnostic tool to diagnose a patient with suspected PE (*Miniati et al 2001*).

4.2.6 Primary pulmonary hypertension (PPH)

Primary pulmonary hypertension (PPH) is a disease of unknown origin. It is characterised by a progressive increase in PA pressures. Despite that the invasive measurement of pulmonary vascular resistance (PVR) by right heart catheterisation remains the gold standard method to evaluate PVR, but echocardiography is still a good screening tool of patients with PH. It can estimate PVR using the ratio of peak tricuspid regurgitant velocity (TRV) to the RV outflow tract time-velocity integral (TVI rvot) or to the LV outflow tract time-velocity integral (TVI lvot). TRV/TVI rvot and TRV/TVI lvot was reported to be correlated significantly with invasively-determined PVR. Echocardiography can also be used to follow-up of PA pressures in patients with pulmonary hypertension to evaluate response to treatment. (*Roule et al 2010*)

4.2.7 Mass in chest

A wide variety of intra-thoracic masses can simulate primary intrinsic cardiac diseases. They can present with various cardiovascular manifestations; an abnormal heart shadow in the X-ray or unusual echoes in close proximity to the heart. Echocardiography can show unusual anterior wall echo which can be misinterpreted to be aneurysmal dilatation of either the RV outflow tract or pulmonary artery. M-mode echocardiography can differentiate between solid and cystic masses by their "sonolucency," which reflects the changes in gain settings. At high gain, the solid masses will "fill-in" with echoes, whereas a cystic structure will not.

An example of cystic masses in the anterior mediastinum is the thymic cyst which may appear as a cystic structure displaced by the great vessels during systole. Contrast echocardiography can help to know whether the cyst originates from the RV or from extra cardiac mediastinal structures (*Child et al 1975*).

In posterior mediastinal mass a wide strong echo, posterior to the posterior LV wall can be seen especially with tumours. An example of posterior mediastinal mass which presents with acute cardiovascular events is hiatus hernia. Hiatus hernia can hinder the sonographic configuration of the cardiac anatomy and can simulate the appearance of a left intra-atrial mass or a posterior mediastinal structure on transthoracic echocardiography. Contrast and transesophageal echocardiography are very helpful for better evaluation and to exclude the intracardiac nature of the mass. Other posterior mediastinal masses are esophageal carcinomas and hematomas, or dissecting aneurysms of the ascending aorta (*Koskinas et al 2008*). Some mediastinal masses can restrict the cardiac filling due to myocardial or pericardial infiltration. Decreased LV compliance impairs left atrial emptying and diminishes anterior mitral valve diastolic closure rate. Diminished ventricular filling may be observed due to decreased venous return as a consequence to compression of vena cava by the mass. So; when the prominent echo in front or behind the heart is seen and no primary cardiac disease can be detected; a mediastinal mass should be suspected and further studies are needed (*Child et al 1975*).

4.2.8 Patients being considered for lung transplantation or other surgical procedure for advanced lung disease to exclude possible cardiac disease

Patients with advanced lung disease need a detailed preoperative echocardiographic examination especially in patient with end stage lung disease (ESLD) who is in need for lung transplantation. Pulmonary hypertension is often detected in those patients. Echocardiography can detect abnormal left atrial filling, abnormal LV relaxation and geometry, RV enlargement, ventricular septal displacement and LV diastolic dysfunction (*Jastrzebski et al 2007*). Increased systolic pulmonary artery pressure, is a significant risk factors for death of patient with ESLD while being on the waiting list. A decrease of ejection fraction below 50% may indicate lower survival (*Jastrzebski et al 2005*).

4.2.9 Acute respiratory infections

There are a number of cardiac complications that occur in cases with pneumonia. Purulent pericarditis, Cardiac tamponade, pulmonary embolism and endocarditis are rare complications but reported specially with *Streptococcus pneumonia*. Congenital heart disease is the predisposing factor in about 22% of cases with recurrent pneumonia in children (*Al-Sabbagh et al 2008, Owayed et al 2000*).

4.2.10 Chronic pulmonary infection/inflammation

Tuberculous pericarditis continues to be a problem in both developed and developing countries. The echocardiography has certain characteristic features of tuberculous pericarditis. There may be pericardial thickening and calcification, intrapericardial fibrin strands, exudative coating with a tendency to form adhesions and in some instances constriction. There may be patchy deposits with "fibrinous" strands criss crossing the pericardial space. Echocardiographic evidence of cardiac tamponade is more common in tuberculous pericardial effusion. Organization of the pericardial tissue may form large pericardial mass or abscess which may obstruct RV free wall (*George et al 2004*).

Sarcoidosis is a granulomatous disease which may affect lungs and may be complicated with pulmonary hypertension. It may develop secondary to granulomatous involvement of pulmonary veins manifesting clinically as pulmonary veno-occlusive disease, extrinsic compression by mediastinal or hilar adenopathy, cardiac involvement including systolic or diastolic dysfunction, increased production of vasoactive endothelin-1 and downstream effects of hypoxemia. Presence of PH is an important risk factor affecting survival. Doppler echocardiography appears to be useful screening tool in the context of sarcoidosis with PH (*Alhamad et al 2010*). Fungal endocarditis has increased in incidence during the last 2 decades and may complicate fungal pulmonary disease especially in presence of prothetic valve or congenital heart disease. Echocardiography is extremely useful to diagnose Candida endocarditis because fungal endocarditis is frequently associated with large vegetations that are easily observed on standard echocardiograms. However, transthoracic echocardiography is less sensitive than transesophageal echocardiography but less invasive. Echocardiography can detect vegetations and intracardiac thrombi which are the most common types but are still rare. It may also demonstrate pericardial effusion, myocardial abscesses, associated myocarditis or pericarditis (*Ellis et al 2001*).

4.2.11 Pulmonary ICU patient

In the chest intensive care setting; echocardiography is a valuable and indispensable bedside diagnostic tool which has the advantage of providing very useful hemodynamic information in a matter of minutes. It is used to establish rapid diagnoses and assessment, to serially monitor the therapeutic interventions and to expect the prognosis in pulmonary/critical care patients with cardiopulmonary dysfunction. It can be used together with clinical assessment and other tools to assess the patient's hemodynamic. It is inevitable and appropriate that the pulmonary intensive care physician should know and have the skills to perform ICU echocardiography. Echocardiography is a useful diagnostic tool in cases with profound hypotension or shock or in whom hypotension or shock fails to respond to the standard treatment. It can confirm the cardiac cause of shock. Global biventricular function, LV myocardial kienetic status (Hypokinetic, hyperkinetic or normokinetic; regional and global) and valve status can be evaluated with standard methods keeping into consideration the amount of inotropic and vasoactive medications givin, the degree of LV filling (by assessement of IVC size); pulmonary vascular resistance and presence of extrinsic compression e.g. cardiac tamponade or effect of mechanical ventilation (*Kaplan & Mayo 2009*).
In septicemia, echocardiography can play a crucial role in the management of the septic ICU patient both by excluding cardiac causes for sepsis, and by monitoring and guiding management of the patient hemodynamics. Despite that septic shock is classically considered as hyperdynamic state, but sepsis can reduce myocardial contractility and ventricular functions and can decrease cardiac output. So, global evaluation of the cardiac functions is of paramount importance. The sepsis-induced cardiomyopathy is classically observed in children and adult patients with meningococcemia. Echocardiography can determine the cardiac source of sepsis e.g. infective endocarditis. It is to be noted that TEE is more sensitive than TTE to detect of small vegetations. However; echocardiography alone cannot be used to make diagnosis of endocarditis and must be used with the other diagnostic criteria. (*Price et al 2008*)
Echocardiography can detect pleural effusion and can differentiate left pleual effusion from the pericardial effusion. With subcostal 2-D echocardiography, right pleural effusion

appears as echo-free mass that is contiguous to the RA but not to any other cardiac chamber. It is also bounded inferiorly by the smooth round surface of the liver. The location of the descending thoracic aorta on 2-D echocardiography serves as a valuable landmark in localizing the pericardial-pleural interface, thereby differentiating pericardial from pleural effusions (*D'Cruz 1984*). However, the right-sided pleural effusion is more difficult to be detected than the left because there is no acoustic window. TEE can detect the echo-free space created by pleural fluid, as well as the appearance of adjacent atelectatic lung. TEE also could be used to quantify the size of effusions. *Howard et al 2011*; could estimate the volume of the pericardial effusion using TEE by applying the following formula:

$$V = 4.5\ CSA(max)(3/2)$$

Where V is the expected pleural effusion volume in milliliters while the CSA(max) is the maximum cross-sectional area in centimeters squared of the pleural effusion recorded by transesophageal echocardiography. Pleural effusion in ICU patient can cause echocardiographic artefacts (called cardiac-mass lung' artefact,) which may give the impression of an intracardiac mass and could be mistaken with mobile components. In presence of hemodynamically unstable patient with significant pleural effusions; echocardiography must be performed to evaluate the cardiac function and to exclude presence of associated pericardial effusion (*Karabinis et al 2008*).

Echocardiography in pulmonary ICU allows immediate evaluation of patients with cardiopulmonary failure, to establish initial diagnosis and serial examinations may be performed to guide ongoing management. It also can evaluate the cardiac function both systolic and diastolic that can be compromised. Echocardiography may not be needed routinely in all patients with respiratory failure, but it is particularly useful when a cardiac cause of acute respiratory failure is suspected. Presence of LV dilation, regional or global myocardial wall motion abnormalities, and/or severe mitral regurgitation are present in cases with cardiogenic pulmonary oedema. On the other hand; a normal heart size and normal systolic and diastolic function in a patient with pulmonary oedema would suggest Adult Respiratory Distress Syndrome (ARDS). Estimation of PA pressure and evaluation of RV function are needed in chronic respiratory failure (*Vieillard-Baron et al 1999*)

Mechanical ventilation may cause potentially detrimental consequences for systemic venous return produced by an increase in pleural pressure. It also decreases RV after-load due to increased positive end expiratory presurre (PEEP), incresed lung volume or both. It also decreases radius of interventricular septum in diastole leading to its leftward shift with impeding filling of the LV and decreased LV cardiac output. However, the effect on the LV is insignificant. On the other hand, continuous positive airway pressure (CPAP) can improve LV afterload by reducing transmural LV pressure (*Huemer et al 1994*). TTE appears as a sensitive noninvasive method which accurately detects changes in central haemodynamics induced by changes in breathing pattern. It is a powerful tool to assess RV function, especially if acute cor pulmonale is a concern, as well as to estimate LV function (*Vieillard-Baron et al 1999*).

Weaning patients from the ventilator remains a crucial issue. TTE helps to identify patients at high risk of weaning failure. TTE findings which expect difficult weaning include: increase of LA pressure, appearance/worsening of mitral regurgitation new/worsening regional wall motion abnormalities, decreased LVEF, shortened deceleration time of mitral Doppler E wave, and increased E/E' ratio (E' is the the maximal velocity of its displacement of the lateral portion of the mitral annulus during early diastole) and reduced tricuspid annular TDI systolic and diastolic velocities. (*Caille et al 2010*)

5. Conclusion

Echocardiography plays a crucial role in diagnosis, monitoring and follow up of many respiratory disorders.

6. References

Aebischer N, Malhotra R, Connors L, Kappenberger L, Parisi AF. (1995). Ventricular interdependence during Valsalva maneuver as seen by two-dimensional echocardiography: new insights about an old method. *J Am Soc Echocardiogr* Vol 8(4):536-42.

Alhamad EH, Idrees MM, Alanezi MO, AlBoukai AA, Shaik SA. (2010) Sarcoidosis-associated pulmonary hypertension: Clinical features and outcomes in Arab patients. *Ann Thorac Med* Vol 5:86-91

Al-Sabbagh A, Catford K, Evans I, Morley SL. (2008). Severe cardiovascular and thromboembolic consequences of pneumococcal infection in a child. *Pediatrics.* Vol 122(4):e945-7.

Aoki T, Iwase M, Watanabe T, Miyaguchi K, Hayashi H, Yokota M. (1994). Left ventricular function in asthmatic children chronically treated with theophylline evaluated by exercise Doppler echocardiography. *Int J Card Imaging.* Vol 10(4):299-304.

Attia G, Ahmad MA, Saleh AB, Elsharkawy A. (2010). Impact of obstructive sleep apnea on global myocardial performance in children assessed by tissue Doppler imaging. *Pediatr Cardiol* Vol 31(7):1025-36.

Baden W, Schaefer J, Kumpf M, Tzaribachev N, Pantalitschka T, Koitschev A, et al. (2008). Comparison of imaging techniques in the diagnosis of bridging bronchus. *Eur Respir J* Vol 31(5):1125-31.

Bhandari AK, Nanda N.C. (1984). Pulmonary arterial aneurysms echocardiographic features in 5 patients. *Am J Cardiol* Vol 53: pp 1438-1441.

Biltagi MA, Maguid MA, Ghafar MA, Farid E. (2008). Correlation of 8-isoprostane, interleukin-6 and cardiac functions with clinical score in childhood obstructive sleep apnoea. *Acta Paediatr* Vol 97(10):1397-405.

Bjørnstad JL, Pillgram-Larsen J, Tønnessen T. (2009). Coronary artery dissection and acute myocardial infarction following blunt chest trauma. *World J Emerg Surg* Vol 14;4:14.

Blum RH, McGowan FX. (2004). Chronic upper airway obstruction and cardiac dysfunction: anatomy, pathophysiology and anesthetic implications. *Paediatr Anaesth* Vol 14: 75–83.

Bohn D. (2002). Congenital Diaphragmatic Hernia. *Am J Respir Crit Care Med* Vol 1;166(7):911-5.

Bosenberg AT, Brown RA. (2008). Management of congenital diaphragmatic hernia. *Curr Opin Anaesthesiol* Vol21(3):323-31

Brenner JI, Waugh RA. (1978). Effect of phasic respiration on left ventricular dimension and performance in a normal population. An echocardiographic study. *Circulation* Vol 57:122-127.

Buda AJ, Pinsky MR, Ingels NJ, Daughters GT, Stinson EB, Alderman EL. (1979). Effect of intrathoracic pressure on left ventricular performance. *N Engl J Med* Vol 30; 301(9):453-9.

Buda AJ, MacKenzie GW, Wigle ED. (1981). Effect of negative intrathoracic pressure on LV outflow tract obstruction in muscular subaortic stenosis. *Circulation* Vol 63;875-881.

Caille V, Amiel JB, Charron C, Belliard G, Vieillard-Baron A, Vignon P. (2010). Echocardiography: a help in the weaning process. *Crit Care* Vol 14(3):R120.

Chicherina EN, Malykh SZ, Shipitsina VV. (2007). The myocardial condition in chronic obstructive pulmonary disease and bronchial asthma. *Klin Med* (Mosk) Vol 85(2):23-6.

Child JS, Abbasi AS, Pearce ML. (1975). Echocardiographic differentiation of mediastinal tumors from primary cardiac disease. *Chest* Vol 67;108-110.

Cioffi G, Russo TE, Stefenelli C, Selmi A, Furlanello F, Cramariuc D. (2010). Severe obstructive sleep apnea elicits concentric left ventricular geometry. *J Hypertens* Vol 28(5):1074-82.

Colombani P. (2009). Preoperative assessment of chest wall deformities. *Semin Thorac Cardiovasc Surg* Vol 21: 58–63.

D'Cruz IA. (1984). Echocardiographic simulation of pericardial fluid accumulation by right pleural effusion. *Chest Vol* 86(3):451-3.

Ellis ME, Al-Abdely H, Sandridge A, Greer W, Ventura W. (2001). Fungal endocarditis: evidence in the world literature, 1965-1995. *Clin Infect Dis* Vol 32(1):50-62.

Falk JA, Kadiev S, Criner GJ, Scharf SM, Minai OA; Diaz P. (2008). Cardiac Disease in Chronic Obstructive Pulmonary Disease. *Proc Am Thorac Soc* Vol 1; 5(4): 543–548.

Fenichel NM, Arora J, Khan R, Antoniou C, AhujaS , Thumpson EJ. (1976). The Effect of Respiratory Motion on the Echocardiogram. *Chest* Vol 69; 655-659.

Ferreira T, Carmo MM, Soares R, Salomão S. (1990). Influence of respiratory cycle on the flows in the entry and exit chambers of the left ventricle. *Rev Port Cardiol* Vol 9(4):329-32.

Fisher MR, Forfia PR, Chamera E, Housten-Harris T, Champion HC, Reda E. Girgis RE, et al. (2009). Accuracy of Doppler Echocardiography in the Hemodynamic Assessment of Pulmonary Hypertension. *Am J Respir Crit Care* Med Vol 1; 179(7): 615–621.

George S, Salama AL, Uthaman B, Cherian G. (2004). Echocardiography in differentiating tuberculous from chronic idiopathic pericardial effusion. *Heart* Vol 90:1338–1339.

Ginghina C, Beladan CC, Iancu M, Calin A, Popescu BA. (2009). Respiratory maneuvers in echocardiography: a review of clinical applications. *Cardiovas Ultrasound* Vol 26; 7:42

Güler N, Sakarya ME, Eryonucu B, Demirbao R. (2003). Transesophageal echocardiographic detection of a pulmonary artery aneurysm complicated by thrombus. *Heart Lung* Vol 32 (3):159-61.

Hasdemir H, Arslan Y, Alper A, Osmonov D, Güvenç TS, Poyraz E, Akyüz S, Yıldız M. (2010). Severe Tricuspid Regurgitation and Atrioventicular Block Caused by Blunt Thoracic Trauma in an Elderly Woman. *J Emerg Med.* Vol 18. [Epub ahead of print].

Higham MA, Dawson D, Joshi J, Nihoyannopoulos P, Morrell NW. (2001). Utility of echocardiography in assessment of pulmonary hypertension secondary to COPD. *Eur Respir J* Vol 17: 350–355.

Howard A, Jackson A, Howard C, Spratt P. (2011). Estimating the Volume of Chronic Pleural Effusions Using Transesophageal Echocardiography. *J Cardiothorac Vasc Anesth.* 22. [Epub ahead of print]

Huemer G, Kolev N, Kurz A, Zimpfer M. (1994). Influence of Positive End-Expiratory Pressure on Right and Left Ventricular Performance Assessed by Doppler Two-Dimensional Echocardiography. *Chest* Vol 106:67-73

Iakovlev VM, Nechaeva GI, Viktorova IA. (1990). Clinical function of the myocardium and cardio- and hemodynamics in patients with pectus carinatum deformity [in Russian]. *Ter Arkh.* Vol 62(4):69-72.

Jastrzebski D, Kozielski J, Nowak J, Zielińska-Leś I, Ziora D, , Szulik B, et al. (2005). Prognostic risk factors in patients with interstitial lung disease referred for lung transplantation. *J Physiol Pharmacol.* Vol 56 Suppl 4:107-13.

Jastrzebski D, Nowak J, Ziora D, Wojarski J, Czyzewski D, Kozielski J, et al. (2007). Left ventricular dysfunction in patients with interstitial lung diseases referred for lung transplantation. *J Physiol Pharmacol.* Vol 58 5(Pt 1):299-305

Kan CD, Yang YJ. (2005). Traumatic aortic and mitral valve injury following blunt chest injury with a variable clinical course. *Heart* Vol 91(5): 568–570.

Kaplan A, Mayo PH. (2009). Echocardiography Performed by the Pulmonary/Critical Care Medicine Physician. *CHEST* Vol 135:529–535

Kara V, Agladioglu K, Ozyol A, Kocer B, Atac K, Oguz S. (2009). ANTERIOR CHEST WALL DEFORMITIES AND ACCOMPANYING CARDIAC PROBLEMS FOR YOUNG MILITARY PERSONNEL *CHEST* Vol 136: 134S-b

Karabinis A, Saranteas T, Karakitsos D, Lichtenstein D, Poularas J, Yang C, Stefanadis C. (2008). The 'cardiac-lung mass' artifact: an echocardiographic sign of lung atelectasis and/or pleural effusion. *Crit Care.* Vol 12:R122. doi: 10.1186/cc7021.

Kennedy MP, Omran H, Leigh MW, Dell S, Morgan L, Molina PL, et al. (2007). Congenital heart disease and other heterotaxic defects in a large cohort of patients with primary ciliary dyskinesia. *Circulation.* Vol 5;115(22):2814-21.

Kircher BJ, Himelman RB, Schiller NB. (1990). Noninvasive estimation of right atrial pressure from the inspiratory collapse of the inferior vena cava. *Am J Cardiol* Vol 66:493-6.

Kirk V, Midgley J, Giuffre M, Ronksley P, Nettel-Aguirre A, Al-Shamrani A. (2010). Hypertension & obstructive sleep apnea in Caucasian children. *World J Cardiol* Vol 2(8): 251-256.

Klingler JW, Begeman MS, Fraker TD Jr, Andrews LT. (1989). Automatic detection of inter-frame motion in echocardiographic images. *Ultrasound Med Biol.* Vol 15(7):683-9.

Koshino Y, Villarraga HR, Orban M, Bruce CJ, Pressman GS, Leinveber P, Saleh HK, et al. (2010). Changes in left and right ventricular mechanics during the Mueller maneuver in healthy adults: a possible mechanism for abnormal cardiac function in patients with obstructive sleep apnea. *Circ Cardiovasc Imaging.* Vol 3(3):282-9.

Koskinas KC, Oikonomou K, Karapatsoudi E; Makridis P. (2008). Echocardiographic manifestation of hiatus hernia simulating a left atrial mass: Case report. *Cardiovasc Ultrasound* Vol 6: 46.

Lang RM, Bierig M, Devereux RB, Flachskampf FA, Foster E, Pellikka PA, Picard MH, et al. (2005). Recommendations for Chamber Quantification: A Report from the American Society of Echocardiography's Guidelines and Standards Committee and the Chamber Quantification Writing Group, Developed in Conjunction with the European Association of Echocardiography, a Branch of the European Society of Cardiology, a Branch of the European Society of Cardiology. *J Am Soc Echocardiogr* Vol 18:1440-1463.

Lee KS, Abbas AE, Khandheria BK, Lester SJ. (2007). Echocardiographic Assessment of Right Heart Hemodynamic Parameters. *J Am Soc Echocardiogr* Vol 20:773-782.

Leigh MW, Pittman JE, Carson JL, Ferkol TW, Dell SD, Davis SD, et al. Clinical and genetic aspects of primary ciliary dyskinesia/Kartagener syndrome. *Genet Med.* 2009; 11(7):473-87.

Lendrum BL, Mondkar AM, Harris JB, Smulevitz B; Carr L. (1979). Respiratory variation in echocardiographic dimensions of left and right ventricles in normal children: The role of the interventricular septum. *Pediatr Cardiol.* Vol 1:39, 39-45.

Marrone O, Bonsignore MR, Insalaco G, Bonsignore G. (1998). What is the evidence that obstructive sleep apnoea is an important illness? *Monaldi Arch Chest Dis* Vol 53: 630–9.

Miniati M, Monti S, Pratali L, Di Ricco G, Marini C, Formichi B, et al. (2001). Value of transthoracic echocardiography in the diagnosis of pulmonary embolism: results of a prospective study in unselected patients. *Am J Med* Vol 110(7):528-35.

Norgård G and Vik-Mo. (1992). Effects of respiration on right ventricular size and function: an echocardiographic study. *Pediatr Cardiol* Vol 13(3):136-40.

Owayed AF, Campbell DM, Wang EEL. (2000). Underlying Causes of Recurrent Pneumonia in Children. *Arch Pediatr Adolesc Med* Vol 154:190-194

Parmley LF, Mantion WC, Mattingly TW. (1958). Nonpenetrating traumatic injury of the heart. *Circulation.* Vol 18(3):371-96.

Pasquier M, Sierro C, Yersin B, Delay D, Carron PN. (2010). Traumatic mitral valve injury after blunt chest trauma: a case report and review of the literature. *J Trauma.* Vol 68(1):243-6. Review.

Peng SM, Sun P, Zeng J, Deng XM. (2006). Cardiac function of children with bronchial asthma. *Zhongguo Dang Dai Er Ke Za Zhi* Vol 8(5):388-90.

Price S, Via G, Sloth E, Guarracino F, Breitkreutz R, Catena E, et al. (2008). Echocardiography practice, training and accreditation in the intensive care: document for the World Interactive Network Focused on Critical Ultrasound (WINFOCUS). *Cardiovascular Ultrasound* Vol 6:49.

Reynolds T, Appleton CP. (1991). Doppler flow velocity pattern of the superior vena cava, inferior vena cava, hepatic vein, coronary sinus, and atrial septal defect: a guide for the echocardiography. *J Am Soc Echo* Vol 4:503.

Riggs TW, Rodriguez R, Snider AR, Batton D. (1989). Doppler echocardiographic evaluation of right and left ventricular diastolic function in normal neonates. *J Am Coll Cardiol* Vol 1; 13(3):700-5.

Riggs TW, Snider AR. (1989). Respiratory influence on right and left ventricular diastolic function in normal children. *Am J Cardiol.* Vol 1; 63(12):858-61.

Romero-Corral; Somers V K, Pellikka PA, Olson EJ, Bailey KR, Korinek J, et al. (2007). Decreased Right and Left Ventricular Myocardial Performance in Obstructive Sleep Apnea. *Chest* Vol 132:1863–1870

Roolvink V, Meursing BTJ, Tummers JKJM, Haarbrink RH, Ernst JMPG. (2004). Arteriovenous fistula after intervertebral disk surgery at L4-L5. *Neth Heart J* Vol 12(6): 295–298.

Roule V, Labombarda F, Pellissier A, Sabatier R, Lognoné T, Gomes S, Et al. (2010). Echocardiographic assessment of pulmonary vascular resistance in pulmonary arterial hypertension. *Cardiovasc Ultrasound* Vol 8: 21.

Pietrzykowski WD, Moll M, Kobielski A, Moll JJ. (2007). Left atrial approach to close the atrial septal defect type II in case of right lung agenesis with extreme dextroversion. *Interact CardioVasc Thorac Surg* Vol 6:126-127.

Said SI. (2001). Neurohumoral aspects of respiratory-cardiovascular interactions. In: Scharf SM, Pinsky MR, Magder S, eds. Respiratory-circulatory interactions in health and disease. New York: Marcel Dekker 427–446.

Shanoudy H, Soliman A, Raggi P, Liu WJ, Russell D C; Jarmukli NF. (1998). Prevalence of Patent Foramen Ovale and Its Contribution to Hypoxemia in Patients with Obstructive Sleep Apnea, *CHEST* Vol 113;91-96

Stoddard MF, Keedy DL, Dawkins PR. (1993). The cough test is superior to the Valsalva maneuver in the delineation of right-to-left shunting through a patent foramen ovale during contrast transesophageal echocardiography. *Am Heart J* Vol 125(1):185-9.

Strutynskiĭ AV, Bakaev RG, Glazunov AB, Banzeliuk EN, Moshkova NK, Reĭsner AA. (2010). The specific features of left cardiac cavity remodeling in patients with chronic obstructive pulmonary disease and chronic cor pulmonale. *Ter Arkh* Vol 82(9):45-9.

Tonks A, Wyldes M, Somerset DA, Dent K, Abhyankar A, Bagchi I, Lander A, et al. (2004). Congenital malformations of the diaphragm: findings of the West Midlands Congenital Anomaly Register 1995 to 2000. *Prenat Diagn* Vol 24:596–604.

Tsai LM, Kuo KJ, Chen J H. (1998). Effects of spontaneous respiration on transmitral Doppler flow patterns in normal subjects and patients with coronary artery disease. *Am Heart J* 136:99-102.

Uiterwaal C, Van Dam I, De Boo T, Van Keulen P, Folgering H, Hopman J, Daniels O. (1989). The effect of respiration on diastolic blood flow velocities in the human heart. *Eur Heart J* Vol 10(2):108-12.

Velibey Y, Altay S, Eren M, Cam N. (2010). Myocardial noncompaction in a patient with kyphoscoliosis. *Turk Kardiyol Dern Ars* Vol 38(7):492-495

Vieillard-Baron A, Loubieres Y, Schmitt JM, Page B, Dubourg O, Jardin F. (1999). Cyclic changes in right ventricular output impedance during mechanical ventilation. *J Appl Physiol* 87:1644-1650.

Weber SA, Montovani JC, Matsubara B, Fioretto JR. (2007). Echocardiographic abnormalities in children with obstructive breathing disorders during sleep. *J Pediatr (Rio J)*. Vol 83(6):518-522.

Weyman AE, Dillon JC, Feigenbaum H, et al. (1973). Echocardiographic patterns of pulmonary valve motion with pulmonary hypertension. *Circulation* Vol 50:910.

Yuan L, Cao T, Duan Y, Yang G, Wang Z, Ruan L. (2004). Noninvasive assessment of influence of resistant respiration on blood flow velocities across the cardiac valves in humans--a quantification study by echocardiography. *Echocardiography*. Vol 21(5):391-8.

Yuan L, Cao T, Zang Y, Pei J, Duan Y, Gao F. (2007). Reversal E/A Value at End-Inspiration Might Be More Sensitive and Accurate for Diagnosing Abnormal Left Ventricular Diastolic Function. *Echocardiography* Vol 24:472-477.

Zagnoev M, Milner S, Levin SL. (1981). Choanal atresia and congenital heart disease. S. *Atr. med. J* Vol 50, 815.

Zeybek C, Yalcin Y, Erdem A, Polat TB, Aktuglu-Zeybek AC, Bayoglu V. (2007). Tissue Doppler echocardiographic assessment of cardiac function in children with bronchial asthma. *Pediatr Int.* Vol 49(6):911-7.

Part 3

Left Ventricular Doppler

5

Tissue Doppler in Ischemic Heart Disease

Ola Gjesdal and Thor Edvardsen
Oslo University Hospital and University of Oslo
Norway

1. Introduction

Tissue Doppler Echocardiography was introduced in the 1960s (Yoshida et al., 1961), and enabled the quantitative assessment of myocardial motion and deformation. The wide use of tissue Doppler as a research tool halted, however, until the early 1990s (Hatle & Sutherland, 2000). Tissue Doppler is now available for high frame rates, wide sector angles and in combination with 2-dimiensional data acquisition. Although widely used in cardiovascular research, the clinical use is limited, probably due to the time consumption associated with special imaging protocols and tedious post processing. Nevertheless, tissue Doppler echocardiography has contributed to most of the available knowledge on the pathophysiology involved in myocardial contraction deficiency.

The experienced cardiologist can easily identify large myocardial infarcts by visual analysis of echocardiograms, but identification of a small MI may be challenging due to the modest changes in tissue properties. In ischemic tissue, the contractility is reduced and reduced deformation and deformation rate is observed. Due to differences in contractility among ischemic and adjacent healthy myocardium, the ischemic myocardium has a characteristic deformation pattern with stretch in early systole, reduced systolic shortening, and a delayed (postsystolic) shortening when the ventricular pressure decays. This early stretch and post systolic shortening pattern has been described both experimentally (Edvardsen, T. et al., 2002; Skulstad et al., 2002) and clinically (Gjesdal et al., 2008; Jamal et al., 1999; Voigt et al., 2004).

2. Deformation indices

Myocardial function was traditionally assessed by tissue Doppler by the measurement of myocardial velocity and displacement indices in directions parallel to the ultrasound beam direction. These indices allowed quantitative assessment of myocardial function in the longitudinal direction, but could not differentiate velocities caused by deformation in the myocardium from velocities caused by displacement and tethering from adjacent structures.

The deforming heart can be assessed by evaluation of tissue velocities or displacement, deformation (strain) or rate of deformation (strain rate).

The Doppler shift utilized for deformational assessment in tissue Doppler echocardiography is a measure directly correlated to tissue velocity, and strain or strain rate measurements are automatically derived by integration or derivation of the spatial velocity distribution (Figure

1). During contraction, the apex is relatively stationary and the strain is relatively equally distributed in the different left ventricular compartments. There is therefore a natural gradient of velocity and displacement in the heart, with higher values observed towards the basal part of the heart. Tethering (pulling) by healthy adjacent myocardium, and translational cardiac motion can thus influence the velocities and displacements of diseased myocardium. When these indices are assessed, the position of the region of interest must therefore be evaluated together with the velocity information (Skulstad et al., 2004).

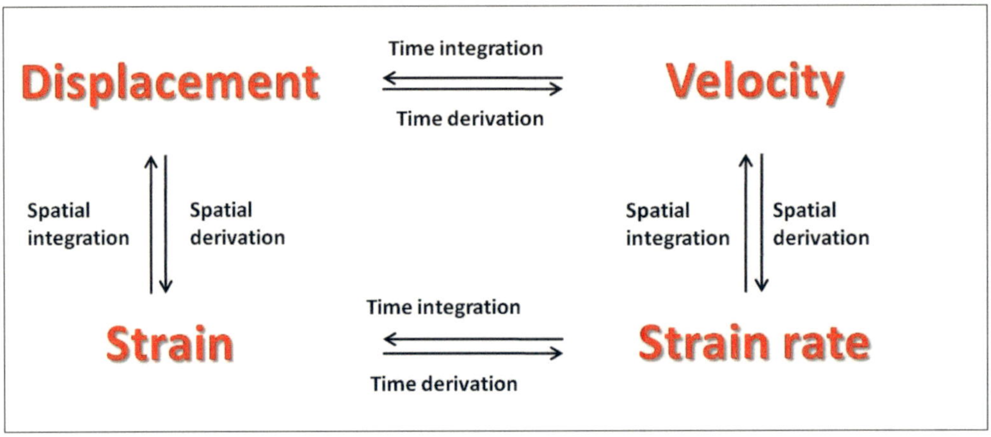

Fig. 1. Mathematical relation between deformation indices

In an attempt to establish a measure that was more specific for myocardial properties the principle of calculating myocardial strain rate from echocardiographic data was introduced (Quinones et al., 1974). This is analogous to the earlier approach to calculate strain rate or "normalized velocities" from apex cardiographic tracings, and the concept of myocardial strain was defined as fractional tissue deformation in response to applied force or stress (Mirsky et al., 1972). In that context, strain represents fractional change of tissue length and is expressed in a dimensionless unit as percent shortening or lengthening (Lagrangian formula). In an effort to improve the ability of TDI to measure regional function, TDI-derived real time *strain rate* was introduced (Heimdal et al., 1998). Strains are more uniformly distributed within the LV myocardium than tissue velocities, and the assessment of myocardial strain by TDI thus simplifies the analysis of regional contractile function by providing an objective parameter of myocardial deformation. Strain is a relatively new index of myocardial function that describes myocardial deformation as the relative change in myocardial segment length over time (D'hooge, J. et al., 2002), and provides information on segmental or global myocardial deformation (Gjesdal et al., 2007). Strain (deformation) or strain rate (rate of deformation) can be assessed in patients by echocardiography using tissue Doppler or speckle tracking echocardiography (Dandel & Hetzer, 2009) or with tagged MRI (Edvardsen & Rosen, 2005), and in experimental studies by sonomicrometry (Urheim et al., 2000). The indices have proven superior to established indices of myocardial function to assess myocardial infarct size (Becker et al., 2006; Chan et al., 2006; Gjesdal et al., 2008; Vartdal et al., 2007), hypertrophic cardiomyopathy (Serri et al., 2006), and in metabolic syndrome (Gong et al., 2009), ads incremental value in predicting outcome in cardiovascular

disease (Ingul, C. B. et al., 2007), and predicts arrhythmic events after myocardial infarct (Haugaa et al., 2009).
Strain and strain rate (SR) were developed as clinical indices of regional myocardial deformation (Edvardsen et al., 2001; Gotte et al., 2001; Mirsky & Parmley, 1973; Rademakers et al., 1994; Zhang et al., 2005) and have been introduced and validated using tagged MRI and sonomicrometry (Derumeaux et al., 2001; Edvardsen, T. et al., 2002; Urheim et al., 2000). Strain is defined as tissue elongation relative to length; usually the length at end diastole (Lagrangian strain) but instantaneous length is also used (Eulerian strain). A positive strain value refers to elongation, whereas a negative strain value describes shortening. Strain and strain rate are related through temporal derivation or integration, respectively. Therefore, negative systolic strain and strain rate values describe a normal contracting myocardial segment. Three main systolic deformation patterns form perpendicular axes in the heart's internal coordinate system (D'hooge et al., 2000); longitudinal shortening, circumferential shortening and radial thickening (Figure 2). In a direct comparison between strain, displacement and ejection velocity, strain by tissue Doppler was found to be superior to describe regional myocardial function, both in an animal model, and in humans(Skulstad et al., 2006).

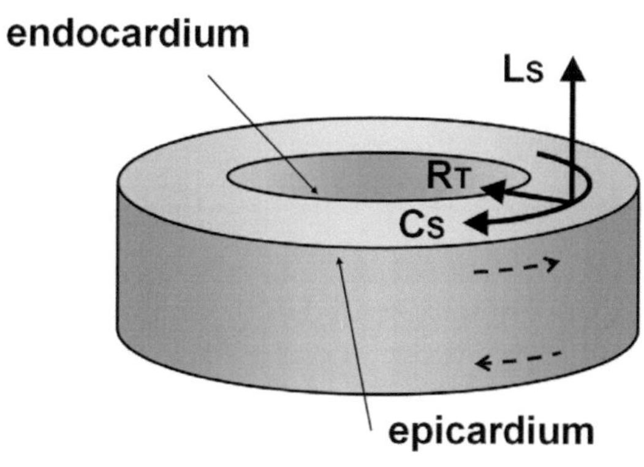

Fig. 2. The heart's coordinate system. Longitudinal shortening (L_S), Circumferential shortening (C_S) and Radial Thickening (R_T) is displayed

Doppler derived measures are angle dependent, and the assessment of global function is limited by angulations of apical segmental myocardium relative to the ultrasound beam direction. To overcome this problem, assessment of mitral plane velocities or displacement has been proposed as an index of global LV function (Alam et al., 1990; Alam, M. et al., 1992; Hoglund et al., 1989; Simonson & Schiller, 1989). Due to tethering from the mid-ventricular and apical segments, the displacement at the base of the left ventricle reflects the average deformation of the LV walls. When opposing walls are evaluated during the same heartbeat, the potential misjudgment caused by apical rocking is reduced to a minimum. Mitral annulus displacement and velocity analyses by TDI has been validated in the clinical setting, is well established and widely available. The method requires dedicated imaging protocols and is angle dependant, but might be more robust compared to speckle tracking imaging when the acoustic window is poor. Mitral annulus displacement has proven to be robust and reproducible (Hayashi et al., 2006), and has demonstrated good ability to predict prognosis following myocardial infarct (Brand et al., 2002). Mitral annulus displacement can also be normalized for end diastolic LV length (normalized Mitral annulus Displacement), an index which corresponds to global strain (Gjesdal et al., 2009).

To eliminate the problem of angle-dependency in Doppler-derived deformation analyses, strain measurement based on two-dimensional speckle-tracking echocardiography (2D-STE) has recently been developed (Amundsen et al., 2006; Cho et al., 2006; D'hooge, J. et al., 2002; Helle-Valle et al., 2005; Leitman et al., 2004). Natural acoustic markers (speckles) visualized by gray scale imaging form patterns within myocardial tissue. Dedicated software identifies the speckle patterns, and myocardial deformation assessed based on deformational changes on a frame-to-frame basis. Strain is calculated for each LV-segment as the average relative deformation in circumferential, longitudinal or radial directions (Becker et al., 2006; Chan et al., 2006; Vartdal et al., 2007) and the method furthermore enables assessment of LV-rotation and twist (Helle-Valle et al., 2005). The method is semi-automatic and relatively independent of angle. Spatial resolution is nearly constant with depth in the direction of the ultrasound beam, while the spatial resolution orthogonal to the beam direction is constant with depth with a linear array transducer, and decreases slightly with depth when a sector or phased array transducer is used. Since speckle tracking echocardiography is a developing methodology for assessment of the same indices that are assessed by tissue Doppler echocardiography, this will also be covered briefly. The implementation of TDI in daily clinical work has been relatively slow and most echocardiographic laboratories do not apply TDI as a routine diagnostic method.

3. Infarct assessment

Direct assessment of myocardial infarct by histopathology is the gold standard for infarct sizing, and is an option in post-mortem studies, in animal studies, and in studies on the explanted heart (Kim et al., 1999; Medrano et al., 1996). Biochemical infarct sizing is based on the correlation between the amount of damaged myocardium and release to the blood pool of specific markers of cardiac necrosis. Peak values correlate to infarct size, but the accuracy of the methods depends on correct timing of the blood sampling in relation to the ischemic event (Gibbons et al., 2004). Visualization of MI by imaging techniques is based on differences in tissue properties among normal and infarcted tissue. In CE-MRI, the infarcted myocardium is highlighted due to retention of contrast medium in the infarcted tissue, while positron emission tomography (PET) and single photon emission computed tomography (SPECT), are based on visualization of viable non-infarcted myocardium due to preserved glucose metabolism and retention of radioactive tracers in viable myocytes, respectively (Gibbons et al., 2004). In echocardiography and in cine- and tagged MRI imaging, changes in cardiac motion pattern, deformation, or changes in LV pumping performance form the basis of infarct sizing.

Myocardial contraction is severely reduced within scars, and systolic deformation of the left ventricle therefore decreases with increasing myocardial scar load (Chan et al., 2006; Hoglund et al., 1989; Skulstad et al., 2006; Vartdal et al., 2007). Assessment of myocardial deformation at a global or segmental level thus represents alternatives to the direct assessment of myocardial scar load by CE-MRI (Figure 3). Echocardiographic scanners are less expensive, widely distributed, and are mastered by most cardiologists, and enables myocardial deformation assessment by a variety of methods. Evaluation of LV-deformation has traditionally been performed by assessment of the relative volume reduction during systole (Left ventricular ejection fraction, LVEF), by visual assessment of the wall thickening in individual LV-segments during systole (Wall motion score, WMS) (Lang et al., 2005), or by assessment of the longitudinal LV-shortening or rate of shortening (mitral annulus displacement or velocity) (Simonson & Schiller, 1989).

Echocardiographic assessment of LVEF is easily available and feasible, but does not provide information on segmental LV-function. Evaluation of regional function by analyses of endocardial motion or local wall thinning and thickening characteristics is user dependent and requires well-trained personnel. Measurement of longitudinal LV-deformation by mitral annulus (MA) displacement or velocity can be performed by tissue Doppler imaging (TDI), pulsed TDI or M-mode echocardiography (Hayashi et al., 2006). Assessment is relatively easy, but the reference values differ among the methods. Furthermore, the methods do not provide information on segmental deformation, and regional deformation may be influenced by tethering or apical rocking. MA-displacement, however, predicts future events in patients with myocardial infarction, heart failure or hypertensive heart disease (Ballo et al., 2008; Hillenbrand et al., 2000; Willenheimer, R. et al., 1997).

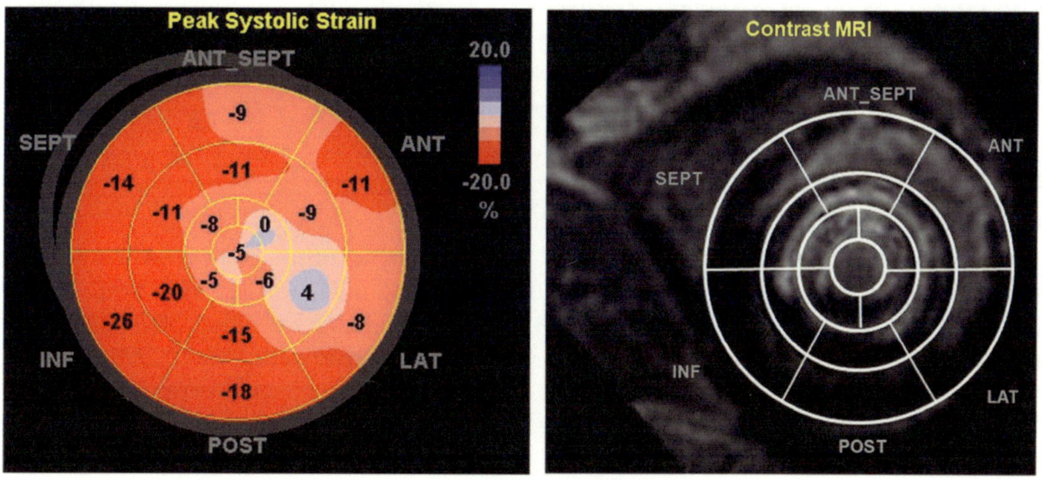

Fig. 3. Bulls eye plot of peak systolic longitudinal strain by speckle tracking echocardiography (left) and gadolinium contrast MRI (right). The center of the plot represents apex, and the rim represents the basal LV segments

Low systolic myocardial velocities in ventricles with myocardial damage, hypertrophy and cardiomyopathy have been demonstrated by several authors (Bach et al., 1996; Gorcsan, III et al., 1996; Miyatake et al., 1995; Uematsu et al., 1995). Mitral annular and myocardial longitudinal velocity measurements have been used in several studies to characterize systole in normal individuals and in different heart diseases (Fukuda et al., 1998; Gulati et al., 1996; Oki et al., 1999; Pai & Gill, 1998; Wilkenshoff et al., 1998). Generally, systolic longitudinal velocity was reduced in most heart diseases. This longitudinal approach has also been useful to describe the diastolic function in normal subjects and patients with LV hypertrophy showing a decrease in VE with age and in LV hypertrophy (Rodriguez et al., 1996). Several conditions are thus responsible for decreased myocardial systolic and diastolic velocities and myocardial single finding of reduced velocity. Based on the available literature, it is likely that focus on the highest systolic velocity or deformation is not sufficient to characterize ischemia from other diseases affecting the contraction of the heart.

4. Validation studies

Tissue Doppler derived strain and strain rate have been validated using tagged MRI and sonomicrometry in humans and in animal studies (Derumeaux et al., 2001; Edvardsen et al., 2002; Urheim et al., 2000). Myocardial longitudinal strain was assessed as the time integral of regional Doppler velocity gradients in a dog model, and compared with strain derived from sonomicrometry crystals placed near the LV apex and base, respectively (Derumeaux et al., 2001; Edvardsen, T. et al., 2002; Urheim et al., 2000).Comparisons during baseline, apical ischemia and preload alterations demonstrated good correlations ($r = 0.92$, $p<0.01$).

In human studies longitudinal myocardial Doppler velocities have been shown to decrease progressively from base to apex, while myocardial strain rates and strains are uniformly distributed among all segments (Edvardsen, T. et al., 2002). Comparisons between myocardial longitudinal strains by SDE and tagged-MRI showed excellent correlations ($r=0.89$ and $r=0.96$, for longitudinal and radial strains respectively ($p<0.001$), in healthy individuals, infarct patients, and during stress echocardiography.

5. Acute ischemic heart disease

5.1 Deformation characteristics

During acute ischemia, the contractility of the ischemic myocardium is reduced. Postsystolic shortening was identified as a sign of viability in a dog model of ischemic heart disease (Takayama et al., 1996), and tissue Doppler enabled the characterization of regional wall motion disturbances during ischemia and reperfusion (Derumeaux et al., 1998). Also in humans, abnormal postsystolic contraction was observed during ischemia (Jamal et al., 1999). Deformation assessment by strain and strain rate demonstrated better ability to evaluate ischemic myocardium compared to velocity based indices in animal models (Hashimoto et al., 2003) and human studies (Edvardsen, T. et al., 2002; Jamal et al., 2002; Zhang et al., 2005), and provide information on small changes in function over time (Ingul et al., 2005),

In a study during and after angioplasty in humans, three major characteristics were identified for the systolic velocity pattern of ischemic myocardium (Edvardsen et al., 2000; Edvardsen et al., 2001). When comparing the ischemic regions of LV with the non-ischemic regions, the ischemic region was recognized by early systolic stretch and reduced peak systolic shortening, followed by a postsystolic shortening when the LV pressure decays during isovolumetric relaxation and early diastole (Figure 4). When the ischemia becomes more severe, the segment gradually becomes passive, and the deformation depends on the passive elastic properties of the myocardial tissue (Skulstad et al., 2002).

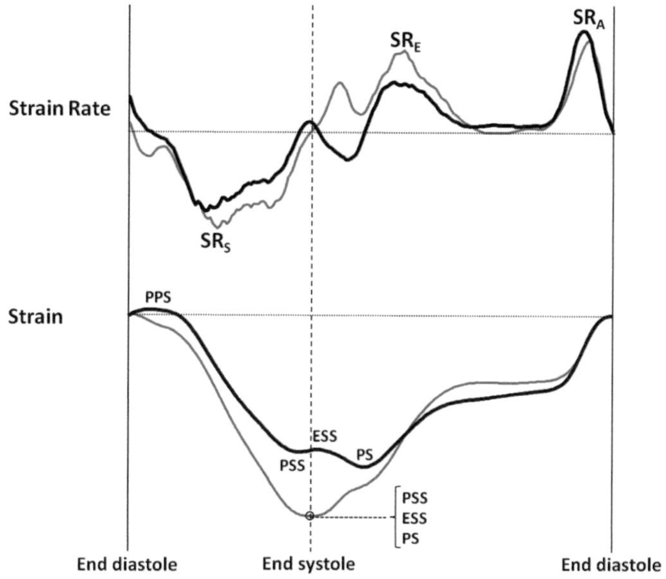

Fig. 4. Strain rate and strain from typical normal (grey) and ischemic (black) myocardium. Ischemic myocardium is characterized by an early peak positive strain (PPS), and peak systolic strain (PSS) is typically lower than end systolic strain (ESS). A post systolic shortening is often seen, and peak strain (PS) therefore occurs after end systole

During ischemia, adjacent myocardium also display altered deformation characteristics. This might be caused by stunning or transient ischemia, but also by alterations in local loading conditions. Remote myocardium generally has been thought to increase the contraction in a compensatory manner to accomplish the demands to cardiac output. This mechanism could be caused by neuro-hormonal activation, but also but the Frank-Starling mechanism secondary to the increased preload of the ischemic heart.

Recently, strain by Doppler and speckle tracking was demonstrated to display similar ability to separate among levels of transmurality in acute ST elevation myocardial infarction, but that reproducibility was somewhat better for speckle tracking derived strain (Sjoli et al., 2009). Postsystolic shortening has also been demonstrated in approximately one third of segments in healthy individuals, and indexation of postsystolic shortening relative to peak systolic shortening has therefore been suggested (Voigt, J. U. et al., 2003). Systolic strain by vector velocity imaging is also found to correlate with infarct in the acute phase, and peak systolic strain was a better predictor of infarct than the post systolic shortening index (Jurcut et al., 2008).

5.2 Identification of area at risk

Strain imaging by tissue Doppler echocardiography shortly after PCI for acute myocardial infarct correlated strongly with global infarct size assessed by delayed enhancement MRI 9 months later (Vartdal et al., 2007). Similar results were also found for speckle tracking echocardiography (Sjoli et al., 2009). Moreover, the strain value correlated with infarct transmurality level, suggesting that this index might be useful for prognostication.

5.3 Non ST elevation infarction

Global strain by speckle tracking deteriorates in non ST-elevation patients while waiting for angiography, and the patients with occlusion did not recover by revascularization, thus suggesting a potential benefit from a more aggressive strategy in these patients (Grenne et al., 2010). Strain measured immediately before revascularization was found to correlate significantly with infarct size assessed by delayed enhancement MRI also in non ST-elevation infarcts (Eek et al., 2010), and presence of reduced function in 4 or more adjacent segments was shown to predict coronary occlusion with high accuracy (Eek et al., 2010).

6. Chronic ischemic heart disease

6.1 Deformation characteristics

In chronic ischemic heart disease, the infarcted area has transformed to scar tissue with increased resistance to passive stretch. As a consequence, early systolic stretch is a less common finding. There is often, however, ischemic areas and areas with subendocardial infarct present adjacent to the infarcted areas, and early stretch can be identified in these areas. In the MESA study, reduced myocardial deformation was found in healthy individuals with increased coronary artery calcification (Edvardsen et al., 2006).

6.2 Estimation of infarct size and level of transmurality

In chronic myocardial infarct, strain values assessed by tissue Doppler or speckle tracking echocardiography are reduced with increasing level of transmural infarct distribution (Becker et al., 2006; Chan et al., 2006; Gjesdal et al., 2007; Sachdev et al., 2006; Weidemann et al., 2003), both at the segmental, at the global, and at a territorial level (Gjesdal et al., 2008). This is interesting, since segments with transmural infarct defined as more than 50% of the segment mass is less likely to benefit from revascularization.

Also the MA-displacement have demonstrated to be reduced both in patients with acute(Hoglund et al., 1989; Skulstad et al., 2006; Stoylen & Skjaerpe, 2003) or chronic infarct (Alam, M. et al., 1992) when compared to controls, and the reduction was greater in infarct-related LV-walls when compared to remote LV-walls. Normalized mitral annulus displacement has also demonstrated good correlation with myocardial infarct size in chronic ischemic heart disease (Gjesdal et al., 2009).

6.3 Risk stratification for arrhythmias

Recently, post myocardial infarct patients with indication for implantable cardioverter-defibrillator (ICD) were followed for arrhythmias requiring appropriate ICD therapy (Haugaa et al., 2009). In the patients with arrhythmia the dispersion of peak strain, calculated as standard deviation of time to maximal strain for all segments, was increased compared to patients who did not require therapy. Moreover, the global strain value was better in the patients without arrhythmia compared to the ones who received ICD therapy.

6.4 Stress testing

Tissue Doppler echocardiography has been used to quantify segmental function during exercise testing by velocity imaging (Pasquet et al., 1999), and has been demonstrated to predict functional recovery from revascularization (Schneider et al., 2005). When comparing deformation imaging and velocity imaging for the detection of regional inducible ischemia during dobutamine stress echocardiography, deformation indices demonstrated superior ability to detect ischemia compared to velocity based indices (Voigt et al., 2004). Moreover, in another study, postsystolic shortening demonstrated the best ability to identify stress induced ischemia after normalization to peak deformation, since postsystolic shortening also occurred to some extent in healthy segments (Voigt, J. U. et al., 2003). Strain and strain rate had been found superior to wall motion score to identify angiographic significant stenoses (Ingul, C. B. et al., 2007), and also to predict outcomes in patients admitted to stress echocardiography for suspected coronary heart disease (Ingul, C. B. et al., 2007).

7. Prognosis

Assessment of strain early following myocardial infarction predicts remodeling defined as more than 15% increase in end diastolic volume (Park et al., 2008). Global LV function assessed by tissue Doppler measurements of the mitral annulus displacement predicts events in chronic infarction (Brand et al., 2002) and congestive heart failure (Willenheimer, R. B. et al., 1997). The addition of strain rate during stress echocardiography added prognostic value over traditional risk factors and echocardiographic parameters (Stanton, T. et al., 2009), and an association between resting deformation indices and events was also demonstrated in people referred to echocardiography (Stanton, T. et al., 2009). Global strain by speckle tracking echocardiography was assessed within 48 hours of myocardial infarct in 659 patients, and found to be superior to LVEF and WMSI to predict mortality and clinical Events (Antoni et al., 2010).

8. Conclusions

All indices of myocardial function demonstrate reduced systolic deformation in infarcted myocardium. The deformation gradually reduces with increasing infarct size and transmural distribution. Ischemic tissue is characterized not only by reduced peak deformation, but also by an altered deformation pattern characterized by early systolic stretch and post systolic shortening.

9. References

Alam M., Hoglund C., Thorstrand C. Longitudinal systolic shortening of the left ventricle: an echocardiographic study in subjects with and without preserved global function. *Clin Physiol* 1992;12:443-52.

Alam M., Hoglund C., Thorstrand C., Hellekant C. Haemodynamic significance of the atrioventricular plane displacement in patients with coronary artery disease. *Eur Heart J* 1992;13:194-200.

Alam M, Hoglund C, Thorstrand C, Philip A. Atrioventricular plane displacement in severe congestive heart failure following dilated cardiomyopathy or myocardial infarction. *J Intern Med* 1990;228:569-75.

Amundsen BH, Helle-Valle T, Edvardsen T, Torp H, Crosby J, Lyseggen E, Stoylen A, Ihlen H, Lima JA, Smiseth OA, Slordahl SA. Noninvasive myocardial strain measurement by speckle tracking echocardiography: validation against sonomicrometry and tagged magnetic resonance imaging. *J Am Coll Cardiol* 2006;47:789-93.

Antoni ML, Mollema SA, Delgado V, Atary JZ, Borleffs CJW, Boersma E, Holman ER, van der Wall EE, Schalij MJ, Bax JJ. Prognostic importance of strain and strain rate after acute myocardial infarction. *European Heart Journal* 2010;31:1640-7.

Bach DS, Armstrong WF, Donovan CL, Muller DW. Quantitative Doppler tissue imaging for assessment of regional myocardial velocities during transient ischemia and reperfusion. *Am Heart J* 1996;132:721-5.

Ballo P, Barone D, Bocelli A, Motto A, Mondillo S. Left ventricular longitudinal systolic dysfunction is an independent marker of cardiovascular risk in patients with hypertension. *Am J Hypertens* 2008;21:1047-54.

Becker M, Hoffmann R, Kuhl HP, Grawe H, Katoh M, Kramann R, Bucker A, Hanrath P, Heussen N. Analysis of myocardial deformation based on ultrasonic pixel tracking to determine transmurality in chronic myocardial infarction. *Eur Heart J* 2006;27:2560-6.

Brand B, Rydberg E, Ericsson G, Gudmundsson P, Willenheimer R. Prognostication and risk stratification by assessment of left atrioventricular plane displacement in patients with myocardial infarction. *Int J Cardiol* 2002;83:35-41.

Chan J, Hanekom L, Wong C, Leano R, Cho GY, Marwick TH. Differentiation of subendocardial and transmural infarction using two-dimensional strain rate imaging to assess short-axis and long-axis myocardial function. *J Am Coll Cardiol* 2006;48:2026-33.

Cho GY, Chan J, Leano R, Strudwick M, Marwick TH. Comparison of two-dimensional speckle and tissue velocity based strain and validation with harmonic phase magnetic resonance imaging. *Am J Cardiol* 2006;97:1661-6.

D'hooge J., Bijnens B., Thoen J., Van de Werf F., Sutherland G. R., Suetens P. Echocardiographic strain and strain-rate imaging: a new tool to study regional myocardial function. *IEEE Trans Med Imaging* 2002;21:1022-30.

D'hooge J, Heimdal A, Jamal F, Kukulski T, Bijnens B, Rademakers F, Hatle L, Suetens P, Sutherland GR. Regional strain and strain rate measurements by cardiac ultrasound: principles, implementation and limitations. *Eur J Echocardiogr* 2000;1:154-70.

D'hooge J., Konofagou E., Jamal F., Heimdal A., Barrios L., Bijnens B., Thoen J., Van de Werf F., Sutherland G., Suetens P. Two-dimensional ultrasonic strain rate measurement of the human heart in vivo. *IEEE Trans Ultrason Ferroelectr Freq Control* 2002;49:281-6.

Dandel M, Hetzer R. Echocardiographic strain and strain rate imaging - Clinical applications. *International Journal of Cardiology* 2009;132:11-24.

Derumeaux G, Loufoua J, Pontier G, Cribier A, Ovize M. Tissue Doppler imaging differentiates transmural from nontransmural acute myocardial infarction after reperfusion therapy. *Circulation* 2001;103:589-96.

Derumeaux G, Ovize M, Loufoua J, ndre-Fouet X, Minaire Y, Cribier A, Letac B. Doppler tissue imaging quantitates regional wall motion during myocardial ischemia and reperfusion. *Circulation* 1998;97:1970-7.

Edvardsen T, Aakhus S, Endresen K, Bjomerheim R, Smiseth OA, Ihlen H. Acute regional myocardial ischemia identified by 2-dimensional multiregion tissue Doppler imaging technique. *J Am Soc Echocardiogr* 2000;13:986-94.

Edvardsen T, Detrano R, Rosen BD, Carr JJ, Liu K, Lai S, Shea S, Pan L, Bluemke DA, Lima JA. Coronary artery atherosclerosis is related to reduced regional left ventricular function in individuals without history of clinical cardiovascular disease: the Multiethnic Study of Atherosclerosis. *Arterioscler Thromb Vasc Biol* 2006;26:206-11.

Edvardsen T., Gerber B. L., Garot J., Bluemke D. A., Lima J. A., Smiseth O. A. Quantitative assessment of intrinsic regional myocardial deformation by Doppler strain rate echocardiography in humans: validation against three-dimensional tagged magnetic resonance imaging. *Circulation* 2002;106:50-6.

Edvardsen T, Rosen BD. Why do we need magnetic resonance imaging in cardiology? *Scand Cardiovasc J* 2005;39:260-3.

Edvardsen T, Skulstad H, Aakhus S, Urheim S, Ihlen H. Regional myocardial systolic function during acute myocardial ischemia assessed by strain Doppler echocardiography. *J Am Coll Cardiol* 2001;37:726-30.

Edvardsen T., Urheim S., Skulstad H., Steine K., Ihlen H., Smiseth O. A. Quantification of left ventricular systolic function by tissue Doppler echocardiography: added value of measuring pre- and postejection velocities in ischemic myocardium. *Circulation* 2002;105:2071-7.

Eek C, Grenne B, Brunvand H, Aakhus S, Endresen K, Smiseth OA, Edvardsen T, Skulstad H. Strain echocardiography predicts acute coronary occlusion in patients with non-ST-segment elevation acute coronary syndrome. *Eur J Echocardiogr* 2010;11:501-8.

Fukuda K, Oki T, Tabata T, Iuchi A, Ito S. Regional left ventricular wall motion abnormalities in myocardial infarction and mitral annular descent velocities studied with pulsed tissue Doppler imaging. *J Am Soc Echocardiogr* 1998;11:841-8.

Gibbons RJ, Valeti US, Araoz PA, Jaffe AS. The quantification of infarct size. *J Am Coll Cardiol* 2004;44:1533-42.

Gjesdal O, Helle-Valle T, Hopp E, Lunde K, Vartdal T, Aakhus S, Smith HJ, Ihlen H, Edvardsen T. Non-Invasive Separation of Large, Medium and Small Reperfused Myocardial Infarcts. A Comprehensive Tissue Doppler and Speckle Tracking Echocardiography Study. *Circ Cardiovascular Imaging* 2008;1:189-96.

Gjesdal O, Hopp E, Vartdal T, Lunde K, Helle-Valle T, Aakhus S, Smith HJ, Ihlen H, Edvardsen T. Global longitudinal strain measured by two-dimensional speckle tracking echocardiography is closely related to myocardial infarct size in chronic ischaemic heart disease. *Clin Sci (Lond)* 2007;113:287-96.

Gjesdal O, Vartdal T, Hopp E, Lunde K, Brunvand H, Smith HJ, Edvardsen T. Left ventricle longitudinal deformation assessment by mitral annulus displacement or global longitudinal strain in chronic ischemic heart disease: are they interchangeable? *J Am Soc Echocardiogr* 2009;22:823-30.

Gong HP, Tan HW, Fang NN, Song T, Li SH, Zhong M, Zhang W, Zhang Y. Impaired left ventricular systolic and diastolic function in patients with metabolic syndrome as assessed by strain and strain rate imaging. *Diabetes Research and Clinical Practice* 2009;83:300-7.

Gorcsan J, III, Gulati VK, Mandarino WA, Katz WE. Color-coded measures of myocardial velocity throughout the cardiac cycle by tissue Doppler imaging to quantify regional left ventricular function. *Am Heart J* 1996;131:1203-13.

Gotte MJ, van Rossum AC, Twisk JWR, Kuijer JPA, Marcus JT, Visser CA. Quantification of regional contractile function after infarction: strain analysis superior to wall thickening analysis in discriminating infarct from remote myocardium. *J Am Coll Cardiol* 2001;37:808-17.

Grenne B, Eek C, Sjoli B, Skulstad H, Aakhus S, Smiseth OA, Edvardsen T, Brunvand H. Changes of Myocardial Function in Patients with Non-ST-Elevation Acute Coronary Syndrome Awaiting Coronary Angiography. *American Journal of Cardiology* 2010;105:1212-8.

Gulati VK, Katz WE, Follansbee WP, Gorcsan J, III. Mitral annular descent velocity by tissue Doppler echocardiography as an index of global left ventricular function. *Am J Cardiol* 1996;77:979-84.

Hashimoto I, Li X, Hejmadi BA, Jones M, Zetts AD, Sahn DJ. Myocardial strain rate is a superior method for evaluation of left ventricular subendocardial function compared with tissue Doppler imaging. *J Am Coll Cardiol* 2003;42:1574-83.

Hatle L, Sutherland GR. Regional myocardial function--a new approach. *Eur Heart J* 2000;21:1337-57.

Haugaa KH, Smedsrud MK, Kongsgaard E, Smiseth OA, Amlie JP, Edvardsen T. Left Ventricular Global Strain Is More Accurate Than EF as a Marker of Arrhythmic Events After Myocardial Infarction. *Journal of the American College of Cardiology* 2009;53:A262.

Hayashi SY, Lind BI, Seeberger A, do Nascimento MM, Lindholm BJ, Brodin LA. Analysis of mitral annulus motion measurements derived from M-mode, anatomic M-mode, tissue Doppler displacement, and 2-dimensional strain imaging. *J Am Soc Echocardiogr* 2006;19:1092-101.

Heimdal A, Stoylen A, Torp H, Skjaerpe T. Real-time strain rate imaging of the left ventricle by ultrasound. *J Am Soc Echocardiogr* 1998;11:1013-9.

Helle-Valle T, Crosby J, Edvardsen T, Lyseggen E, Amundsen BH, Smith HJ, Rosen BD, Lima JA, Torp H, Ihlen H, Smiseth OA. New noninvasive method for assessment of left ventricular rotation: speckle tracking echocardiography. *Circulation* 2005;112:3149-56.

Hillenbrand HB, Lima JA, Bluemke DA, Beache GM, McVeigh ER. Assessment of myocardial systolic function by tagged magnetic resonance imaging. *J Cardiovasc Magn Reson* 2000;2:57-66.

Hoglund C, Alam M, Thorstrand C. Effects of acute myocardial infarction on the displacement of the atrioventricular plane: an echocardiographic study. *J Intern Med* 1989;226:251-6.

Ingul C. B., Rozis E., Slordahl S. A., Marwick T. H. Incremental value of strain rate imaging to wall motion analysis for prediction of outcome in patients undergoing dobutamine stress echocardiography. *Circulation* 2007;115:1252-9.

Ingul CB, Stoylen A, Slordahl SA. Recovery of stunned myocardium in acute myocardial infarction quantified by strain rate imaging: a clinical study. *J Am Soc Echocardiogr* 2005;18:401-10.

Ingul C. B., Stoylen A., Slordahl S. A., Wiseth R., Burgess M., Marwick T. H. Automated analysis of myocardial deformation at dobutamine stress echocardiography: an angiographic validation. *J Am Coll Cardiol* 2007;49:1651-9.

Jamal F, Kukulski T, D'hooge J, De S, I, Sutherland G. Abnormal postsystolic thickening in acutely ischemic myocardium during coronary angioplasty: a velocity, strain, and strain rate doppler myocardial imaging study. *J Am Soc Echocardiogr* 1999;12:994-6.

Jamal F, Kukulski T, Sutherland GR, Weidemann F, D'hooge J, Bijnens B, Derumeaux G. Can changes in systolic longitudinal deformation quantify regional myocardial function after an acute infarction? An ultrasonic strain rate and strain study. *J Am Soc Echocardiogr* 2002;15:723-30.

Jurcut R, Pappas CJ, Masci PG, Herbots L, Szulik M, Bogaert J, Van de Werf F, Desmet W, Rademakers F, Voigt JU, D'hooge J. Detection of regional myocardial dysfunction in patients with acute myocardial infarction using velocity vector imaging. *J Am Soc Echocardiogr* 2008;21:879-86.

Kim RJ, Fieno DS, Parrish TB, Harris K, Chen EL, Simonetti O, Bundy J, Finn JP, Klocke FJ, Judd RM. Relationship of MRI delayed contrast enhancement to irreversible injury, infarct age, and contractile function. *Circulation* 1999;100:1992-2002.

Lang RM, Bierig M, Devereux RB, Flachskampf FA, Foster E, Pellikka PA, Picard MH, Roman MJ, Seward J, Shanewise JS, Solomon SD, Spencer KT, Sutton MS, Stewart WJ. Recommendations for chamber quantification: a report from the American Society of Echocardiography's Guidelines and Standards Committee and the Chamber Quantification Writing Group, developed in conjunction with the European Association of Echocardiography, a branch of the European Society of Cardiology. *J Am Soc Echocardiogr* 2005;18:1440-63.

Leitman M, Lysyansky P, Sidenko S, Shir V, Peleg E, Binenbaum M, Kaluski E, Krakover R, Vered Z. Two-dimensional strain-a novel software for real-time quantitative echocardiographic assessment of myocardial function. *J Am Soc Echocardiogr* 2004;17:1021-9.

Medrano R, Lowry RW, Young JB, Weilbaecher DG, Michael LH, Afridi I, He ZX, Mahmarian JJ, Verani MS. Assessment of myocardial viability with 99mTc sestamibi in patients undergoing cardiac transplantation. A scintigraphic/pathological study. *Circulation* 1996;94:1010-7.

Mirsky I, Parmley WW. Assessment of passive elastic stiffness for isolated heart muscle and the intact heart. *Circ Res* 1973;33:233-43.

Mirsky I, Pasternac A, Ellison RC. General index for the assessment of cardiac function. *Am J Cardiol* 1972;30:483-91.

Miyatake K, Yamagishi M, Tanaka N, Uematsu M, Yamazaki N, Mine Y, Sano A, Hirama M. New method for evaluating left ventricular wall motion by color-coded tissue Doppler imaging: in vitro and in vivo studies. *J Am Coll Cardiol* 1995;25:717-24.

Oki T, Tabata T, Mishiro Y, Yamada H, Abe M, Onose Y, Wakatsuki T, Iuchi A, Ito S. Pulsed tissue Doppler imaging of left ventricular systolic and diastolic wall motion velocities to evaluate differences between long and short axes in healthy subjects. *J Am Soc Echocardiogr* 1999;12:308-13.

Pai RG, Gill KS. Amplitudes, durations, and timings of apically directed left ventricular myocardial velocities: I. Their normal pattern and coupling to ventricular filling and ejection. *J Am Soc Echocardiogr* 1998;11:105-11.

Park YH, Kang SJ, Song JK, Lee EY, Song JM, Kang DH, Kim YH, Lee CW, Hong MK, Kim JJ, Park SW, Park SJ. Prognostic value of longitudinal strain after primary reperfusion therapy in patients with anterior-wall acute myocardial infarction. *J Am Soc Echocardiogr* 2008;21:262-7.

Pasquet A, Armstrong G, Beachler L, Lauer MS, Marwick TH. Use of segmental tissue Doppler velocity to quantitate exercise echocardiography. *J Am Soc Echocardiogr* 1999;12:901-12.

Quinones MA, Gaasch WH, Alexander JK. Echocardiographic assessment of left ventricular function with special reference to normalized velocities. *Circulation* 1974;50:42-51.

Rademakers FE, Rogers WJ, Guier WH, Hutchins GM, Siu CO, Weisfeldt ML, Weiss JL, Shapiro EP. Relation of regional cross-fiber shortening to wall thickening in the intact heart. Three-dimensional strain analysis by NMR tagging. *Circulation* 1994;89:1174-82.

Rodriguez L, Garcia M, Ares M, Griffin BP, Nakatani S, Thomas JD. Assessment of mitral annular dynamics during diastole by Doppler tissue imaging: comparison with mitral Doppler inflow in subjects without heart disease and in patients with left ventricular hypertrophy. *Am Heart J* 1996;131:982-7.

Sachdev V, Aletras AH, Padmanabhan S, Sidenko S, Rao YN, Brenneman CL, Shizukuda Y, Lie GR, Vincent PS, Waclawiw MA, Arai AE. Myocardial strain decreases with increasing transmurality of infarction: a Doppler echocardiographic and magnetic resonance correlation study. *J Am Soc Echocardiogr* 2006;19:34-9.

Schneider C, Bahlmann E, Malisius R, Hertting K, Antz M, Kuck KH. Tissue velocity imaging during dobutamine stimulation for assessment of myocardial viability: Segmental analysis in patients after myocardial infarction. *Int J Cardiol* 2005.

Serri K, Reant P, Lafitte M, Berhouet M, Le B, V, Roudaut R, Lafitte S. Global and regional myocardial function quantification by two-dimensional strain: application in hypertrophic cardiomyopathy. *J Am Coll Cardiol* 2006;47:1175-81.

Simonson JS, Schiller NB. Descent of the base of the left ventricle: an echocardiographic index of left ventricular function. *J Am Soc Echocardiogr* 1989;2:25-35.

Sjoli B, Orn S, Grenne B, Vartdal T, Smiseth OA, Edvardsen T, Brunvand H. Comparison of left ventricular ejection fraction and left ventricular global strain as determinants of infarct size in patients with acute myocardial infarction. *J Am Soc Echocardiogr* 2009;22:1232-8.

Skulstad H, Andersen K, Edvardsen T, Rein KA, Tonnessen TI, Hol PK, Fosse E, Ihlen H. Detection of ischemia and new insight into left ventricular physiology by strain Doppler and tissue velocity imaging: assessment during coronary bypass operation of the beating heart. *J Am Soc Echocardiogr* 2004;17:1225-33.

Skulstad H, Edvardsen T, Urheim S, Rabben SI, Stugaard M, Lyseggen E, Ihlen H, Smiseth OA. Postsystolic shortening in ischemic myocardium: active contraction or passive recoil? *Circulation* 2002;106:718-24.

Skulstad H, Urheim S, Edvardsen T, Andersen K, Lyseggen E, Vartdal T, Ihlen H, Smiseth OA. Grading of myocardial dysfunction by tissue Doppler echocardiography: a comparison between velocity, displacement, and strain imaging in acute ischemia. *J Am Coll Cardiol* 2006;47:1672-82.

Stanton T., Ingul C. B., Hare J. L., Leano R., Marwick T. H. Association of myocardial deformation with mortality independent of myocardial ischemia and left ventricular hypertrophy. *JACC Cardiovasc Imaging* 2009;2:793-801.

Stanton T., Leano R., Marwick T. H. Prediction of all-cause mortality from global longitudinal speckle strain: comparison with ejection fraction and wall motion scoring. *Circ Cardiovasc Imaging* 2009;2:356-64.

Stoylen A, Skjaerpe T. Systolic long axis function of the left ventricle. Global and regional information. *Scand Cardiovasc J* 2003;37:253-8.

Takayama Y, Holmes JW, LeGrice I, Covell JW. Enhanced regional deformation at the anterior papillary muscle insertion site after chordal transsection. *Circulation* 1996;93:585-93.

Uematsu M, Miyatake K, Tanaka N, Matsuda H, Sano A, Yamazaki N, Hirama M, Yamagishi M. Myocardial velocity gradient as a new indicator of regional left ventricular contraction: detection by a two-dimensional tissue Doppler imaging technique. *J Am Coll Cardiol* 1995;26:217-23.

Urheim S, Edvardsen T, Torp H, Angelsen B, Smiseth OA. Myocardial strain by Doppler echocardiography. Validation of a new method to quantify regional myocardial function. *Circulation* 2000;102:1158-64.

Vartdal T, Brunvand H, Pettersen E, Smith HJ, Lyseggen E, Helle-Valle T, Skulstad H, Ihlen H, Edvardsen T. Early prediction of infarct size by strain Doppler echocardiography after coronary reperfusion. *J Am Coll Cardiol* 2007;49:1715-21.

Voigt J. U., Exner B., Schmiedehausen K., Huchzermeyer C., Reulbach U., Nixdorff U., Platsch G., Kuwert T., Daniel W. G., Flachskampf F. A. Strain-rate imaging during dobutamine stress echocardiography provides objective evidence of inducible ischemia. *Circulation* 2003;107:2120-6.

Voigt J. U., Lindenmeier G., Exner B., Regenfus M., Werner D., Reulbach U., Nixdorff U., Flachskampf F. A., Daniel W. G. Incidence and characteristics of segmental postsystolic longitudinal shortening in normal, acutely ischemic, and scarred myocardium. *J Am Soc Echocardiogr* 2003;16:415-23.

Voigt JU, Nixdorff U, Bogdan R, Exner B, Schmiedehausen K, Platsch G, Kuwert T, Daniel WG, Flachskampf FA. Comparison of deformation imaging and velocity imaging for detecting regional inducible ischaemia during dobutamine stress echocardiography. *Eur Heart J* 2004;25:1517-25.

Weidemann F, Dommke C, Bijnens B, Claus P, D'hooge J, Mertens P, Verbeken E, Maes A, Van de WF, De S, I, Sutherland GR. Defining the transmurality of a chronic myocardial infarction by ultrasonic strain-rate imaging: implications for identifying intramural viability: an experimental study. *Circulation* 2003;107:883-8.

Wilkenshoff UM, Sovany A, Wigstrom L, Olstad B, Lindstrom L, Engvall J, Janerot-Sjoberg B, Wranne B, Hatle L, Sutherland GR. Regional mean systolic myocardial velocity estimation by real-time color Doppler myocardial imaging: a new technique for quantifying regional systolic function. *J Am Soc Echocardiogr* 1998;11:683-92.

Willenheimer R., Cline C., Erhardt L., Israelsson B. Left ventricular atrioventricular plane displacement: an echocardiographic technique for rapid assessment of prognosis in heart failure. *Heart* 1997;78:230-6.

Willenheimer R. B., Erhardt L. R., Cline C. M., Rydberg E. R., Israelsson B. A. Prognostic significance of changes in left ventricular systolic function in elderly patients with congestive heart failure. *Coron Artery Dis* 1997;8:711-7.

Yoshida T, Mori M, Nimura Y, Hikita G, Takagishi S, Nakanishi K, Satomura S. Analysis of heart motion with ultrasonic Doppler method and its clinical application. *Am Heart J* 1961;61:61-75.

Zhang Y, Chan AK, Yu CM, Yip GW, Fung JW, Lam WW, So NM, Wang M, Wu EB, Wong JT, Sanderson JE. Strain rate imaging differentiates transmural from non-transmural myocardial infarction; a validation study using delayed-enhancement magnetic resonance imaging. *J Am Coll Cardiol* 2005;46:864-71.

6

Evaluation of Left Ventricular Diastolic Function by Echocardiography

Juan Lacalzada et al.*
Hospital Universitario de Canarias, La Laguna, Santa Cruz de Tenerife
Spain

1. Introduction

The normal cardiac cycle consists of two phases, systole and diastole, which are repeated over time to maintain an adequate cardiac output. The systole has been traditionally regarded as the main capital phase, leaving at diastole as a secondary process and almost forgotten. However, today we know that diastole is a crucial stage in the functioning of the heart. Its dysfunction can lead even in cases with preserved systolic function in heart failure. About half of patients with new diagnoses of heart failure have normal or near normal global ejection fractions. These patients are diagnosed with "diastolic heart failure" or "heart failure with preserved ejection fraction" (Zipes et al., 2011).

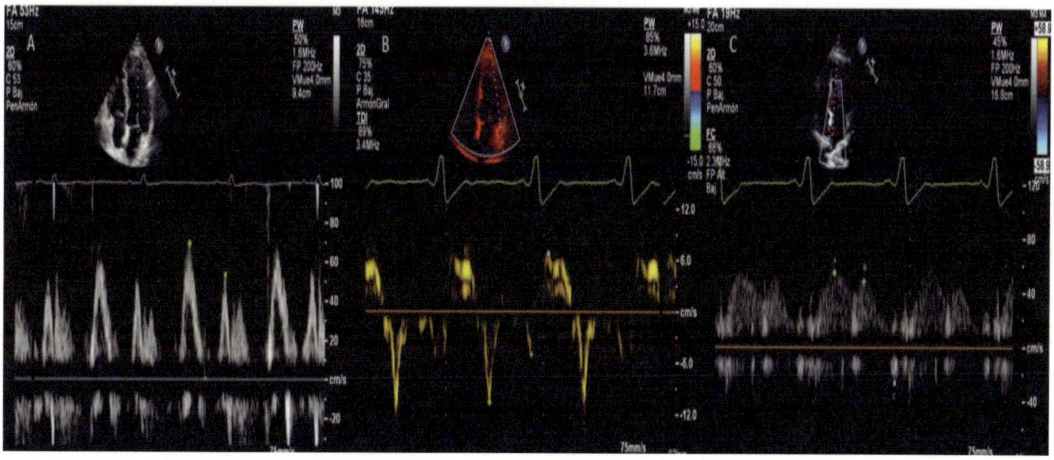

Fig. 1. Normal diastolic Doppler patterns: A) Mitral inflow. B) Mitral annular tissue Doppler. C) Pulmonary venous flow

* Amelia Duque, Alejandro de la Rosa, Antonio Barragan, María Manuela Izquierdo, Eduardo Arroyo and Ignacio Laynez
Hospital Universitario de Canarias, La Laguna, Santa Cruz de Tenerife, Spain
Ana Laynez
Medstar Health Research Institut, Washington Hospital Center, Washington, DC, U.S.A.

Echocardiography has played a central role in the evaluation of left ventricular diastolic function over the past two decades. Alterations in diastolic function may be transient (eg acute ischemia) or persistent (myocardial necrosis, left ventricular hypertrophy or myocardial infiltration). The indices of diastolic function can be organized into three groups: measures of isovolumetric relaxation, indices of passive left ventricular (LV) characteristics derived from the diastolic LV pressure-volume relations, and measurements of the pattern of LV diastolic filling obtained from Doppler echocardiography (figure 1) or radionuclide angiography. Nowdays, echocardiography is the technique of choice for the estimation of diastolic function.

1.1 Normal heart cycle

The ventricle has two alternating functions: systolic ejection and diastolic filling. The optimal performance of the LV depends on its ability to cycle between two states: first a compliant chamber in diastole that allows the LV to fill from low left atrium pressure and second a stiff chamber (rapidly rising pressure) in systole that ejects the stroke volume at arterial pressures. Diastole can be divided into four phases: isovolumetric diastolic relaxation period, the rapid filling phase, slow filling phase and atrial systole. Ventricular relaxation energy consumed primarily in the first two phases, while in the latter two processes have more influence the ventricular-compliance.

The Valsalva maneuver can be used to decrease preload and unmask the seemingly normal pattern of pseudonormal filling to reveal a pattern characteristic of relaxation abnormality. The pulmonary venous flow pattern, the tissue Doppler mitral annular velocity profile, left atrial (LA) size, and color M-mode, all contribute to the assessment of diastolic function and filling pressures, allowing classification of diastolic function and left ventricular filling pressures.

The first pressure crossover corresponds to the end of isovolumic relaxation and mitral valve opening. In the first phase, LA pressure exceeds LV pressure, accelerating mitral flow. Peak mitral E roughly corresponds to the second crossover. Thereafter, LV pressure exceeds LA pressure, decelerating mitral flow. These two phases correspond to rapid filling. Slow filling, with almost no pressure differences, follows this. During atrial contraction, LA pressure again exceeds LV pressure.

At baseline, the majority of filling occurs in early diastole ventricular after mitral valve opening, giving rise to the E wave mitral Doppler signal (figure 1). The filling rate is high turn. In meso and diastolic signal originates small and anterograde diastasis, followed by a wave in diastole. The peak velocity ratio E / A is usually greater than 1. There are situations such as tachycardia or arrhythmias such as atrial fibrillation which may affect ventricular filling.

1.2 Mechanisms of diastolic dysfunction

Although diastolic dysfunction is not uncommon in patients with normal wall thickness, left ventricular hypertrophy (LVH) is among the important reasons for it. In patients with diastolic heart failure, concentric hypertrophy (increased mass and relative wall thickness), or remodeling (normal mass but increased relative wall thickness), can be observed. In contrast, eccentric LVH is usually present in patients with depressed ejection fractions. Because of the high prevalence of hypertension, especially in the older population, LVH is common, and hypertensive heart disease is the most common abnormality leading to diastolic heart failure. Left ventricular mass may be best measured using 3-dimensional echocardiography. Nevertheless, it is possible to measure it in most patients using 2-

dimensional (2D) echocardiography, with the recently published guidelines of the American Society of Echocardiography (Oh et al., 2006).

The measurement of LA volume is highly feasible and reliable in most echocardiographic studies, with the most accurate measurements obtained using the apical 4-chamber and 2-chamber views, but it is important to consider left atrium volume measurements in conjunction with a patient's clinical status, other chambers' volumes, and Doppler parameters of left ventricular relaxation (Oh et al., 2006).

Symptomatic patients with diastolic dysfunction usually have increased pulmonary artery pressures. Therefore, in the absence of pulmonary disease, increased pulmonary artery pressures may be used to infer the presence of elevated LV filling pressures. Indeed, a significant correlation was noted between pulmonary artery systolic pressure and noninvasively derived LV filling pressures (Rodríguez-Padial et al., 2002).

The assessment of LV diastolic function and filling pressures is of paramount clinical importance to distinguish this syndrome from other diseases such as pulmonary disease resulting in dyspnoea, to assess prognosis, and to identify underlying cardiac disease and its best treatment. The criterion standard for demonstrating LV diastolic dysfunction is cardiac catheterization to obtain pressure-volume curves to measure the rate of pressure decay during isovolumic relaxation (Murphy et al., 2006). However, this measurement is imperfect because of the additional effect of transmyocardial pressure on the LV; routine invasive cardiac catheterization is also not feasible. Noninvasive modalities should thus include routine measurements of diastolic function. Echocardiography has played a central role in the evaluation of LV diastolic function over the past two decades.

2. Mitral inflow

2.1 Recording technique

Doppler mitral inflow velocity-derived variables remain the cornerstone of the evaluation of diastolic function. To evaluate the early and late filling phases, mitral inflow velocities are obtained by placing the pulsed-wave Doppler at the tips of the mitral valve leaflets in the apical 4-chamber view. This is the point at which the mitral inflow velocities are maximal and maximal accuracy and reproducibility of measurement are obtained. Normal mitral inflow consists of biphasic flow from the LA into the LV: rapid filling wave at the beginning of diastole, after mitral valve opening, when the transmitral gradient is higher (E-wave), followed by A-wave corresponding to a further increase in mitral flow velocity after atrial contraction (figure 1 A).

The ultrasound beam needs to be in parallel with the direction of blood flow to obtain an optimal flow signal and can be used to place the color Doppler sample volume in the predominant direction of mitral filling flow. With left ventricular dilatation, as in patients with dilated cardiomyopathy, the heart becomes more spherical, which causes the mitral inflow is directed progressively more lateral and beyond. Therefore, the optimal position of the transducer is approximately 20 degrees lateral to the apex in normal subjects and more lateral in those with growth of the left ventricle. The sample volume should be small (1-2 mm), resulting in a more contrasted flow record (Appleton et al, 1997).

2.2 Mitral inflow velocities

Primary measurements of mitral inflow include the peak early filling (E-wave) and late diastolic filling (A-wave) velocities, the E/A ratio, deceleration time (DT) of early filling velocity, and the isovolumetric relaxation time (IVRT) (figure 1). Secondary measurements include mitral A-wave duration, diastolic filling time, the A-wave velocity-time integral, and the total mitral inflow velocity-time integral (and thus the atrial filling fraction) with the sample volume at the level of the mitral annulus.

It is well established that the mitral E-wave velocity primarily reflects the LA- LV pressure gradient during early diastole and is therefore affected by preload and alterations in left ventricle relaxation (Appleton et al, 1988). The mitral A-wave velocity reflects the LA- LV ventricle pressure gradient during late diastole, which is affected by LV compliance and LA contractile function. E-wave DT is influenced by left ventricle relaxation, left ventricle diastolic pressures following mitral valve opening, and left ventricle compliance (i.e., the relationship between left ventricle pressure and volume). Patients with conditions associated with increased left ventricle stiffness have more rapid rates of deceleration of early left ventricle filling and shorter deceleration times (Ohno et al, 1994). In summary, mitral deceleration time is an important parameter that should be considered in drawing conclusions about operative left ventricle stiffness, particularly in patients without marked slowing of left ventricle relaxation.

Factors that affect mitral inflow include heart rate, rhythm, PR interval, cardiac output, mitral annular size, left atrium function, left ventricle end-systolic or end-diastolic volumes, and left ventricle elastic recoil.

2.3 Diastolic filling patterns

The initial classification of diastolic filling is based on the measurement of E-wave and A-wave velocities and E/A ratio (figure 2). Mitral valve inflow patterns, which have been attributed in varying degree to diastolic dysfunction, include normal pattern, impaired LV relaxation pattern, restrictive LV filling pattern and pseudonormal LV filling pattern.

2.3.1 Normal pattern

In healthy, young, disease-free individuals the E-wave exceeds the A-wave, and therefore the E/A ratio is more than 1 (Figure 1-A). In adolescents and young adults, there may be a disproportionate contribution of active ventricular relaxation to ventricular filling, which results in a markedly accentuated E-wave velocity. In this instance, E/A ratio can exceed a value of 2 in a normal, disease-free individual. With advancing age, there is natural stiffening of the ventricle, which results in delayed relaxation and therefore a progressive decrease in E-wave velocity and an increase in A-wave velocity with age so that the E/A ratio in a disease-free individual older than 60 years is often less than 1 (Klein et al, 1994).

2.3.2 Impaired left ventricle relaxation pattern

In almost every type of heart disease, the initial alteration of diastolic filling is impaired or slowed myocardial relaxation (figure 2 A). When myocardial relaxation is markedly delayed, patients have a mitral filling pattern with prolonged isovolumetric relaxation time (> 200 ms) and deceleration time (> 220 ms), decreased E-wave velocity and increased A-wave, since more of the ventricular filling happens to occur at the beginning of diastole to do at the end of it, with atrial contraction. This produces an E/A ratio <1 (figure 2). In addition, in the presence of bradycardia, a characteristic low meso-diastolic (after early filling) mitral inflow velocity may be seen, due to a progressive fall in LV diastolic pressure related to slow LV relaxation. However, increased filling pressure can mask these changes in mitral velocities. Therefore, an E/A ratio < 1 and deceleration time > 240 ms have high specificity for abnormal LV relaxation, but can be seen with either normal or increased filling pressures, depending on how delayed LV relaxation is (Oh et al, 1997).

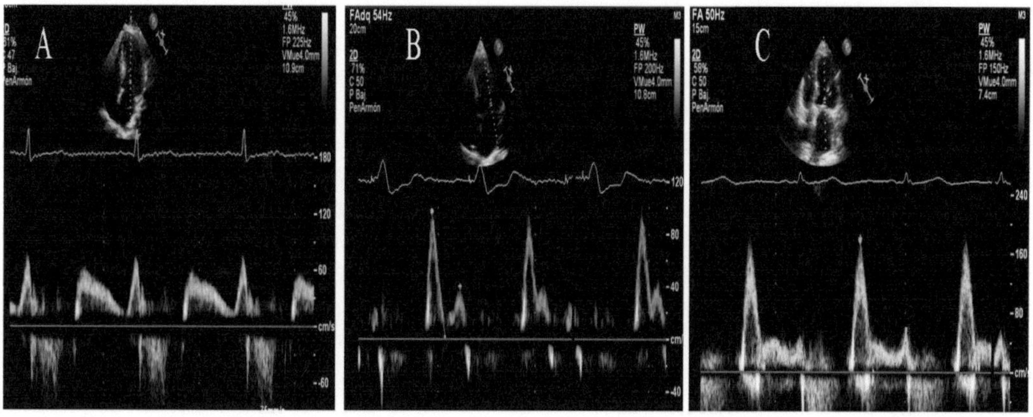

Fig. 2. Pulsed Doppler mitral filling flow showing: A) Impaired relaxation pattern, B) Pseudonormal pattern C) Restrictive pattern

2.3.3 Restrictive left ventricle filling pattern

This pattern (figure 2C) represents a combination of a stiff, noncompliant ventricle and elevated LV end-diastolic pressure. Increased left atrial pressure produces an earlier opening of the mitral valve, a shortening of IVRT and increased initial transmitral gradient (high E-wave velocity). Early diastolic filling in a non-distensible ventricle cause a rapid increase in LV early diastolic pressure with a rapid equalization of LV and LA pressures which produce a shortening of the deceleration time. Atrial contraction increases the pressure of the LA, but the speed and duration are shortened because LV pressure is increases even faster. Therefore, the restrictive physiology is characterized by increased E-wave velocity, decreased A-wave velocity, E/A ratio >2, shortened deceleration time (<160 ms) and isovolumetric relaxation time (<70 ms) (figure 2). A restrictive physiology pattern identifies advanced, usually symptomatic disease, with a poor prognosis (figure 2).

2.3.4 Pseudonormal left ventricular filling pattern

Pseudonormalization is a transitional phase between abnormal relaxation and restrictive physiology (figure 2 A). During this transition, the incoming mitral flow pattern is going through a phase that resembles the normal diastolic filling pattern, ie, E / A ratio of 1-1.5 and a normal deceleration time (160-200 ms). This is the result of a moderate increase of filling pressure superimposed on a decreased compliance. This pattern represents a moderate stage of diastolic dysfunction .The determination of pseudonormal filling may be difficult by mitral inflow velocities alone. Monitoring mitral inflow patterns during the Valsalva maneuver, wich reduces LV preload, may change the "normal" E/A ratio and unmask evidence of delayed relaxation. Changes of mitral inflow during Valsalva maneuver have a moderate diagnostic value for the differentiation of normal and pseudonormal pattern. Increased duration of atrial phase but not increase in atrial velocity allowed the diagnosis of pseudonormalization (Wierzbowska-Drabik et al, 2007). Reflex tachycardia during the Valsalva maneuver and subsequent fusion of the E velocity and A velocity waves on the mitral velocity curves is a sign of normal left ventricular filling pressures (Maniu et al, 2004). There are several other techniques for separating the pseudonormal from a truly normal pattern, which are discussed subsequently.

2.4 Variations in mitral inflow patterns

Not all patterns of mitral flow velocity fit into one of these three patterns (figure 2). The spectrum is broad as a result of different contributions and degree of underlying pathology, abnormal relaxation, and changes in compliance and volume status. The same degree of decreased compliance will result in different curves of mitral flow velocity depending on whether there is impaired relaxation. In the presence of significant LVH, deceleration time can be elongated even with increased pressure in the LA, while a similar increase in pressure in other patients leads to a shortening of the deceleration time. In severe LVH, it can see a pattern of meso-tele-diastolic prominent triphasic mitral flow as a result of markedly prolonged relaxation that continues in the meso-diastole. Even though the initial slope present a short deceleration time, continued filling indicate that the main problem is an abnormal relaxation and not a decrease in distensibility. A counter example is the constrictive pericarditis, in which a normal relaxation and a decrease in compliance may result in a markedly shortened mitral deceleration time without a significant increase in filling pressures (Oh et al, 1994).

In patients with dilated cardiomyopathies, Doppler mitral flow velocity variables and filling patterns correlate better with cardiac filling pressures, functional class, and prognosis than left ventricle ejection fraction (Vanoverschelde et al, 1990). A restrictive filling pattern is associated with a poor prognosis, especially if it persists after preload reduction.

In patients with coronary artery disease (Yamamoto et al, 1997) or hypertrophic cardiomyopathy (Nishimura et al, 1996) in whom left ventricle ejection fractions are ≥ 50%, mitral variables correlate poorly with hemodynamics. This may be related to the marked variation in the extent of delayed LV relaxation seen in these patients, which may produce variable transmitral pressure gradients for similar LA pressures. A restrictive filling pattern and LA enlargement in a patient with a normal ejection fraction are associated with a poor prognosis similar to that of a restrictive pattern in dilated cardiomyopathy. This is most commonly seen in restrictive cardiomyopathies, especially amyloidosis (Klein, 1990, 1991) and in heart transplant recipients (Valantine et al, 1989).

3. Pulmonary Venous Flow

3.1 Pulmonary flow assessment

The pulmonary venous flow (PVF) is a very useful tool in the study of LV function (figure 1 C). The arrival of blood to the atrium occurs throughout the cardiac cycle and is highly dependent on the filling conditions. For this reason PVF a useful tool in studying diastolic function and is closely related to the LA pressure and pulmonary capillary pressure (Skagseth et al, 1976). The positive components of pulmonary flow are generated during ventricular systole and early diastole, while the negative cash flow are generated by the contraction of the LA (Rajagopalan et al, 1979). This flow can be obtained by transthoracic

echocardiography, though the records are more accurate by Transesophageal study (Bartzokis et al, 1991).
There are many applications for which the study has found utility of PVF: differentiation between constrictive prericarditis and restrictive cardiomyopathy (Schiavone et al, 1989), the estimation of filling pressures of LV (Kuecherer et al, 1990), the assessment of diastolic function (Klein et al, 1989), the function of the LA and the assessment of mitral insufficiency and stenosis (Castello et al, 1991).

3.1.1 Recording technique

The clearest record of flows is achieved by transesophageal study. Generally, from an angle of 45 to 60 degrees and rotating the probe to the left. From this point appears below the right pulmonary veins and superior. To get the left venous flow probe must be rotated 110 degrees. Transthoracic echo also allows in most cases (90%) the obtaining of PVF (Klein et al, 1994). To achieve an adequate flow, must be placed the sample volume or two centimeters into the vein. Usually, achieved in this way flow pattern consistent in: a first positive wave called S1 wave, which coincides with early ventricular systole, a second systolic wave S2 and diastolic wave D. Then, there is a reverse wave corresponding to atrial contraction wave A (figure 3). In relation to the wave pressure in the left atrium records S1 corresponds to the waves a, c and the decrease x. S2 wave is from the peak decrease x to v. (Klein et al, 1991).

3.1.2 Factors affecting the pulmonary flow

There are numerous physiological circumstances that may affect the PVF. These include: the age, conditions of preload, left ventricular contractility or conduction disturbances and frequency. All these circumstances should be taken into account when assessing appropriate paths. In any case seems to be a direct relationship between the S2 wave and atrial pressure (Hoit et al, 1992). Changes in LV filling and compliance affect D velocity. Ar velocity, and duration are impacted by LV late diastolic pressures, atrial preload, and LA contractility. The S/D ratio and Ar velocities increase with older age, but Ar velocities higher than 35 cm/s suggest increased LV end-diastolic pressure. (Hoit et al, 1992). Volume overload influence LA pressure and is in the ratio S2/D in the presence of a normal live systolic function of the LA. Therefore there is a relationship between atrial contractile reserve and the ratio S2/D. So that, in the absence of left ventricular dysfunction mean atrial pressure can be estimated by the PVF (Hoit et al, 1992).

3.2 Diastolic dysfunction

The PVF is an excellent models proper instrument for differentiating normal filling patterns and pseudo normal (Kuecherer et al, 1990; Appleton et al, 1997) (figure 3). The subjects with diastolic dysfunction slows early ventricular filling while the wave is increased, in these cases increases the ratio S2/D, while extending the deceleration speed of the wave D (Hofmann et al, 1995).
Increased LA pressure normalizes the mitral flow pattern of filling. This phenomenon known as pseudo normalization can be differentiated using the PVF. S2 wave D wave decreases and increases with decreasing the ratio S2/D. At the same time there is an increase in the flow rate back to more than 35 cm /sec (Rakowski et al, 1996). The main difficulty of this method consists in obtaining an adequate record atrial reverse flow.

The restrictive pattern is characterized by increased early filling velocity with rapid deceleration and poor filling late contribution. The PVF in this situation shows a small wave S2 and a D wave, however, very high. Similarly increases atrial reverse flow velocity (Klein et al, 1989).

3.3 Estimation of ventricular filling pressure

PVF can be used to estimate LA pressure (Castello et al., 1995). The mean atrial pressure has a negative correlation with S2 systolic wave, in patients with ventricular dysfunction to reduce the displacement of the ring (Hoit et al., 1992). On the other hand the duration of the reverse wave is correlated with increased LV end-diastolic pressure (Dini et al., 2000). At duration of greater than 30 ms has a high sensitivity and specificity for the detection of atrial pressure greater than 20 mm Hg. (Dini et al., 2000).

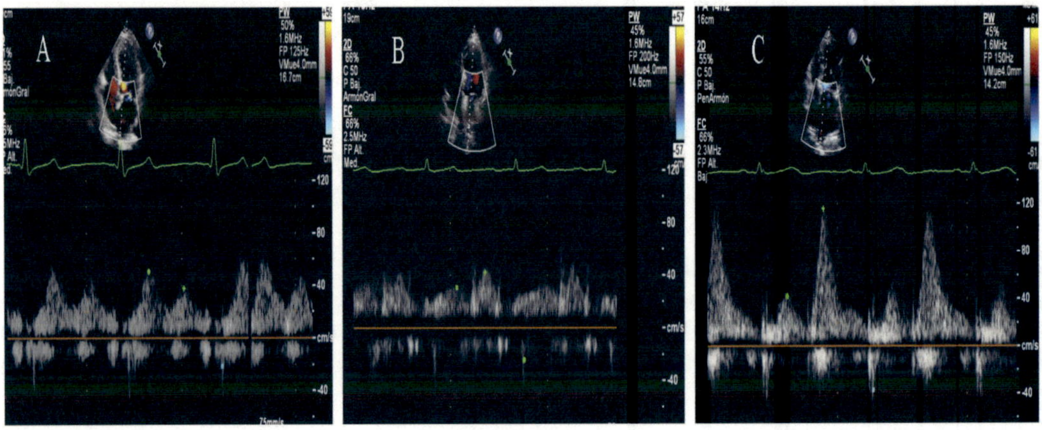

Fig. 3. Pulsed Doppler pulmonary blood flow showing: A) Impaired relaxation pattern, B) Pseudonormal pattern C) Restrictive pattern

4. Color M-mode flow propagation velocity

4.1 Introduction

One of the most important physiologic parameters that allows LV filling at relatively low pressure is the rate of relaxation. This is best defined by the time constant of isovolumic pressure decay (τ, tau). LV relaxation is an important determinant of early transmitral pressure gradients which in turn determine transmitral Doppler filling patterns. The propagation velocity of early flow into the LV cavity measured by color M-mode Doppler was first proposed by Brun (Brun et al., 1992) as an index of LV relaxation (Garcia et al., 1997).

Flow propagation velocity evaluation and interpretation of LV filling in clinical practice is complicated by the multitude of variables that determine intraventricular flow: preload, stroke volume, cardiac output, driving pressure, inertial forces, and viscous friction, but geometry, systolic function, and contractile dyssynchrony play major roles (Nagueh et al., 2009). Taking advantage of this property, color M-mode Doppler indexes have been used for solving the problem of differentiating normal from pseudonormal pulsed Doppler patterns.

4.2 Recording technique

Doppler recordings are obtained in apical four chambers view. We must display the color Doppler sector map of the mitral inflow and make some adjustments to obtain the longest column of color flow from the mitral annulus to the apex. The M-mode scan line is placed through the center of the left ventricular inflow blood column, aligning the cursor in the same direction, from the mitral valve to the left ventricular to the apex. Then the color flow baseline is shifted to lower the Nyquist limit so that the central highest velocity jet is blue. Flow propagation velocity is determined by the slope of the first aliasing line during early filling, from the mitral plane to 4 cm distally into the left ventricle cavity (figure 4). The velocity of the M-mode spectra must be 100 mm/s. Flow propagation velocity (Vp) > 50 cm/s is considered normal (Garcia et al., 1997 ; Nagueh et al., 2009).

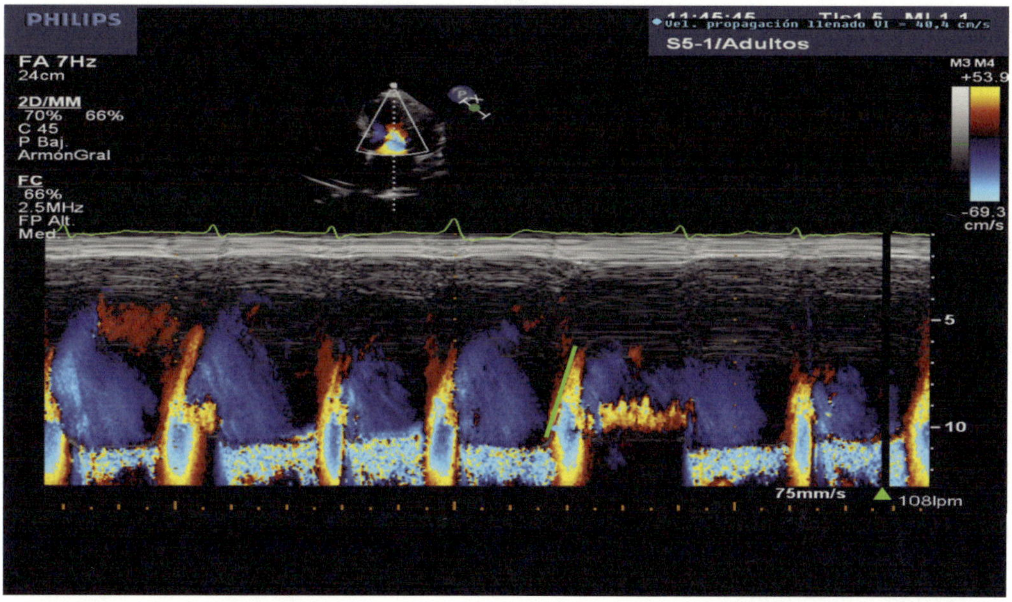

Fig. 4. Color M-mode flow propagation velocity from a patient with depressed ejection fraction and impaired LV relaxation

4.3 Clinical settings

Noninvasive estimation of LV filling pressures is currently utilized using Doppler echocardiography. Flow propagation velocity has been used to solve the problem of differentiating normal from pseudonormal pulsed Doppler patterns and to determine mean pulsed capillary wedge pressure.

It´s known that flow propagation velocity, as assessed by color M-mode Doppler, has a good correlation with the time constant of isovolumic relaxation (τ, tau) and, along with isovolumetric relaxation time, is a key parameter for the prediction of pulmonary wedge pressure and such methods are useful for the estimation of left ventricular filling pressure, both in patients with depressed and preserved systolic function (Gonzalez-Vilchez et al., 1999). In the same way, García (Garcia et al.,1997), based on the relation among peak E wave velocity, tau and LA pressure, have reported a strong correlation between dimensionless, have been confirmed too in patients with atrial fibrillation (Nagueh et al., 1997).

Flow propagation velocity correlates with the rate of myocardial relaxation. However, caution should be with patients with high filling pressures and normal ejection fraction because flow propagation velocity can be increased in these patients, despite impaired relaxation. Flow propagation velocity is inversely related to end systolic volume but directly to ejection fraction, stroke volume, and cardiac output (Rivas-Gotz et al., 2003). Accordingly, it is possible for the flow propagation velocity to fall in the normal range in patients with normal ejection fraction despite the presence of impaired relaxation. In most of patients with depressed ejection fractions exists a lot of signs of impaired diastolic function and measure flow propagation velocity it could be redundant. However, if other Doppler indices appear inconclusive, flow propagation velocity can provide useful information for the prediction of LV filling pressures. Thus $E/Vp \geq 2{,}5$ predicts pulsed capillary wedge pressure >15 mm Hg, with reasonable accuracy in patients with low ejection fraction (Rivas-Gotz et al., 2003). Then, flow propagation velocity is most reliable as an index of LV relaxation in patients with depressed ejection fractions and dilated left ventricles. In the other patient groups, it is preferable to use other indices.

5. Tissue Doppler annular early and late diastolic velocities

5.1 Introduction

Tissue Doppler imaging (TDI) is a ultrasound modality which has become an essential part of the echocardiography evaluation of diastolic function. This technique allows the assessment of the movement and the velocities within the myocardium and the mitral annulus. The velocity of annular motion reflects shortening and lengthening of the myocardial fibers along the longitudinal plane and provides information about segmental and global cardiac function. These data, when coupled with more traditional mitral inflow velocity data can be used to predict diastolic function and LV filling pressures. Normally, three different annular velocities can be recognized as a mirror image of the transmitral inflow pattern: the systolic (S), early diastolic (e´) and late diastolic (a´) velocities (figure 1 B).

5.2 Recording technique

These velocities are obtained from the apical four-chamber view by placing a 2 to 5-mm pulsed Doppler sample volume at the lateral and medial (septal) borders of the mitral annulus, ensuring the coverage of the longitudinal excursion of the mitral annulus in both systole and diastole (Waggoner et al., 2001). For a correct acquisition, angulation between the ultrasound beam and the annular plane of motion should be minimized, and gain and filter settings must be optimized to allow for a clear tissue signal with minimal background noise. Although annular velocities can also be obtained by color-coded tissue Doppler image (TDI), this method is not recommended, because there is a paucity of studies and the validation studies were performed using pulsed wave Doppler.

Occasionally, an additional mid-diastolic flow velocity can be recorded by tissue Doppler imaging demonstrating a mid-diastolic component (L´), resulting in triphasic mitral inflow filling pattern, it suggests advanced diastolic dysfunction (Jong-Won Ha et al., 2006).

For the assessment of global LV diastolic function, it is recommended to acquire and measure tissue Doppler signals at the septal and lateral sides of the mitral annulus and their average, given the influence of regional function on these velocities and time intervals (Rivas-Gotz et al., 2003).

5.3 Clinical settings

Several studies in animals and humans have demonstrated significant correlation between e´ and the LV relaxation so its value is a good indicator of the cardiac function. Usually, e´ from the lateral annulus is higher than a´ so different cut off values, should be applied. A value ≥ 10 cm/s (septal) or ≥ 15 cm/s (lateral) are consistent with normal function. The e´ velocity is determined by LV relaxation, preload, systolic function and LV pressure whereas the main hemodynamic determinants of the a´ velocity are left atrial systolic function and LV end-diastolic pressure. The early diastolic velocity (e´) decreases progressively with age and also is reduced in patients with other conditions leading to an impaired relaxation such as LVH or restrictive cardiomyopathy, where e´ decreases as LV filling pressure increases (Ommen et al., 2000). This velocity is essential for classifying the diastolic filling pattern (Figure 5) and estimating filling pressures and furthermore, it is useful to distinguish between constrictive pericarditis and other forms of diastolic dysfunction. In constrictive pericarditis, the impairment in ventricular filling occurs as a result of an external constriction, whereas in restrictive cardiomyopathy there is an inherent abnormality in ventricular relaxation. Therefore, e´ will be normal or even above normal in patients with pure constrictive pericarditis as compared to those with restriction where e´ will be lower.

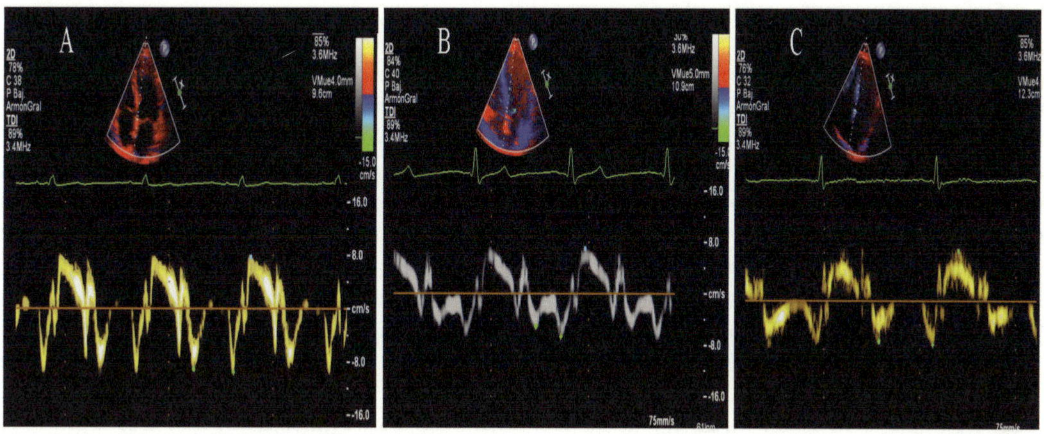

Fig. 5. Doppler tissue imaging of mitral annular motion: A) Impaired relaxation pattern, B) Pseudonormal pattern C) Restrictive pattern

In addition and interestingly, it should be noted that TDI mitral annular velocities are considered less load-dependent than other conventional Doppler parameters (Dae-Won Sohn et al., 1997). For this reason, its assessment appears to be useful to correct the effect of LV relaxation on mitral inflow E velocity in patients with cardiac disease, especially in the detecting a pseudonormalization pattern of mitral inflow. In these cases, the annular e´/a´ ratio and the mitral E velocity to TDI Doppler e´ (E/e´ ratio) can predict LV filling pressures and correlates well with pulmonary capillary wedge pressure (Rivas-Gotzet al., 2003; Ommen et al., 2000) (figure 5 B). For the diagnosis of diastolic dysfunction, the E/e´ ratio has been identified as the best parameter for diagnosis when compared to other Doppler measures (Nagueh et al., 2009; Kasner et al., 2007). This ratio is also clinically very useful in patients with atrial fibrillation where a´ is not present.

An E/e´ ratio < 8 is associated with normal filling pressures and a ratio > 15 is associated with increased filling pressures (Ommen et al., 2000). When values are between 8 and 15, other echocardiography indices should be used and it is recommended that e´ and the E/e´ ratio should not be used as the sole data in drawing conclusions about LV diastolic function. TDI derived velocities also have some limitations. There are some conditions where this E/e´ ratio is not accurate to estimate the LV filling pressures: in normal patients e´ is directly related to preload (Firstenberg et al., 2000), so this index may not provide a reliable information, patients with localized disease process, such as lateral myocardial infarction or patients with mitral valve disease and heavy lateral annular calcification can result in mitral annulus velocities being lower at the lateral annulus than at the septal annulus, patients with constrictive pericarditis have an inverse relationship between E/e´ and with pulmonary capillary wedge pressure (Garcia et al., 1997) additionally, e´ velocity can be increased in patients with moderate to severe mitral regurgitation due to increased flow.
To summarize, Tissue Doppler imaging provides accurate and valuable information and should be included as part of an echocardiography study when studying myocardial diastolic function.

6. Deformation measurements

6.1 Deformation measurements assessment

Doppler tissue (DT) and speckle tracking echocardiography (STE) has been introduced as quantitative method for measuring systolic and diastolic function. DT can measure myocardial functional parameters such as speed, acceleration, displacement, velocity of myocardial deformation and deformation. The STE can measure the twist of the LV.
Strain means deformation and can be calculated using different formulas. In clinical cardiology, strain is most often expressed as a percentage or fractional strain (Lagrangian strain). Systolic strain represents percentage shortening when measurements are done in the long axis and percentage radial thickening in the short axis. Systolic strain rate (SR) represents the rate or speed of myocardial shortening or thickening, respectively. Myocardial strain and SR are excellent parameters for the quantification of regional and global contractility and may also provide important information in the evaluation of diastolic function. Until recently, the only clinical method to measure myocardial strain has been magnetic resonance imaging with tissue tagging, but complexity and cost limit this methodology to research protocols.
The longitudinal motion of the heart shows a descent of the base toward the apex during systole, with a reverse movement during the phases of early filling (E) and atrial systole (A), whereas the apex remains virtually stationary throughout the heart cycle. Both longitudinal M-mode and Doppler tissue imaging (DTI) of the mitral annulus have demonstrated this. (Rodriguez et al., 1996). Thus the velocities increase from zero at the apex to a maximum at the base of the ventricle for all phases, with a longitudinal velocity gradient. It can be shown that the longitudinal velocity gradient is a measure of the rate of longitudinal deformation, or SR. (Støylen et al., 1999). The unit of SR is centimeters per second per centimeter, or s^{-1}, and the values of SR can be displayed in the same manner as velocities: as color mapping or digital curves, as shown in figure 6. This method is termed strain rate imaging (SRI). In SRI, velocities are converted to regional velocity differences, showing regional systolic and diastolic dysfunction in coronary disease and also temporal distribution of deformation in normal ventricles. The velocities caused by contraction of more apical segments or by

translation of the whole heart are subtracted. SRI provides quantitative measurement of local deformation rates, whereas color mapping provides semiquantitative data and information about the spatial-temporal relations between events in the ventricle during the heart cycle.

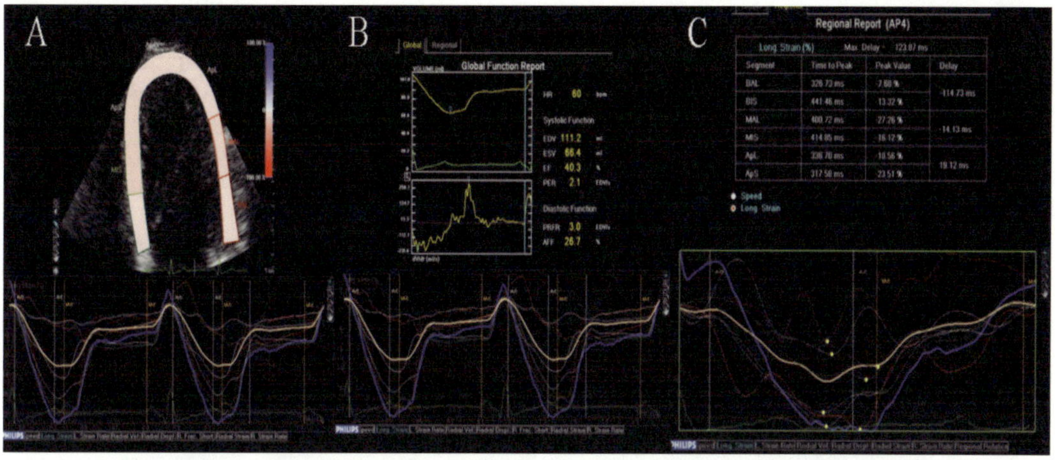

Fig. 6. Digital curves of strain rate (A), global function (B), regional function (C)

Lengthening during isovolumic relaxation generally is seen first in the midwall, and at the same time, reciprocal shortening is seen in neighboring segments, whereas stretching starts later in the apex. M mode or DTI of the mitral ring can demonstrate a slight lengthening of the whole ventricle during this phase, mainly in the basal parts. In addition, SRI is subject to misinterpretation as a result of angle deviation (Støylen et al., 2000) and this effect is especially pronounced in the apex.

The peak velocity of the mitral annulus is determined not only by the rate of deformation (the local strain rate), but also by the propagation of the stretch wave. DTI and tissue Doppler-derived measurements are sensitive measures of diastolic function. Strain rate imaging shows a complex pattern of deformation during diastole because of its high sampling frequency, compared with all other methods, including MR. The main deformations during early and late filling phases are the result of both local relaxation rate and the propagation of the stretching wave from base to apex. This provides new physiologic and pathophysiologic information. The present application, however, seems to overestimate true peak strain rate. In contrast to regional systolic function, the DTI measurements are quicker and may be more practical for clinical work, whereas the level of detail in SRI data enables deeper insight into diastolic physiology. (Courtois et al., 1990).

SRI shows the ventricular deformation during early filling to be a dynamic event that is slowed in subjects with delayed relaxation. The strain rate propagation is the main determinant of the filling rate, and is consistent with filling time.

6.2 Recording technique

Tissue Doppler-based myocardial strain has been introduced as a bedside clinical method and has undergone comprehensive evaluation for the assessment of regional systolic function (Heimdal et al., 1998). Myocardial motion in DT (Figure 7) is shown as color-coded speeds along a series of ultrasound scan lines within a 2D sector. The frequency of pictures for DT must be 80 to 200 frames per second, depending on the width of the ultrasound sector, and is usually set higher than for the simultaneous images in grayscale. Myocardial velocities are decoded into numerical values that can be stored digitally for "off-line" analysis. By convention, since the flat apical long-axis motion is dominated by red-coded velocities during systole and diastole in blue. Dysfunctional myocardium, however, may show abnormal movements with reversed velocities during systole. Myocardial function is rarely assessed 2D color but postprocessing can be done with mode M, but the usual method is the analysis of rates from multiple regions within a 2D image. Tissue velocities can be assessed, integrated tissue displacement or velocity, SR and myocardial SR integrated. Limitations are noise signal, angle dependence and the reverberations.

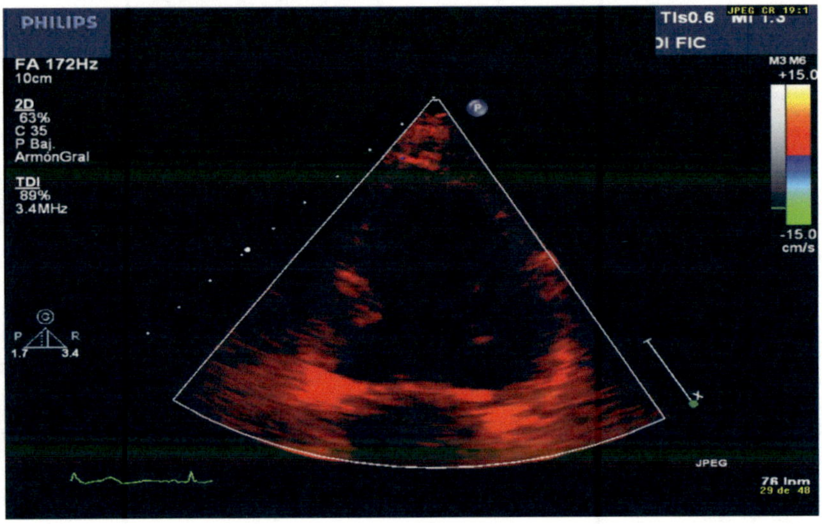

Fig. 7. Myocardial motion in DT shown as color-coded speeds of ultrasound scan lines within a 2D sector

Strain may also be measured by 2D STE, an emerging technology that measures strain by tracking speckles in grayscale echocardiography images of the LV, obtained in the apical 2, 3-and 4-chamber views and short-axis basal, mid, apical-ventricular views. The LV radial and circumferential functions must be determined in the short-axis views (figure 8) and longitudinal function in the 3 apical views (figure 6) using grey-scale acquisition at a frame rate over 80 s^{-1} (Amundsen et al., 2006). The glare is created by interference of ultrasound beams in the myocardium and are observed in B-mode images in gray scale, functioning as natural acoustic markers can be tracked in their motion frame by frame, measuring the distance automatically between shine on a piece defined myocardial deformation, independently of myocardial insonation angle and translational heart. In contrast with strain DT-based, STE can measure the deformation of the LV short-axis circumferential, radial and longitudinal multiple segments in areas near the apex. Another promising feature is the ability to measure the rotation and twisting of the LV. This is in contrast to tissue Doppler–based strain, which is very sensitive to misalignment between the cardiac axis and the ultrasound beam. Problems with tissue Doppler–based strain include significant signal noise and signal drifting. STE is limited by relatively lower frame rates.

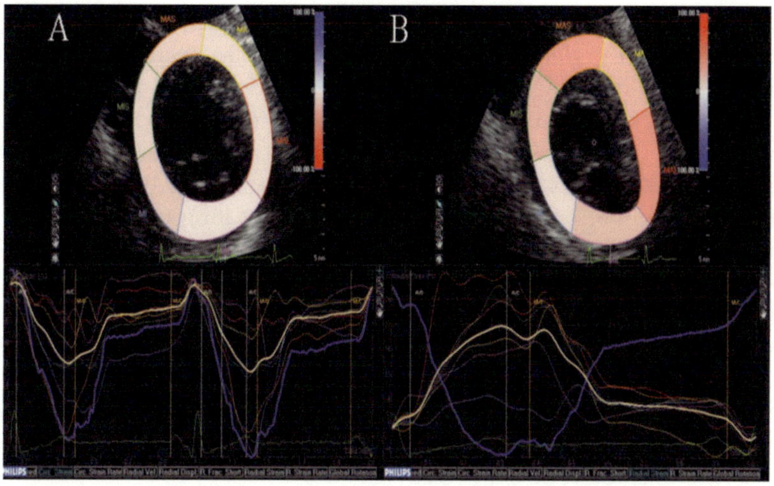

Fig. 8. Strain measured by 2D speckle-tracking echocardiography. The LV circumferential (A) and radial (B) functions shown as digital curves in the short-axis views

Similarly, regional Recommendations for the Evaluation of Left Ventricular Diastolic Function by Echocardiography differences in the timing of transition from myocardial contraction to relaxation, with SRI can identify ischemic segments. (McMahon et al.,2004). Currently, Doppler flow velocity and myocardial velocity imaging are the preferred initial echocardiography methodologies for assessing LV diastolic function.

6.3 Clinical settings

Analysis of diastolic function for assessment of myocardial viability has been evaluated (Hoffmann et al., 2005). SR analysis allows quantitative segmental analysis of myocardial function and has been used during dobutamine stimulation for assessment of systolic functional reserve and related to F18-fluorodeoxyglucose positron emission tomography. Early and late diastolic function during dobutamine stimulation is impaired for nonviable segments compared with viable segments. Diastolic SR analysis during dobutamine stimulation may be added to systolic function analysis in the assessment of myocardial viability.

STE may be helpful for the detection of early changes in LV diastolic function in patients with essential hypertension. Hypertensive patients had a lower mean relaxation based on SRE and SRE/A at the basal, mid, and apical regions, with the basal parts appearing more compromised and with higher segmental diastolic dysfunction compared with controls. Abnormal segmental relaxation might also be present in individuals with 'normal' mitral annular early diastolic velocities (Pavlopoulos & Nihoyannopoulos, 2009).

Myocardial shortening after aortic valve closure, i.e. PSS (Post-systolic shortening), has been suggested as a sensitive marker of regional myocardial dysfunction (Voigt et al., 2003). However, PSS may also occur in healthy subjects. To discriminate between pathological and physiological PSS, Voigt et al. (Voigt et al., 2003) described that the timing and the magnitude are different between these two situations. In this study PSS was significantly larger and reduced in diabetic patients compared with control subjects. The precise mechanism is unknown, but not related to myocardial ischemia induced by epicardial coronary artery stenosis, thus they described the first signs of systolic dysfunction following established diastolic dysfunction in diabetic patients. This study reinforces that LVEF is not a sensitive indicator for the detection of subclinical systolic dysfunction. 2D STE has the potential for detecting subclinical LV systolic dysfunction, and it might provide useful information for the risk stratification of an asymptomatic diabetic population.

Diastolic dysfunction in diabetic patients can be also assessed with more novel echocardiography techniques such as STE. Despite a normal LV mass, LV volume, and LVEF, the diabetic population show impairment of LV longitudinal strain and SR but preserve circumferential and radial strain and SR. Using 2D STE to assess all myocardial segments it has been demonstrated a reduced longitudinal strain and SR (predominantly derived form epicardial/endocardial fiber contraction) but preserved circumferential and radial strain and SR (predominantly derived from mid-wall circumferential fibers contraction) in diabetic patients. This finding suggests that myocardial dysfunction in early diabetic cardiomyopathy might start in the subendocardium (Arnold et al., 2009). The novel aspect of the present study was the multidirectional strain and SR analysis using 2D STE in patients with uncomplicated type 2 diabetes mellitus.

In other study Shanks M and cols. examined the prognostic value of novel diastolic indexes in ST-elevation acute myocardial infarction (AMI), derived from strain and SR analysis using 2-dimensional STE and only mean SRIVR was an independent predictor of outcome in patients with AMI. This could be in part because SR measured during the isovolumic relaxation period (before mitral valve opens) reflects the rate of myocardial expansion that is least influenced by LV loading conditions (Shanks et al., 2010).

7. Left ventricuar untwisting

7.1 Introduction

2-D STE has been successfully applied to the relatively simple and accurate measurement of LV torsion during systole and untwisting at early diastole. In addition, LV untwisting is commonly seen at the LA contraction, whereas its determinants and clinical significance have not been clarified. Both parameters may provide an additional noninvasive insight into LV systolic and diastolic function (Buchalter et al., 1990). Given the angle independence of speckle tracking and its higher reproducibility, this technique is preferred for measuring rotation. LV twist is calculated as the difference between basal and apical rotation.

LV twisting motion (torsion) is due to contraction of obliquely oriented fibers in the subepicardium, which course toward the apex in a counterclockwise spiral. The moments of the subepicardial fibers dominate over the subendocardial fibers, which form a spiral in opposite direction. Therefore, when viewed from apex toward the base, the LV apex shows systolic counterclockwise rotation and the LV base shows a net clockwise rotation. Untwisting starts in late systole but mostly occurs during the isovolumetric relaxation period and is largely finished at the time of mitral valve opening. Diastolic untwist represents elastic recoil due to the release of restoring forces that have been generated during the preceding systole. LV twist appears to play an important role for normal systolic function, and diastolic untwisting contributes to LV filling through suction generation. It has been assumed that the reduction in LV untwisting with attenuation or loss of diastolic suction contributes to diastolic dysfunction in diseased hearts. (Bell et al., 2000). Diastolic dysfunction associated with normal aging, however, does not appear to be due to a reduction in diastolic untwist. (Hees et al., 2004).

7.2 Recording technique

With the recent introduction of STE, it is feasible to quantify LV rotation, twist, untwist clinically. Wang et al (Wang et al., 2007) demonstrated that, in patients with diastolic dysfunction, the LV torsion and peak untwisting rate are preserved, as opposed to patients with systolic dysfunction in which the measurements are reduced. Thus, the assessment of torsional recoil, or untwisting, should provide an accurate estimate of LV relaxation. Stuber et al (Stuber et al., 1999) found that early diastolic untwisting and untwisting rates were significantly reduced in parallel to the degree of LVH in hypertensive patients.

7.3 Clinical settings

In the present study (Appleton et al., 1988), was identified that the late diastolic LV untwisting rate is related to peak A velocity of the transmitral flow, E/e, and LA volume index in patients with cardiovascular risk factors and mild to moderate LV diastolic dysfunction (E/A <1). In addition, multivariate equation for predicting late diastolic untwisting was highest for LA volume index. This provide the correlation between LV untwisting during LA contraction and LA size, suggesting "disease history" in patients with LV diastolic dysfunction.

Measurements of LV twist and untwisting rate, although not currently recommended for routine clinical use and although additional studies are needed to define their potential clinical application, may become an important element of diastolic function evaluation in the future.

8. Future directions

Diastolic strain rate

Myocardial strain and SR are excellent parameters for the quantification of regional contractility and may also provide important information in the evaluation of diastolic function (Nagueh et al., 2009). Signal noise, signal drifting and angel dependency are included in the potential problems of tissue Doppler derived strain and SRI.

The speckles function as natural acoustic markers that can be obtained simultaneously from multiple regions within an image plane (Nagueh et al., 2009). It has a number of advantages over established methods. It is acquired directly from LV myocardium, as opposed to indirect data of annulus and blood flow velocities. It is not affected by mitral annulus or valvular disease. It occurs during IVRT when valves are closed and therefore is not exposed to transmitral pressure gradient. It is derived from all myocardial segments and thus is a true global index. It is not affected by translation and tethering and takes into consideration the initial resting length (Wang & Nagueh, 2009). It is demonstrated that in patients with diastolic dysfunction, the LV torsion and peak untwisting rate are preserved, as opposed to patients with systolic dysfunction in which the measurements are reduced (Wang et al., 2007). STE also allows for appreciation of accentuated regional myocardial rotation, torsion and twist during positive inotropic stimulation with dobutamine or during ischemia (Helle-Valle et al., 2005). Assessment of post-systolic strain and early diastolic untwist by echocardiography provides important insights into mechanisms of diastolic function.

Limitation of this technique include the dependence on 2D image quality and frame rates, difficulty of selection of image plane, and the reproducibility and variability of measurements from ventricles with different geometries. It also includes the longer time needed for analysis and the lower frame rate (80 per second) which can lead to an underestimation of peak SR, although the concept itself is not affected by this limitation.

The development of 3D speckle tracking may assist with these limitations. The newly developed 3D-STE imaging used with real-time 3D echocardiography data sets has the potential to avoid the limitations of 2D-STE imaging in the assessment of LV wall motion, because it tracks the motion of speckles within the scan volume, regardless of the direction of motion (Maffessanti et al., 2009). 3D-STE shows more homogenous color distribution in normal ventricles, consistent with the expected normal patterns of LV wall motion, compared to 2D-STE in the same subject. The regional time curves allow better quantitative discrimination between normal and abnormal segments. In segments with normal wall motion, 3D-STE demonstrates a larger magnitude of displacement, likely reflecting the ability to register all 3 components of the motion vector compared to the 2D-STE single-plane analysis. The relatively smaller normal variability of measurements using 3D-STE compared with those using 2D-STE provide additional support to the superiority of 3D-STE in imaging the complexity of 3D wall motion. The limitations of the 3D-STE technique are the relatively low temporal and spatial resolution, both affecting the accuracy of endocardial tracking in a considerable proportion of the segments.

Left ventricular twisting and untwisting

The clinical value of assessing LV untwisting rate is not defined. When LV twist and untwisting rate were assessed in patients with diastolic dysfunction or diastolic heart failure, both twist and untwisting rate were preserved, and no significant relation was noted with the time constant of LV relaxation. The complex interplay between preload, afterload and contractility determines twist values in diastolic heart failure (DHF).

In patients with LVH, Takeuchi et al (Takeuchi et al., 2007) showed a normal LV torsion, without intergroup differences based on its extent. In another study (Park et al., 2008), observed that LV twist was increase in patients with early diastolic dysfunction and normal in patients with advanced grades. The independent predictors of LVEF in DHF patients were circumferential strain and LV twist, and it is possible that normal twist is a compensatory mechanism in DHF that can help maintain a normal LVEF (Wang et al., 2008). The limitation of this technique is the selection of the image plane, and further clinical testing of STE in patients is needed to determine whether reproducible measurements can be obtained from ventricles with different geometries. STE can be suboptimal at the LV base, showed in the significant variability in the measurements.

Left atrial volume measurements

LA volume index is a more robust marker than LA area or LA diameter, in patients with suspected heart failure and normal LVEF. For these reasons, in a recent consensus document LA volume index >40 ml/m2 is considered to provide sufficient evidence of diastolic LV dysfunction when the E/e' ration is non-conclusive or when plasma levels of natriuretic peptides are elevated (Paulus et al., 2007); and a LA volume index <29 ml/m2 is proposed as a prerequisite to exclude heart failure with normal LVEF.

In another study (Park et al., 2011) evaluated the LA volume index (LAVi) over late diastolic mitral annulus velocity (A') ratio (LAVi/A') as a useful parameter to identify advance diastolic dysfunction and predict clinical outcomes in patients with dyspnea. They showed that LAVi/A' is a useful new echo index to discriminate advanced diastolic dysfunction in dyspneic patients with a wide range of LVEF. They also added that this ratio has the additional benefit in the assessment of the gray zone diastolic dysfunction with 8≤ E/e'≤15, concluding that a LAVi/A'≥4.0 was an independent predictor of clinical outcomes.

Diastolic stress test

During exercise, to maintain adequate LV filling and stroke volume, the filling pressures raise provoking symptoms to patients with diastolic dysfunction. Therefore, it is useful to evaluate LV filling pressure with exercise. The E/e' ratio has been applied for that objective. E and e' velocities increase proportionally in subjects with normal myocardial relaxation, and the E/e' ratio remains unchanged or is reduced (Ha et al., 2003). In patients with impaired myocardial relaxation, however, the increase in e' with exercise is lower than that of mitral E velocity, such that the E/e' ration increases (Ha et al., 2005). Furthermore, mitral DT decreases slightly in normal individuals with exercise, but shortens >50 ms in patients with a marked elevation of filling pressures. Mitral E velocity increases with exertion and, after the termination of exercise, stays increased for a few minutes, in cardiac patients. In these patients, at baseline, exercise, and recovery, e' velocity remains reduced. Therefore, E and e' velocities can be recorded after exercise. Exercise is usually performed using a supine bicycle protocol or with dobutamine infusion (Duncan et al., 2005).

This test is most useful in patients with unexplained exertional dyspnea who have mild diastolic dysfunction and normal filling pressures at rest. However, the potential limitations in patients with mitral valve disease, atrial fibrillation and regional LV dysfunction, and the lack of clinical data, diminish recommendations for its routine clinical use.

9. References

Arnold C.T., Delgado V, Bertini M, Rutger W, Rijzewijk L, Shanks M, Nucifora G, Smit J, Diamant M, Romijn J, Roos A, Leung D, Lamb H, Bax J. Findings from Left Ventricular Strain and Strain Rate Imaging in Asymptomatic Patients With Type 2 Diabetes Mellitus *Am J Cardiol* 2009;104: 1398–1401. ISSN 0002-9149.

Amundsen BH, Helle-Valle T, Edvardsen T, Torp H, Crosby J, Lyseggen E et al. Noninvasive myocardial strain measurement by speckle tracking echocardiography: validation against sonomicrometry and tagged magnetic resonance imaging. *J Am Coll Cardiol* 2006; 47:789–93. ISSN 0735-1097.

Appleton CP, Jensen JL, Hatle LK & Oh JK. Doppler evaluation of left and right ventricular diastolic function a technical guide for obtaining optimal flow velocities recordings. *J Am Soc Echocardiogr* 1997; 10 : 271-292. ISSN: 0894-7317.

Appleton CP, Hatle LK & Popp RL.Relation of transmitral flow velocity patterns to left ventricular diastolic function: new insights from a combined hemodynamic and Doppler echocardiographic study.*J Am Coll Cardiol* 1988; 12:426–40. ISSN 0735-1097.

Bartzokis T, Lee R, Yeoh TK, Grogin H, Schnittger I. Transesophageal echo-Doppler echocardiographic assessment of pulmonary venous flow patterns. *J Am Soc Echocardiogr* 1991; 4:457–64. ISSN: 0894-7317.

Bell SP, Nyland L, Tischler MD, McNabb M, Granzier H, LeWinter M.Alterations in the determinants of diastolic suction during pacing tachycardia. *Circ Res 2000*; 87:235-40. ISSN: 00097330.

Brun P. Left ventricular flow propagation during early filling is related to wall relaxation: a color M-mode Doppler analysis.*J Am Coll Cardiol*.1992;20: 420-432.ISSN:0735-1097.

Buchalter MB, Weiss JL, Rogers WJ, Zerhouni EA, Weisfeldt ML, Beyar R, Shapiro EP. Noninvasive quantification of left ventricular rotational deformation in normal humans using magnetic resonance imaging myocardial tagging. *Circulation* 1990;81:1236—44. ISSN 0009-7322.

Castello R, Pearson AC, Lenzen P, Labovitz AJ. Effect of mitral regurgitation on pulmonary venous velocities derived from transesophageal echocardiography color guided pulsed Doppler imaging. *J Am Coll Cardiol* 1991; 17:1499–506.ISSN: 0735-1097.

Castello R, Vaughn M, Dressler FA, et al. Relation between pulmonary venous flow and pulmonary wedge pressure: influence of cardiac output. *Am Heart J* 1995; 130:127–34. ISSN: 0002-8703.

Courtois M, Kovacs SJ Jr, Ludbrook PA. Physiological early diastolic intraventricular pressure gradient is lost during acute myocardial ischemia. *Circulation* 1990; 81:1688–96. ISSN 0009-7322.

Dae-Won Sohn, In-Ho Chai, Dong-Jum Lee, Hee-Chan Kim et al.Assessment of Mitral annulus velocity by Doppler Tissue Imaging in the evaluation of the left ventricular diastolic function. *J Am Coll Cardiol* 1997;30 :470-80. ISSN: 0735-1097.

Duncan, A.M., Lim, E., Gibson, D.G. and Henein, M.Y. Effect of dobutamine stress on left ventricular filling in ischemic dilated cardiomyopathy: pathophysiology and prognostic implications. *J Am Coll Cardiol.* 2005; 46: 488-96. ISSN 0735-1097.

Firstenberg MS, Levine BD, Garcia MJ, Greenberg NL, Cardon L, Morehead AJ et al. Relationship of echocardiographic indices to pulmonary capillary wedge pressures in healthy volunteers. *J Am Coll Cardiol* 2000; 36:1664–9. ISSN: 0735-1097.

Garcia MJ, Ares MA, Asher C et al. An index of early left ventricular filling that combined with pulsed Doppler peak E velocity may estimate capillary wedge pressure. *J Am Coll Cardiol* 1997; 29:448. ISSN: 0735-1097.

Gonzalez-Vilchez F. Combined use of pulsed and color M-mode Doppler echocardiography for the estimation of pulmonary capillary wedge pressure: an empirical approach based on an analytical relation. *J Am Coll Cardiol.* 1999; 34: 515-523. ISSN: 0735-1097.

Ha, J.W., Lulic, F., Bailey, K.R., Pellikka, P.A., Seward, J.B., Tajik, A.J., et al. Effects of treadmill exercise on mitral inflow and annular velocities in healthy adults. *Am J Cardiol.* 2003; 91: 114-5. ISSN 0002-9149.

Ha, J.W., Oh, J.K., Pellikka, P.A., Ommen, S.R., Stussy, V.L., Bailey, K.R., et al. Diastolic stress echocardiography: a novel noninvasive diagnostic test for diastolic dysfunction using supine bicycle exercise Doppler echocardiography. *J Am Soc Echocardiogr.* 2005; 18: 63-8. ISSN: 0894-7317.

Hees PS, Fleg JL, Dong SJ, Shapiro EP. MRI and echocardiographic assessment of the diastolic dysfunction of normal aging: altered LV pressure decline or load?. *Am J Physiol Heart Circ Physiol* 2004; 286: H782–8. ISSN: 0363-6135.

Helle-Valle, T., Crosby, J., Edvardsen, T., Lyseggen, E., Amundsen, B.H., Smith, H.J., et al. New noninvasive method for assessment of left ventricular rotation: speckle tracking echocardiography. *Circulation.* 2005; 112: 3149-56. ISSN 0009-7322.

Heimdal A, Stoylen A, Torp H, Skjaerpe T. Real-time strain rate imaging of the left ventricle by ultrasound. *J Am Soc Echocardiogr* 1998; 11: 1013–9. ISSN: 0894-7317.

Hoffmann T, Keck A, van Ingen G, Simic O, Ostermeyer J, Meinertz T. Simultaneous measurement of pulmonary venous flow by intravascular catheter Doppler velocimetry and transesophageal Doppler echocardiography: relation to left atrial pressure and left atrial and left ventricular function. *J Am Coll Cardiol* 1995; 26:239-49. ISSN: 0735-1097.

Hoffmann R, Altiok E, Nowak B, Kühl H, Kaiser HJ, Buell U, Hanrath P. Strain rate analysis allows detection of differences in diastolic function between viable and nonviable myocardial segments. *J Am Soc Echocardiogr* 2005;18:330-5. ISSN: 0894-7317.

Hoit BD, Shao Y, Gabel M, Walsh RA. Influence of loading conditions and contractile state on pulmonary venous flow: validation of Doppler velocimetry. *Circulation* 1992 ;86:651–9. ISSN 0009-7322.

Jong-Won Ha, Jeong-Ah Ahn, Jae-Yun Moon et al. Triphasic mitral inflow velocity with mid-diastolic flow: The presence of mid-diastolic mitral annular velocity indicates advanced diastolic dysfunction. *Eur J Echocardiography* 2006; 7: 16-21. ISSN: 1525-2167.

Kasner M, Westermann D, Steendijk P et al. Utility of Doppler echocardiography and tissue fraction: a comparative Doppler conductance catheterization study. *Circulation* 2007; 116:637. ISSN 0009-7322.

Klein AL, Hatle LK, Burstow DJ, et al. Doppler characterization of left ventricular diastolic function in cardiac amyloidosis.*J Am Coll Cardiol* 1989;13:1017–26.ISSN: 0735-1097.

Klein AL, Hatle LK, Taliercio CP, Taylor CL, Kyle RA, Bailey KR et al. Serial Doppler echocardiographic follow-up of left ventricular diastolic function in cardiac amyloidosis. *J Am Coll Cardiol* 1990; 16:1135–41. ISSN 0735-1097.

Klein AL, Tajik AJ. Doppler assessment of pulmonary venous flow in healthy subjects and in patients with heart disease.*JAmSocEchocardiogr* 1991; 4:379–92. ISSN: 0894-7317.

Klein AL, Burstow DJ, Tajik AJ, Zachariah PK, Bailey KR, Seward JB. Effects of age on left ventricular dimensions and filling dynamics in 117 normal persons. *Mayo Clin Proc* 1994; 69:212–24. ISSN: 0025-6196.

Kuecherer HF, Muhiudeen IA, Kusumoto FM, et al. Estimation of mean left atrial pressure from transesophageal pulsed Doppler echocardiography of pulmonary venous flow. *Circulation* 1990; 82:1127–39. ISSN 0009-7322.

Maniu CV, Nishimura RA & Tajik AJ. Tachycardia during the Valsalva maneuver: a sign of normal diastolic filling pressures. *J Am Soc Echocardiogr* 2004 Jun;17(6):634-7. ISSN: 0894-7317.

McMahon CJ, Nagueh SF, Pignatelli RH, Denfield SW, Dreyer WJ, Price JF et al. Characterization of left ventricular diastolic function by tissue Doppler imaging and clinical status in children with hypertrophic cardiomyopathy. *Circulation* 2004;109: 1756–62. ISSN 0009-7322.

Maffessanti, F., Nesser, H.J., Weinert, L., Steringer-Mascherbauer, R., Niel, J., Gorissen, W., et al. Quantitative evaluation of regional left ventricular function using three-dimensional speckle tracking echocardiography in patients with and without heart disease. *Am J Cardiol.* 2009; 104: 1755-62. ISSN 0002-9149.

Murphy, J. et al, *Mayo Clinic Cardiology: Concise Textbook*, 2006, Third Edition, Informer Healthcare, 0849390575, USA.

Nagueh S. Doppler tissue imaging: a noninvasive technique for evaluation of left ventricular relaxation and estimation of filling pressures. *J Am Coll Cardiol.* 1997; 30: 1527-1533. ISSN: 0735-1097.

Nagueh, S.F., Appleton, C.P., Gillebert, T.C., Marino, P.N., Oh, J.K., Smiseth, O.A., et al. Recommendations for the evaluation of left ventricular diastolic function by echocardiography. *Eur J Echocardiogr.* 2009; 10: 165-9 ISSN: 1525-2167.

Nishimura RA, Appleton CP, Redfield MM, Ilstrup DM, Holmes DR Jr & Tajik AJ. Noninvasive Doppler echocardiographic evaluation of left ventricular filling pressures in patients with cardiomyopathies: a simultaneous Doppler echocardiographic and cardiac catheterization study. *J Am Coll Cardiol* 1996; 28: 1226–33. ISNN 0735-1097.

Oh JK, Hatle LK, Seward JB et al. Diagnostic role of Doppler echocardiography in constrictive pericarditis. *J Am Coll Cardiol* 1994 ; 23 : 154-162. ISSN 0735-1097.

Oh JK, Appleton CP, Hatle LK, Nishimura RA, Seward JB & Tajik AJ. The noninvasive assesment of left ventricular diastolic function with two-dimensional and doppler echocardiography. *J Am Soc Echocardiogr* 1997 ; 10 : 246-70. ISSN: 0894-7317.

Oh, J. et al, *The Echo Manual*, October 2006, 3rd Edition, Lippincott Williams & Wilkins, 0781748534, USA.

Ohno M, Cheng CP & Little WC. Mechanism of altered patterns of left ventricular filling during the development of congestive heart failure. *Circulation 1994*; 89: 2241–50. ISSN 0009-7322.

Ommen SR, Nishimura RA, Appleton CP et al. Clinical utility of Doppler echocardiography and tissue Doppler imaging in the estimation of left ventricular filling pressures: A comparative simultaneous Doppler-catheterization study. *Circulation* 2000;102:1788. ISSN 0009-7322.

Park, S.J., Miyazaki, C., Bruce, C.J., Ommen, S., Miller, F.A. and Oh, J.K. Left ventricular torsion by two-dimensional speckle tracking echocardiography in patients with diastolic dysfunction and normal ejection fraction. *J Am Soc Echocardiogr.* 2008; 21: 1129-37. ISSN: 0894-7317.

Park, H.J., Jung, H.O., Min, J., Park, M.W., Park, C.S., Shin, D.I., et al. Left Atrial Volume Index Over Late Diastolic Mitral Annulus Velocity (LAVi/A') Is a Useful Echo Index to Identify Advanced Diastolic Dysfunction and Predict Clinical Outcomes. *Clin Cardiol.* 2011; 34: 124-30. ISSN: 1205-6626.

Paulus, W.J., Tschope, C., Sanderson, J.E., Rusconi, C., Flachskampf, F.A., Rademakers, F.E., et al. How to diagnose diastolic heart failure: a consensus statement on the diagnosis of heart failure with normal left ventricular ejection fraction by the Heart Failure and Echocardiography Associations of the European Society of Cardiology. *Eur Heart J.* 2007; 28: 2539-50. ISSN 0195-668x.

Pavlopoulos H & Nihoyannopoulos P. Regional left ventricular distribution of abnormal segmental relaxation evaluated by strain echocardiography and the incremental value over annular diastolic velocities in hypertensive patients with normal global diastolic function. *European Journal of Echocardiography* 2009; 10: 654–662. ISSN: 1525-2167.

Rajagopalan B, Friend JA, Stallard T, Lee GD. Blood flow in pulmonary veins. I. Studies in dog and man. *Cardiovasc Res* 1979;13: 667–76. ISSN: 0008-6371.

Rakowski H, Appleton CP, Chan KL, et al. Canadian consensus recommendations for the measurement and reporting of diastolic dysfunction by echocardiography: from the Investigators of Consensus on Diastolic Dysfunction by Echocardiography. *J Am Soc Echocardiogr* 1996; 9:736–60. ISSN: 0894-7317.

Rivas-Gotz C. Impact of left ventricular ejection fraction on estimation of left ventricular filling pressures using tissue Doppler and flow propagation velocity. *The American Journal of Cardiology*. 91(6): March 2003; 780-783. ISSN:0002-9149

Rodriguez L, Garcia M, Ares M, et al. Assessment of mitral annular dynamics during diastole by Doppler tissue imaging: comparison with mitral Doppler inflow in subjects without heart isease and in patients with left ventricular hypertrophy. *Am Heart J* 1996;131:982-7. ISSN: 0002-8703.

Rodríguez-Padial, L., *Ecocardiografía clínica*, 2002, 1st Edition, Aula médica, 9788478852949, Spain.

Schiavone WA, Calafiore PA, Salcedo EE. Transesophageal Doppler echocardiographic demonstration of pulmonary venous flow velocity in restrictive cardiomyopathy and constrictive pericarditis. *Am J Cardiol* 1989; 63:1286–8. ISSN: 0002-9149.

Shanks M, Arnold C.T., van de Veire N, Antoni L, Bertini M, Delgado V, Nucifora G, Holman E , Choy J, Schalij M , Bax J. Incremental Prognostic Value of Novel Left Ventricular Diastolic Indexes for Prediction of Clinical Outcome in Patients With ST-Elevation Myocardial Infarction. *Am J Cardiol* 2010;105:592–597. ISSN 0002-9149.

Skagseth E. Pulmonary vein flow pattern in man during thoracotomy. *Scand J Thorac Cardiovasc Surg* 1976; 10:36–42. ISSN: 0036-5580.

Støylen A, Heimdal A, Bjornstad K, et al. Strain rate imaging by ultrasound in the diagnosis of regional dysfunction of the left ventricle. *Echocardiography* 1999;16:321-9. ISSN: 1540-8175.

Støylen A, Heimdal A, Bjørnstad K, et al. Strain rate imaging by ultrasonography in the diagnosis of coronary artery disease. *J Am Soc Echocardiogr* 2000;13:1053-64). ISSN: 0894-7317.

Stuber M, Scheidegger M, Fischer S, Nagel E, Steinemann F, Hess O, Boesiger P. Alterations in the local myocardial motion pattern in patients suffering from pressure overload due to aortic stenosis. *Circulation* 1999; 100:361–368.) ISSN 0009-7322.

Takeuchi, M., Borden, W.B., Nakai, H., Nishikage, T., Kokumai, M., Nagakura, T., et al. Reduced and delayed untwisting of the left ventricle in patients with hypertension and left ventricular hypertrophy: a study using two-dimensional speckle tracking imaging. *Eur Heart J*. 2007; 28: 2756-62. ISSN 0195-668x.

Valantine HA, Appleton CP, Hatle LK, Hunt SA, Billingham ME, Shumway NE et al. A hemodynamic and Doppler echocardiographic study of ventricular function in long-term cardiac allograft recipients. Etiology and prognosis of restrictive-constrictive physiology. *Circulation* 1989; 79: 66–75. ISSN 0009-7322

Vanoverschelde JL, Raphael DA, Robert AR & Cosyns JR. Left ventricular filling in dilated cardiomyopathy: relation to functional class and hemodynamics. *J Am Coll Cardiol* 1990; 15:1288–95. ISSN 0735-1097.

Voigt JU, Lindenmeier G, Exner B, Regenfus M, Werner D, Reulbach U et al. Incidence and characteristics of segmental postsystolic longitudinal shortening in normal, acutely ischemic, and scarred myocardium. *J Am Soc Echocardiogr* 2003;16:415–23.ISSN: 0894-7317.

Waggoner AD, Bierig SM. Tissue Doppler imaging: a useful echocardiographic method for the cardiac sonographer to assess systolic and diastolic left ventricular function. *J Am Soc Echocardiogr 2001;* 14:1143–52. ISSN: 0894-7317.

Wang, J., Khoury, D.S., Yue, Y., Torre-Amione, G. and Nagueh, S.F. Left ventricular untwisting rate by speckle tracking echocardiography. *Circulation*. 2007; 116: 2580-6. ISSN 0009-7322.

Wang, J., Khoury, D.S., Yue, Y., Torre-Amione, G. and Nagueh, S.F. Preserved left ventricular twist and circumferential deformation, but depressed longitudinal and radial deformation in patients with diastolic heart failure. *Eur Heart J*. 2008; 29: 1283-9. ISSN 0195-668x.

Wang, J. and Nagueh, S.F. Current perspectives on cardiac function in patients with diastolic heart failure. Circulation. 2009; 119: 1146-57. ISSN 0009-7322.

Wierzbowska K, Drozdz J, Plewka M, Kurpesa M, Krzemińska M & Kasprzak JD. Assessment of mitral inflow during standardized Valsalva maneuver in stratification of diastolic function. *Echocardiography* 2007 May;24(5):464-71. ISSN 1540-8175.

Yamamoto K, Nishimura RA, Chaliki HP, Appleton CP, Holmes DR Jr & Redfield MM. Determination of left ventricular filling pressure by Doppler echocardiography in patients with coronary artery disease: critical role of left ventricular systolic function. *J Am Coll Cardiol* 1997; 30:1819–26. ISSN 0735-1097.

Zipes, D. et al, *Braunwald's Heart Disease: A Textbook of Cardiovascular Medicine*, 2011, 9th edition, Saunders, 9781437703986, USA.

7

Left Ventricle Postinfarction Aneurism: Comparison Between Diagnostic Value of Different Methods of Visualization

Maryna N. Dolzhenko, Sergey V. Potashev and Natalia N. Nosenko
The P.L.Shupik National Medical Academy Of Postgraduate Education/Cardiology And Functional Diagnosis Department
Ukraine

1. Introduction

Today method of coronary angiography and ventriculography (CVG) is a "golden standard" in diagnosis of coronary arteries atherosclerosis (Masaki Y. et al., 2005). Besides, CVG is successfully used for left ventricle (LV) global contractility evaluation and LV aneurism diagnosis in the patients after acute myocardial infarction (AMI) before surgeon revascularization and decision about LV surgeon plastics. But being invasive, this method has certain limitations and cannot be suitable for dynamic medical supervision afterwards (Schuijf J.D. et al., 2004). It should be mentioned, that possibility of coronary atherosclerosis diagnosis is not necessarily connected with arterial lumen narrowing. Atherosclerotic plague prolapses into arterial lumen, causing its narrowing and relevant clinical symptoms. But early stages of atherosclerosis usually do not lead to hemodynamically significant patency decrease and may not be seen by means of CVG. That is why design of new methods of coronary pathology, especially non-invasive, is of great importance. Among the demands to up-to-date examination methods high specificity, sensitivity, accuracy and safety should be mentioned, as well as high repeatability and economical suitability. All these features are attributes of multislice spiral computed tomography (MSCT) (Laissy et al., 2007; Masaki et al., 2005), what explains constantly growing interest to this method. Main advantage of Doppler echocardiography (EchoCG) is that it allows non-invasively and in real time to evaluate dimensions and behaviour of cardiac structures, to obtain characteristics of heart hemodynamics and indirect impression of chamber and main vessels pressures. Significant comparability of EchoCG results with chambers catheterization data has been long proven (Becher et al., 2004; Swedberg et al, 2005). Postinfarction LV aneurism promotes LV remodeling, worsens its systolic and diastolic function. LV myocardial function may improve in case of adequate vascularization revival due to surgeon procedure, for instance coronary arteries bypass graft (CABG) (Becher et al., 2004; Budoff, 2004; Dirksen et al., 2002; Dolzhenko et al.. 2007). Aneurism resection significantly influences LV remodelling, promotes chamber pressures decrease and slows down heart failure (HF) progression (Dolzhenko et al., 2008). That is why cardiologist and cardiac surgeon need maximum of objective information not only about coronary arteries patency, but also about LV structural and functional changes in order to adequately evaluate severity of operational

risk and long-term postoperational prognosis (Budoff, 2004; Dirksen et al., 2002; Dolzhenko et al., 2008). Up to now there were few attempts to compare informative diagnostic value of invasive and non-invasive methods of LV structural anomalies in the patients after AMI.
Among those, there are promising data regarding high correlation (r=0.76) of non-invasive evaluation of left ventricle (LV) ejection fraction (EF) between resting echocardiographic EFs and single photon emission computed tomography (SPECT) resting gated sestamibi images in patients with single-vessel disease, and a moderate correlation (r=0.68 and r=0.68) in patients with 2- and 3-vessel disease, respectively, while patients with two and 3-vessel disease were statistically more likely to have RWMAs detected by gated SPECT sestamibi than by echo (Fleming, 2002).
It has also been shown, that changes in resting LVEF and high-dose dipyridamole pharmacologically induced stress LVEF (SEF) provide a valuable diagnostic marker as to the number of significantly diseased coronary arteries and can be acquired from gated SPECT sestamibi images (Fleming&Boyd, 2002).
The aim of this study was to compare the efficacy of modern methods of heart left chambers visualization in the patients after acute myocardial infarction (AMI) with LV aneurism before coronary arteries bypass graft (CABG) combined with LV aneurismectomy (CABG+AE) in LV global contractility evaluation and reliability in LV chronic aneurism and its thrombosis diagnosis.

2. Methods

The study was approved by local ethics committee.
In the study we prospectively included 116 patients after AMI with LV postinfarction aneurism (LVA) without significant valvular dysfunction eligible for CABG combined with LVA resection. Exclusion criteria were a history of recent myocardial infarction (4 weeks before pre-operative angiography), atrial fibrillation, significant valvular heart disease or previous CABG. During and after the CABG, standard laboratory markers for myocardial infarction were obtained and none of the patients was diagnosed with perioperative myocardial infarction. Medication treatment in all the post-infarction patients included aspirin, statin, beta-blocker, ACE inhibitor and nitrates, if indicated. All patients underwent EchoCG and MSCT prior to the operation. Fourty age-matched subjects with CAD and without AMI history, who underwent CVG, EchoCG and contrast MSCT for coronary revascularization decision, served as controls. Program of the study included X-ray contrast CVG, MSCT with chambers contrast and Doppler EchoCG.

2.1 Coronary angiography

Coronary angiography with ventriculography was conducted and interpreted by trained physicians 1 week preceding CABG+AE. A 50% or more reduction of the luminal diameter in 2 orthogonal projections of a major coronary artery or one of its major branches or a bypass graft was considered to be significant for CAD. It is known, that LV postinfarction aneurism is a transmural scar with typical smooth inner surface without trabecular structures. LV wall is usually very thin in this place, causing inner and outer wall surfaces bulging. During systole the involved LV segment are akynetic or dyskinetic (showing paradox bulging movement) (Fleisher et al., 2007). LV aneurism and its thrombosis diagnosis during CVG with further confirmation *ad oculus* during operation was used as diagnostic "golden standard" (Fleisher et al., 2007). LV global contractility was evaluated by ejection fraction (EF) calculation by Simpson disc method in right anterior oblique 300 projection (Fleisher et al., 2007; Scanlon et al., 1999).

2.2 Echocardiography

A standard clinical echocardiographer, equipped with pulsed-wave TDI option (Medison "SonoAce" 9900) was used. Recordings and calculations of different parameters, including LV chamber volumes and EF, were performed according to the recommendations of the American Society of Echocardiography(Scanlon et al., 1999). LV global contractility was evaluated by by Simpson disc method in 4- and 2-chamber apical positions by calculating end-diastolic (EDV, ml) and end-systolic (ESV, ml) volumes with their indices to body surface area (EDI and ESI, ml/m^2) and LV EF, %. LV aneurism was defined as transmural a- or dyskinetic scar tissue with distinct smooth inner surface involving two or more LV segments (Dolzhenko et al., 2008; Fleisher et al., 2007).

2.3 Multislice computed tomography

MSCT was performed on tomographer «Light Speed-16» («General Electric Company», USA) using cardiological «Advantage Workstation 4.2» («General Electric Company», USA). Spiral mode of tomography with 2,5 mm thick slice and retrospective ECG synchronization was intravenous ed with 6-8 seconds scanning time and 360^0 rotation. Study was performed at breath held after infusomat "Omnipac" intravenous infusion. Exposure dose constituted 2,2 mSv per one study at 16 slices per 200 frames. LV global contractility was evaluated by LV EF calculation by Simpson disc method in 4-chamber projection. LV aneurism was defined as transmural a- or dyskinetic fibrous scar tissue with distinct smooth inner surface without trabecular structures involving two or more LV segments (Dirksen et al., 2002; Swedberg et al., 2005).

2.4 Statistics

Comparison of different methods was performed using multiple regression analysis with 95% confidence interval and correlation analysis. In comparison of diagnostic value of the studied methods we evaluated the following characteristics: accuracy (diagnostic efficacy) – percentage of correct test results out of general quantity of both positive and negative results; sensitivity (Se) – percentage of subjects with positive test results in the population with the studied pathology; specificity (Sp) – percentage of subjects with negative test results in the population with the studied pathology; positive predictive value (+PV) – probability of symptom or disease in case of positive test result; negative predictive value (-PV) – case of negative (normal) test result.

The above numbered indices were calculated by formulas:

$$Se=N(TP)/(N(TP)+N(FN))x100\%;$$

$$Sp=N(TN)/(N(TN)+N(FP)x100\%;$$

$$+PV=N(TP)/(N(TP)+N(FP) \times 100\%;$$

$$-PV= (TN)/(N(TN)+N(FN)x100\%;$$

where N is the quantity of studied patients; TP – truly positive diagnosis; FP – false positive diagnosis; TN - truly negative diagnosis; FN - false negative diagnosis[12,13]. The results are expressed as the mean and 1 standard deviation. The parameters of patients and healthy subjects were compared using an unpaired t-test. A paired t-test was used to compare results within the same group. A P-value of <0,05 was considered significant.

3. Results

The main clinical features of the study group patients are presented in Table 1.

Index	Abs.	%
LV EF (%)	37,1±12,4	-
LV EDI (ml/m^2)	112,4±28,2	-
LV ESI (ml/m^2)	73,8±27,6	-
Diabetes mellitus (n)	14	12,1%
Hypertension (n)	75	64,7%
Angina pectoris	107	92,3%
Functional class I	15	12,9%
Functional class II	23	19,8%
Functional class III	64	55,2%
Functional class IV	14	12,1%
Heart failure (NYHA functional class)		
I (LV > 45%)	17	14,7%
II (LV < 45%)	86	74,1%
I (LV < 45%)	13	11,2%
Lesions localization		
3-vessels disease and/or left main (n)	41	35,3%
2-vessels disease (n)	43	37,1%
1 -vessel disease (n)	32	27,6%
Aneurism localization		
Predominantly anterior LV aneurism (n)	28	24,1%
Anterior + apical aneurism + inferior (n)	38	32,8%
Anterior + septal + apical aneurism (n)	50	43,1%
*Data are presented as total (n) or M±SD (n=116)		

Table 1. Clinical features of the patients studied

As it is seen from the table, according to CVG data there were predominantly patients with 2- and 3-vessels disease of left main coronary artery lesion. Aneurisms according to CVG, MSCT and EchoCG data were mainly located in the anterior LV segments with frequent propagation to interventricular septum (IVS) and LV apex (43,1% cases) and LV apex with propagation to inferior apical segments (32,8% cases).

At comparison of results of LV global contractility (LV EF) data of different visualization methods significantly correlated between each other. EchoCG data highly correlated both with CVG (r=0,80) and MSCT (r=0,71, p<0,0001). Comparison of LV EF results according to CVG and MSCT also showed good correlation (r=0,73, p<0,0001 compared to EchoCG data) (Fig. 1, 2.). Thus, in LV global contractility evaluation all three methods were equally precise, while EchoCG is the method of preference, as having the least limitations, which corresponds to existing guidelines (Scanlon et al., 1999).

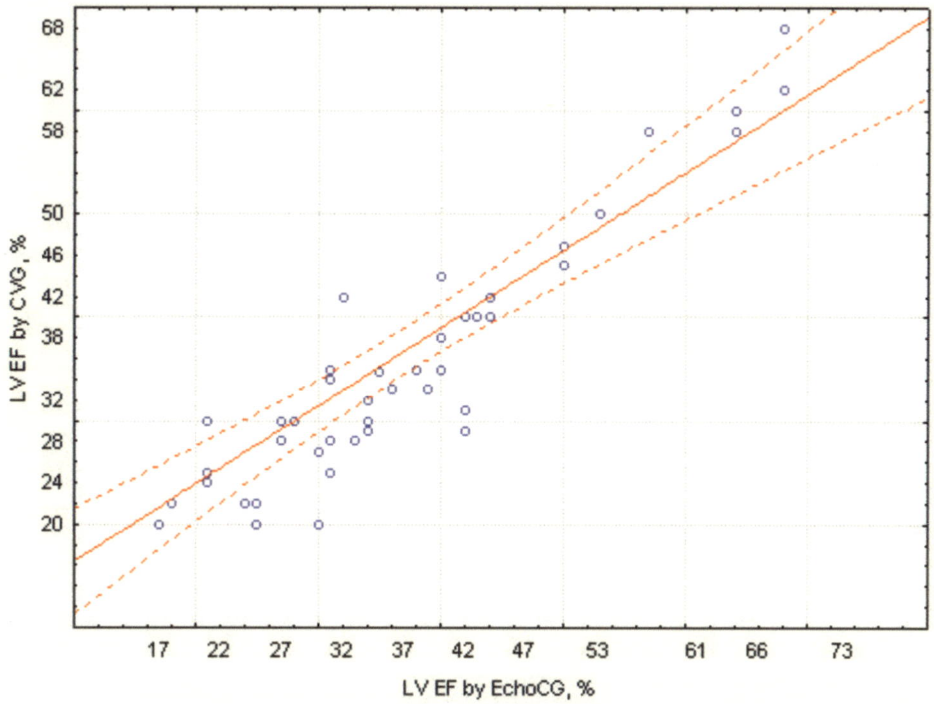

Fig. 1. Correlation of LV EF calculation according to CVG and EchoCG

At LV chronic aneurism diagnosis MSCT was the most sensitive method, which allowed diagnosis of aneurism in 100% cases. During EchoCG false negative result was obtained in 1 (0,09%) case, but there were no false positive results. At CVG there were 7 false negative (6,0%) cases but no false positive cases (accuracy - 86,2%, p<0,0001 compared both to MSCT and EchoCG).

MSCT sensitivity in aneurism diagnosis compared to CVG was 90,8%, while EchoCG sensitivity equaled 89,5% (p=0,74), while methods' specificity constituted 60% and 65%, respectively (p=0,43). Positive predictive value of methods was 89,6% and 90,7% (p=0,78), while negative predictive value was 63,2% and 61,9% (p=0,84), respectively (Table 2).

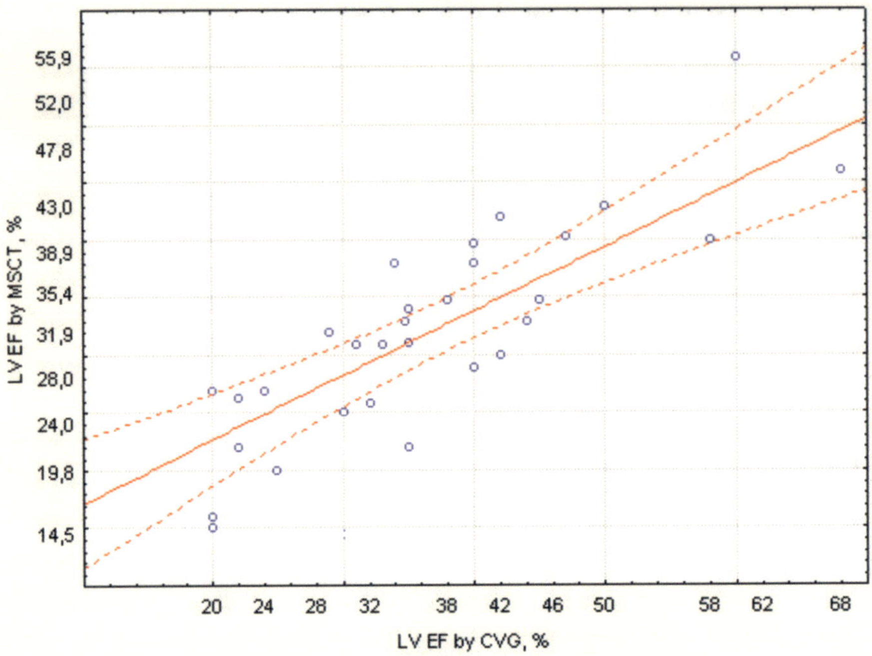

Fig. 2. Correlation of LV EF calculation according to CVG and MSCT

MSCT	EchoCG	p
Se = 90,8%	Se = 89,5%	0,74
Sp = 60,0%	Sp = 65,0%	0,43
+PV = 89,6%	+PV = 90,7%	0,78
- PV = 63,2%	- PV = 61,9%	0,84

Table 2. Comparison of diagnostic value of the studied methods in LV chronic aneurism diagnosis compared to CVG and post operation results

Frequency of aneurism diagnosis according to CVG data significantly correlated both with MSCT ($r=0,62$, $p<0,0001$) and EchoCG ($r=0,63$, $p<0,0001$).
Aneurism thrombosis during operation was found in 37 (31,9%) cases. Before operation according to CVG there were 14 (12,1%) false negative and 8 (6,9%) false positive aneurism thrombosis cases (accuracy - 81,0% of post operation findings). According to EchoCG data there were 5 (4,3%) false negative and 2 (1,7%) false positive cases (accuracy - 94,0%, $p=0,0031$ compared to CVG). At MSCT exams there were no false negative or false positive results (accuracy - 100%, $p<0,0001$ compared to CVG). Frequency of simultaneous correct LV aneurism thrombosis diagnosis was 48,7% (18 cases).
Data regarding diagnostic value of MSCT and EchoCG compared to CVG is presented in Table 3.

MSCT	EchoCG	p
Se = 69,2%	Se = 61,5%	0,22
Sp = 79,7%	Sp = 76,8%	0,59
+ PV = 56,3%	+ PV = 50,0%	0,34
- PV = 87,3%	- PV = 84,1%	0,49

Table 3. Comparison of diagnostic value of the studied methods in LV aneurism thrombosis diagnosis compared to CVG and post operation results

Frequency of LV aneurism thrombosis diagnosis by CVG correlated both with MSCT (r=0,52, p<0,0001) and EchoCG (r=0,36, p<0,0001). Still, the highest correlation was found between LV aneurism thrombosis diagnosis provided by MSCT and EchoCG (r=0,86, p<0,0001 compared to CVG in both cases) (Fig. 3).

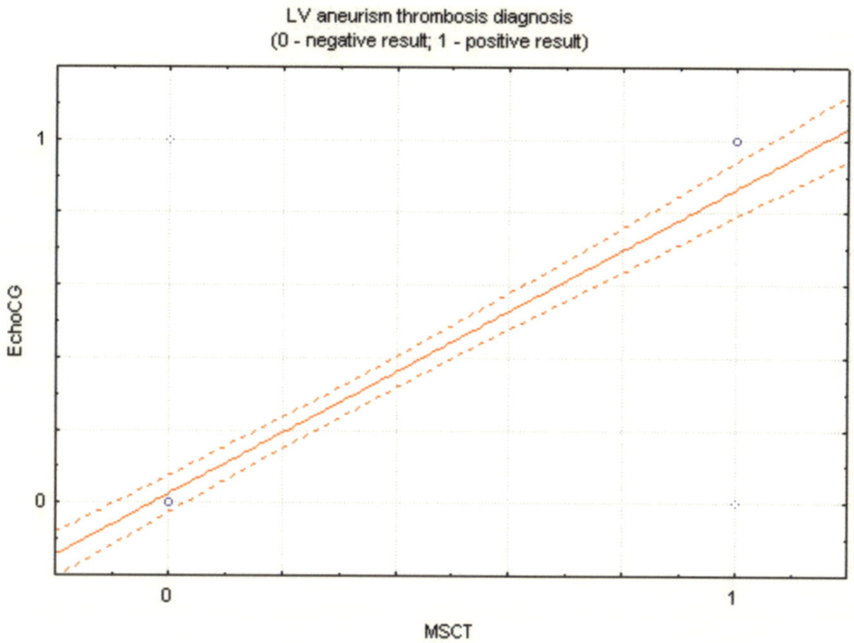

Fig. 3. Correlation of LV aneurism thrombosis diagnosis according to MSCT and EchoCG data

4. Discussion

According to the results of our study, MSCT showed the highest accuracy in diagnosis of LV chronic aneurism, as well as its thrombosis, compared to CVG and EchoCG. MSCT and EchoCG also showed high sensitivity and positive predictive value in diagnosis of LV chronic aneurism and high specificity and negative predictive value in diagnosis of LV aneurism thrombosis compared to CVG. On the other hand, results of CVG significantly correlated with both MSCT and EchoCG results data. Despite the fact that CVG is considered to be an invasive "golden standard" in diagnosing LV structural pathology, high accuracy of MSCT and EchoCG is explained due to visualization of the whole LV wall with characteristic myocardial signal. During CVG invasive cardiologist sees only endocardial contour outlined by contrast, which might be a cause of false positive or false negative diagnosis, especially in case of a small aneurism, which is shown by our study data by intraoperational findings of LV aneurism and its thrombosis and corresponds to reference data (Budoff, 2004; Dirksen et al., 2002; Dolzhenko et al., 2007; Masaki et al., 2005; Schuijf et al., 2004). Besides, during MSCT or EchoCG thrombotic tissue has certain structural texture, significantly visually different from one of myocardium, which explains higher accuracy of these methods in aneurism thrombosis diagnosis compared to CVG, especially in case of flat and thin parietal clot (Laissy et al., 2007), when CVG does not show significant contrast filling defect. These considerations are confirmed by results of our study and may explain high accuracy, sensitivity and positive predictive value of MSCT in LV aneurism thrombosis diagnosis. MSCT and EchoCG show identical positive and negative predictive value in LV aneurism thrombosis diagnosis, while EchoCG shows significantly higher specificity and positive predictive value in LV chronic aneurism diagnosis compared to MSCT.

4.1 Study limitations

In case of defining LV volumes and EF EchoCG is the method of preference being reliable, non-invasive and, thus, having minimum of limitations (Becher et al., 2004; Budoff, 2004; Dolzhenko et al., 2007; Swedberg et al., 2005). Despite good correlations between all methods of visualization, MSCT seemed to give seriously lower absolute values of LV EF compared to EchoCG. Higher accuracy in defining LV global contractility by EchoCG may be explained by the fact, that LV volumes quantification by EchoCG is performed in two perpendicular planes under visual and manual control of sonographist. On the other hand, in CVG or MSCT EDV and ESV quantification is performed automatically by installed software in one fixed projection, which may lead to inaccuracy, especially in case of marked LV eccentric remodeling and aneurism presence (Budoff, 2004; Dirksen et al., 2002; Fleisher et al., 2007; Scanlon et al., 1999).

5. Conclusion

In the patients with LV chronic postinfarction aneurism data of non-invasive methods highly correlate with CVG data. In LV chronic aneurism diagnosis transthoracic EchoCG and MSCT have high accuracy compared to CVG due to high sensitivity and positive predictive value of these methods. There was no significant difference between prognostic value of MSCT and transthoracic EchoCG in LV chronic aneurism and its thrombosis diagnosis, which allows to consider MSCT a reliable alternative to EchoCG in LV structural anomalies diagnosis in the patients after AMI prior to planned CABG+AE. Data provided by MSCT and transthoracic EchoCG in LV chronic aneurism and its thrombosis significantly highly correlate with "golden standard" CVG results, which allows to consider these non-invasive methods highly reliable in defining the discussed myocardial structural anomalies.

6. Acknowledgment

Authors thank Prof. Anatoliy Rudenko, Head of Coronary Heart Disease Surgeon Treatment Department of The N.M.Amosov Institute Of Cardiovascular Surgery Of AMS Of Ukraine, and Dr. Oleg Sharayevskiy, Head of MSCT Department of NSC "The N.D.Strazhesko Institute Of Cardiology" Of AMS Of Ukraine, for the provided CCA and MSCT results data for the studied patients.

7. References

Becher H. et al. BSE procedure guidelines for the clinical application of stress echocardiography, recommendations for performance and interpretation of stress echocardiography: A report of the British Society of Echocardiography Policy Committee. *Heart,* Vol. 90 (December 2004), pp. vi23 - vi30.

Budoff M.J. Tracking Progression of Heart Disease with Cardiac Computed Tomography. *Journal of Cardiovascular Pharmacology and Therapeutics,* Vol. 9 (April 2004), pp. 75 - 82.

Dirksen M.S., et al. Usefulness of dynamic multislice computed tomography of left ventricular function in unstable angina pectoris and comparison with echocardiography. *Am. J. Cardiol,* Vol. 90 (February 2002), pp. 1157-1160.

Dolzhenko M.N. et al. Left ventricle diastolic function in the patients after coronary arteries bypass graft combined with left ventricle aneurismectomy according to tissue doppler imaging: one year follow-up. *Postgrad. Med. J,* Vol. 83 (May 2007), pp. 320-324.

Dolzhenko M.N. et al. Changes in left ventricle myocardial function in patients with postinfarction cardiosclerosis according to tissue Doppler imaging after coronary arteries bypass graft combined with left ventricle aneurismectomy. *Heart and vessels,* No. 2 (Aptil 2008), pp. 34-41.

Fleisher Lee A. et al. ACC/AHA 2007 Guidelines on Perioperative Cardiovascular Evaluation and Care for Noncardiac Surgery: A Report of the American College of Cardiology/American Heart Association Task Force on Practice Guidelines (Writing Committee to Revise the 2002 Guidelines on Perioperative Cardiovascular Evaluation for Noncardiac Surgery. *Circulation,* Vol. 116 (October 2007), pp. e418 - e500.

Fleming R.M. A Tate-en-Tate Comparison of Ejection Fraction and Regional Wall Motion Abnormalities as Measured by Echocardiography and Gated Sestamibi SPECT. *Angiology,* Vol. 53, 3 (May 2002), pp. 313-321.

Fleming R.M., Boyd L.D. High-Dose Dipyridamole and Gated Sestamibi SPECT Imaging Provide Diagnositic Resting and Stress Ejection Fractions Useful for Predicting the Extent of Coronary Artery Disease. *Angiology,* 53, 4 (July 2002), pp. 415-421.

Kasner M. et al. Utility of Doppler Echocardiography and Tissue Doppler Imaging in the Estimation of Diastolic Function in Heart Failure With Normal Ejection Fraction: A Comparative Doppler-Conductance Catheterization Study. *Circulation,* Vol. 116 (August 2007), pp. 637 - 647.

Kyung-Jong Yoo, et al. The comparison of the graft patency after coronary artery bypass grafting using coronary angiography and multi-slice computed tomography. *Eur. J. Cardiothorac. Surg.,* Vol. 24 (July 2003), pp. 86.

Laissy Jean-Pierre et al. Comprehensive evaluation of preoperative patients with aortic valve stenosis: usefulness of cardiac multidetector computed tomography. *Heart*, Vol. 93 (September 2007), pp. 1121 - 1125.

Masaki Y. et al. Cardiac Functional Analysis with Multi–Detector Row CT and Segmental Reconstruction Algorithm: Comparison with Echocardiography, SPECT, and MR Imaging. *Radiology*, Vol. 234 (October 2005), pp. 381 - 390.

Mok C.K., Cheung K.L., WangR.Y. Unruptured right coronary sinus to left ventricle aneurysm diagnosed by cross sectional echocardiography. *Heart*, Vol. 53 (February 1985), pp. 226 – 229.

Petry A., Sabin K. (2003). *Demonstrable statistics in medicine*, GAOTAR-MED, Moscow

Rebrova O.Y. (2002). *Statistical analysis of medical data*, Media Sphere, Moscow

Scanlon P.J. et al. ACC/AHA Guidelines for Coronary Angiography: Executive Summary and Recommendations. *Circulation*, Vol. 99 (May 1999), pp. 2345-57.

Schuijf J.D. et al. Noninvasive Angiography and Assessment of Left Ventricular Function Using Multislice Computed Tomography in Patients With Type 2 Diabetes. *Diabetes Care*, Vol. 27 (December 2004), pp. 2905 - 2910.

Swedberg K. et al. Guidelines for Diagnosis and Treatment of Chronic Heart Failure. *Eur. Heart Journ.*, Vol. 26 (June 2005), pp. 1115-1140.

Part 4

Special Considerations

8

Doppler Contrast Echocardiography

Vincent L. Sorrell and Sachin Kumar
University of Arizona and the Sarver Heart Centre, Tucson
United States of America

1. Introduction

The advent and evolution of 2D echocardiography with Doppler gave a new dimension to the evaluation of valvular heart disease (VHD) and noninvasive cardiovascular hemodynamics. Extending from basic M-mode evaluation to the more sophisticated Doppler techniques, the way one looks at the valve anatomy and physiology has changed significantly. Doppler echocardiography has become the everyday tool for diagnosing valve pathology and for the serial evaluation of VHD (van de Brink et al, 1991). Despite significant technical advancements in image quality, spatial and temporal resolution, suboptimal image quality has not been entirely eliminated. Often due to body habitus (both obesity and markedly underweight individuals), chronic obstructive lung diseases or mechanically ventilated patients, 2D echocardiography suffers from poor signal to noise ratio (SNR). In these circumstances, the spectral Doppler signals are also weak due to high acoustic impedance. Harmonic imaging, power Doppler, low mechanical index pulsing and contrast echocardiography (CE) are some of the methods to improve image quality (Allen MR et al, 1999; Kitzman DW et al, 2000).

Gramiak and Shah, often considered pioneers in the use of contrast agents, demonstrated the use of indocyanine dye to improve visualization of cardiac chambers (Gramiak & Shah, 1969). Several authors have compared the application of contrast use against second harmonic imaging in assessing endocardial definition and proven its superiority (Kornbluth M et al, 2000). The American Society of Echocardiography (ASE) has recommended the use of contrast for the purposes of improving endocardial visualization in all subjects with >2 suboptimal contiguous wall segments, to reduce interpreter's variability and augment accuracy (Mulvagh SL et al, 2008). They also recommend using contrast agents to diagnose pathologic conditions that occur predominantly in the left ventricular (LV) apex, since this near-field region is better visualized after CE. This would include diseases such as apical variant of hypertrophic cardiomyopathy, isolated left ventricular noncompaction, apical thrombus and left ventricular aneurysm or pseudoaneurysm.

Contrast agents have also been used for enhancing the spectral Doppler signals required for evaluation of LV diastolic function, cardiovascular hemodynamic assessment, and comprehensive valvular analysis. Despite these standard national guidelines and recommendations, it has been estimated that <1% of warranted patients ever receive contrast. These authors believe that CE is underutilized across the globe. In this chapter, we focus our attention to one particular use of contrast agents-the augmentation of continuous and pulse wave spectral Doppler to assist in the evaluation of valvular function and the estimation of cardiovascular hemodynamics.

Evaluation of valve function rests on acquiring accurate spectral and color Doppler signals. Not infrequently, physicians are asked to interpret echo studies with inadequate Doppler signal jets which may result in either the underestimation(lack of signal) or overestimation (excess noise) of the true flow gradients. In such instances, one can effectively utilize contrast agents to better define the Doppler signal to increase SNR, translating into optimized assessment of VHD. Contrast agents have been used to increase the sensitivity of Doppler signals for the assessment of tricuspid regurgitation, pulmonary venous flow, aortic and mitral regurgitation and stenosis.

Contrast agents have evolved tremendously from their initial use by Gramiak and Shah. Initial agents used by these authors were Indocyanine green, normal saline, and 5% dextrose in water (Gramiak & Shah, 1969). Currently, 2nd generation contrast agents are routinely available for use. Prior to understanding the role of contrast agents in Doppler echocardiography; the reader should have some insight into the properties, behavior and evolution to the current generation of contrast agents. In the United States (US), the Federal Drug and Administration (FDA) agency has approved two contrast agents for the indications of left ventricular opacification (LVO) and endocardial border delineation (EBD). Definity (Lantheus Medical Imaging, North Bellerica, MA) has a phospholipid shell and Optison (GE Healthcare, Princeton, NJ) has a human albumin shell. Both of these agents were designed to allow relative diffusion and permeability and ultimate dissolution of the encapsulated gas, which is perflouropropane (PFC). There are several other agents, (Levovist, SonoVue, CARDIOsphere and Imagify) used all across the globe but haven't yet gained FDA approval. SonoVue has been approved and recommended by the European Society of Echocardiography (ESE) for similar LVO indications as recommended by the ASE. These agents are used primarily for LVO and EBD, but there is evidence to support their utility for other indications, including spectral Doppler augmentation. Unlike contrast for LVO, the use of contrast specifically for Doppler enhancement requires a smaller amount of contrast and care in decreasing the Doppler gain settings (sometimes to the zero baseline) to avoid excess noise ("blooming" effect). If one was to measure this noise, then the estimated velocity will be incorrect and the calculated pressure gradient inaccurate. To minimize this potential, these authors perform the Doppler analysis after the 2D LVO study so the contrast is less intense. Also, be certain to measure only along the normal Doppler spectral contour and avoid small irregularities or 'spikes' within the modal velocity display.

2. Right heart

Initial use of contrast agents was confined to right-sided pathology as the initial agents did not have the ability to cross the pulmonary circulation. The first attempt at using traditional contrast agents like agitated saline, dextrose and sonicated albumin was to improve tricuspid regurgitation (TR) spectral Doppler signals to establish the diagnosis of pulmonary hypertension (PH). Sonicated albumin (Albunex, Molecular Biosystems, Inc., San Diego, California) has the ability to traverse the pulmonary circulation. Noninvasive estimation of pulmonary arterial pressures is crucial to monitor patients with heart disease and to make screening diagnosis of PH. Besides, the relevance of exercise response to pulmonary pressures cannot be ignored as it adds prognostic importance. The ability to capture accurate tricuspid regurgitation Doppler signals in patients with or without pulmonary hypertension, at rest or immediately after exercise, is highly variable even with optimum system gain, filters, compression and patient (multiple views, variable patient positions, breath holding) settings.

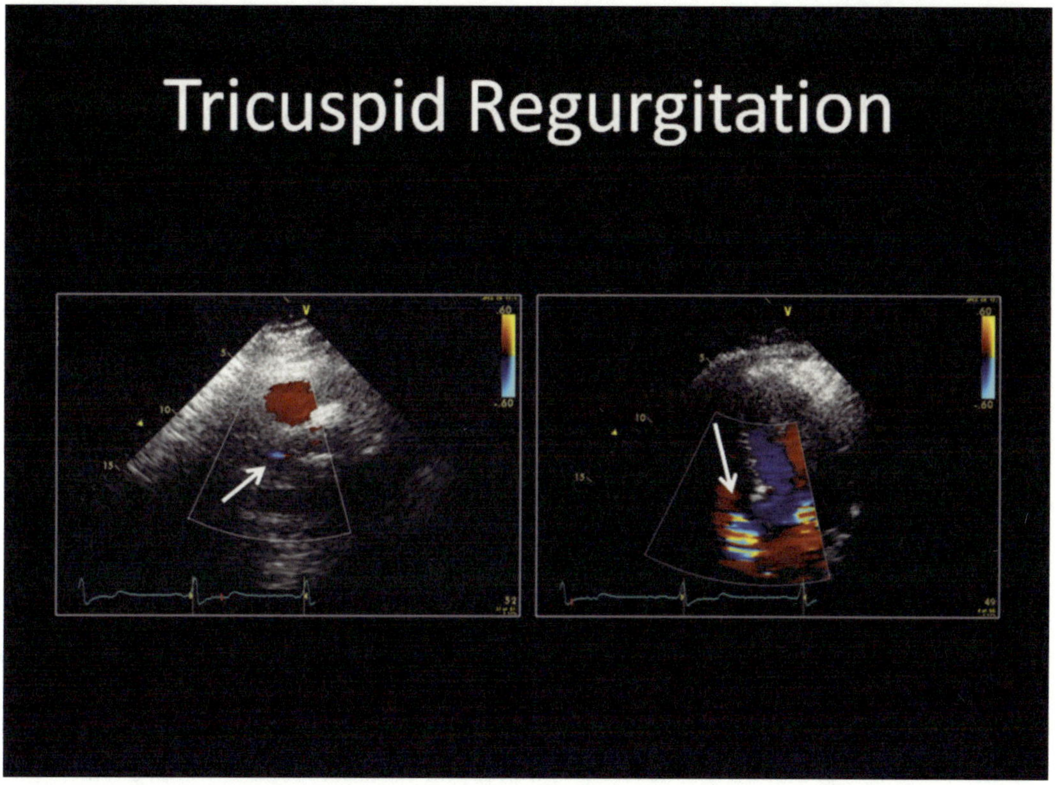

Fig. 1. Color flow Doppler display of tricuspid regurgitation (TR). Left. Unenhanced systolic image with very weak color flow demonstrating minimal TR (arrow). Right. Contrast enhanced image with gains set at zero to minimize noise artifact. Note the enhanced systolic color flow Doppler signal (arrow) allowing for an increased likelihood to measure the conventional spectral Doppler tracing

The idea to improve TR Doppler signal began with a simple experiment of intravenous injection of agitated normal saline. Beard and Byrd, analyzed 38 patients referred to their echocardiography laboratory (in addition to 7 normal subjects), looking for enhancement of the TR spectral Doppler signals (Beard and Byrd, 1988). They concluded that agitated saline significantly improved the TR jet if the jet was inadequately visualized before contrast enhancement. Importantly, it did not impact the results if there was no Doppler signal seen prior to saline enhancement. This is important, since in the absence of any TR, taking the time to perform a contrast-enhanced Doppler evaluation may not be warranted. However, it has been reported that TR is present in >50% of normal young individuals and this percentage is significantly greater in patients with cardiovascular pathology (Shah & Raney, 2008). In this study, many of patients had pulmonary artery catheters in place and the enhanced spectral Doppler TR gradient estimated PA pressures was able to be corroborated with the invasive PA pressure measurements.

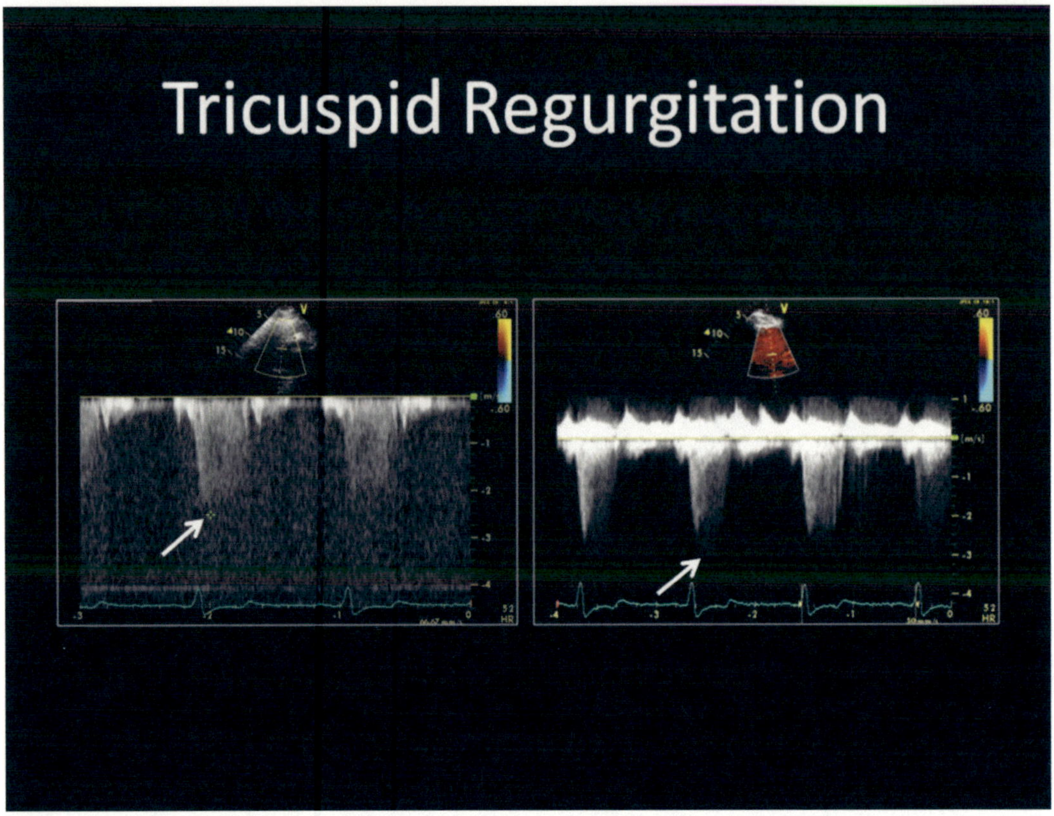

Fig. 2. Continuous wave spectral Doppler display of tricuspid regurgitation (TR). Left. Unenhanced systolic image with weak Doppler display demonstrating a maximal TR velocity of 2.5M/s or 25mmHg gradient (arrow). Right. Contrast enhanced image with increased signal to noise ratio able to confirm the maximal systolic velocity approaching 3.0M/s or 36mmHg (arrow)

Himelman et al reported similar findings in patients with chronic obstructive pulmonary disease and demonstrated similar results at rest and with exercise (Himelman et al, 1988). However, the criticism of agitated saline has been that the Doppler signal obtained tends to be noisy and rough ("fish bone like") and only marginally better than unenhanced spectral or color flow Doppler. Terasawa et al compared agitated saline with sonicated albumin in patients with invasive hemodynamic data to assess the right ventricular systolic pressure (RVSP) (Terasawa et al, 1993). The authors observed that both contrast agents enhanced the spectral Doppler signals, but possibly due to cursor angle errors, they both underestimated the invasively determined RVSP. Several other investigators also noted that the sonicated albumin findings were significantly more accurate relative to the agitated saline findings (Beppu et al, 1991). Despite these results, owing to its universal availability and ease of administration, agitated saline remains the contrast agent primarily used for enhancement of right sided spectral Doppler signals such as the maximal TR velocity. Modern contrast agents (Definity and Optison) have not been extensively studied for the purposes of right sided conditions including TR spectral Doppler signal optimization. Investigators at Mayo clinic conducted retrospective analysis of a large number of patients who received Definity for the purposes of RVSP estimation and suggested its utility for this indication (Abdelmoneim et al, 2010). However, the intention of the study was to demonstrate the safety of this contrast agent in patients with pulmonary hypertension undergoing stress echocardiography. Second generation contrast agents improve the spectral Doppler envelope of TR by increasing the SNR and increasing the likelihood that the actual peak TR velocity is identified.

In addition to the estimation of the RVSP (as a surrogate of the pulmonary artery systolic pressure), Doppler echocardiography is also able to estimate the pulmonary artery diastolic pressure (PADP) using the spectral Doppler envelope of pulmonary regurgitation (PR). The pulmonary capillary wedge pressure (PCWP), also the PADP (a surrogate of the left atrial pressure), has shown to correlate well with the sum of PR end diastolic pressures gradients and the estimated right atrial (RA) pressure ,also known as the central venous pressure. RA pressure can be estimated using inferior vena cava dimensions and phasic respiratory changes. To determine the PR end diastolic gradient, the spectral Doppler velocity profile of the PR jet must be accurately measured, but is often suboptimal due to a weak signal. This has been shown to improve with use of sonicated albumin by several authors (Masuyama T et al, 1986). Analyzing the overall evidence, it appears that use of modern contrast is safe and useful as a screening tool for the diagnosis of PH in suspected patients, particularly when there is a hint that the spectral Doppler is weak and an underestimation of the true maximal velocity. Contrast enhanced Doppler echocardiography appears to be a promising option for the serial follow up of patients with PH, thus obviating the need for frequent invasive testing. Furthermore, exercise Doppler echocardiography with contrast may help unmask the diagnosis of PH in asymptomatic individuals. To date, the routine use of contrast agents for the purposes of enhancing the Doppler signals on the right side is not recommended and should be considered an option on an individual patient basis.

3. Left heart

Development of transpulmonary agents has expanded the horizon and potential for use of contrast agents. These agents tend to be stable, have an excellent acoustic profile, and tend to be biologically inert. 5% sonicated albumin was the first to be FDA approved for LVO and EBD. Due to concerns with pressure sensitivity, resulting in a very short effective half life, it was not been a widely used agent. Newer 2nd generation agents, like Definity and Optison, have properties of ideal transpulmonary agents and hence gained FDA approval in US.

Left ventricular filling pressure, compliance and diastolic function is assessed by a composite of multiple measurements and each component has its own value. Contrast agents are very effective for augmenting the pulmonary venous (PV) Doppler flow pattern which adds value to the assessment of diastolic function of the heart. Due to the distance of left atrium and the PV from the transducer, the spectral Doppler display of the PV flow is often suboptimal. Even if one is able to acquire signals, these usually have low SNR causing challenges in accurate assessment. A normal PV inflow displays a systolic phase and diastolic phase. There is another short, low velocity reversal of flow coinciding with atrial contraction, called the AR-wave (atrial reversal). In normal individuals systolic phase dominates. In patients with abnormal diastolic function, as the left ventricle gets stiffer, majority of emptying of the PV occurs in diastole which results in blunting of the systolic phase with relative augmentation of the diastolic phase. The width and the velocity of the AR wave is also exaggerated (Rossvoll O et al, 1993; Tabata T et al, 2003). The systolic and diastolic phases of the PV tend to be well displayed, using PV flows obtained with TEE as the reference standard (Castello R et al, 1991). However, the atrial reversal phase is the most often suboptimal, but importantly has the highest correlation with LA pressure. It has been demonstrated that with the use of contrast agents, the visualization of the PV flow Doppler spectrum can be improved, particularly, the atrial reversal phase, translating into improved diastolic performance assessment (William MJ et al, 1995). Contrast increases the likelihood of identifying the actual peak systolic, diastolic and the atrial velocities, although the ratios of the systolic/diastolic velocities may remain unchanged (Izumi C et al, 1996). There are other reported studies which suggest that the peak systolic and diastolic PV velocities are augmented, but the atrial reversal flow might not be as robust as expected (von Bibra H et al, 1994). However, majority of published reports do come to the agreement that contrast agents improve the overall sensitivity of accurately measuring the different phases of PV spectral Doppler flow pattern. Importantly, the PV flow pattern also aids in the assessment of the severity of mitral stenosis and regurgitation.

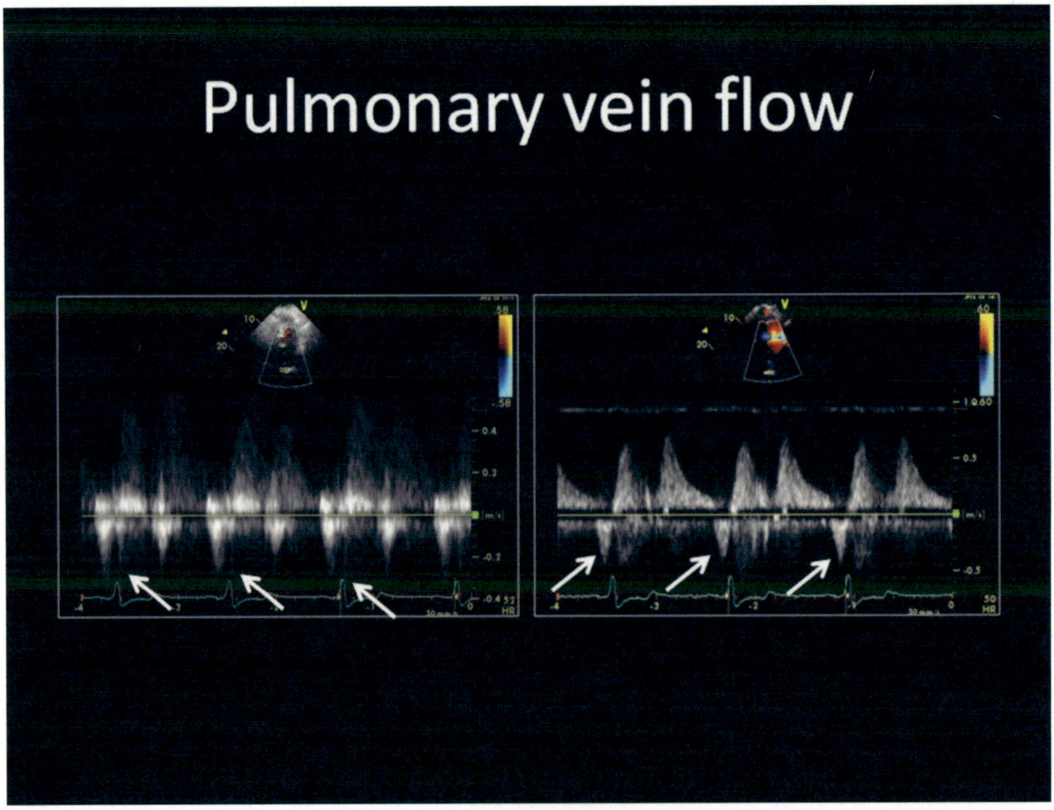

Fig. 3. Pulsed wave spectral Doppler display of pulmonary venous flow. Left. Unenhanced image with adequate tracing of the systolic (S) and diastolic (D) waves, but difficult to discern the atrial reversal (AR) velocity (arrow). Right. Contrast enhanced image with optimal spectral Doppler tracing confirming the AR maximal velocity is abnormally increased at >40cm/s (arrow)

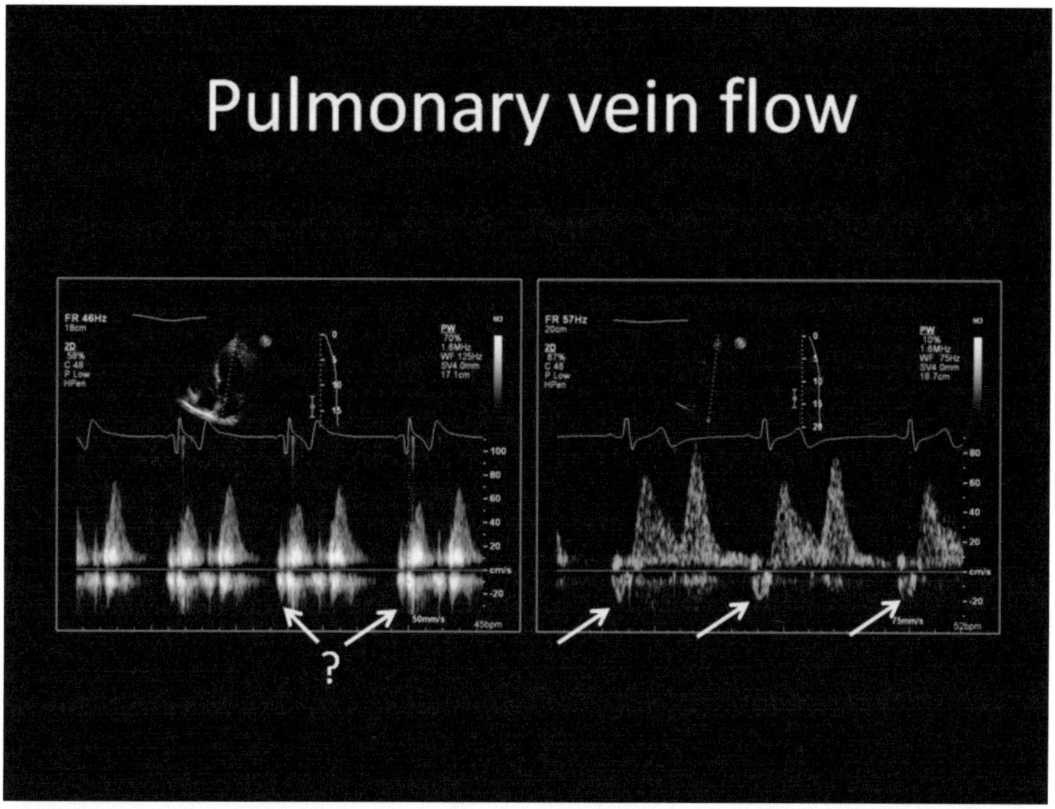

Fig. 4. This is a different patient demonstrating the ability to use contrast to improve pulmonary venous flow assessment. Pulsed wave spectral Doppler display of pulmonary venous flow. Left. Unenhanced image with adequate tracing of the systolic (S) and diastolic (D) waves, but difficulty in discerning the atrial reversal (AR) velocity (arrow). Right. Contrast enhanced image with optimal spectral Doppler tracing confirming the AR maximal velocity is normal and <20cm/s (arrow)

Evaluation of severity of mitral regurgitation (MR) rests on obtaining adequate spectral and color flow Doppler across the mitral valve as well as observing the changes in pulmonary venous flow. In eccentric jets, where one can easily underestimate the severity of MR using the color flow Doppler pattern alone, additional parameters are vital. Contrast agents have previously been employed and have demonstrated their ability to assist in the evaluation of MR. Terasawa et al, demonstrated an improvement in the Doppler velocity profile in all study patients (N=17) with a good reproducibility (Terasawa A et al, 1993). These authors analyzed the velocity profile in detail to elucidate the mechanism for the noted augmentation of spectral Doppler display and suggested that the velocity in the centre of the jet remained unchanged before and after the contrast. However the marginal velocities along the edges of the spectral Doppler envelope were better seen due to improved signal-to-noise ratio. Unlike the effect of contrast which increases the identified peak velocity of the maximal TR spectral Doppler profiles, the peak mitral regurgitation spectral Doppler velocity was not significantly altered in this report. This finding should have important ramifications in the accurate determination of the spectral profile trace, which is used in quantitative evaluation of the MR regurgitant volume (Enriquez-Sarano M etal, 1995; Hall SA et al, 1997; Pu M et al, 2001) .This finding should add value and improve the ability to accurately measure other spectral Doppler parameters beyond the peak velocity. A number of spectral Doppler analyses have been reported as having significant clinical value and may benefit from contrast enhancement when the Doppler signal is weak (table 1).

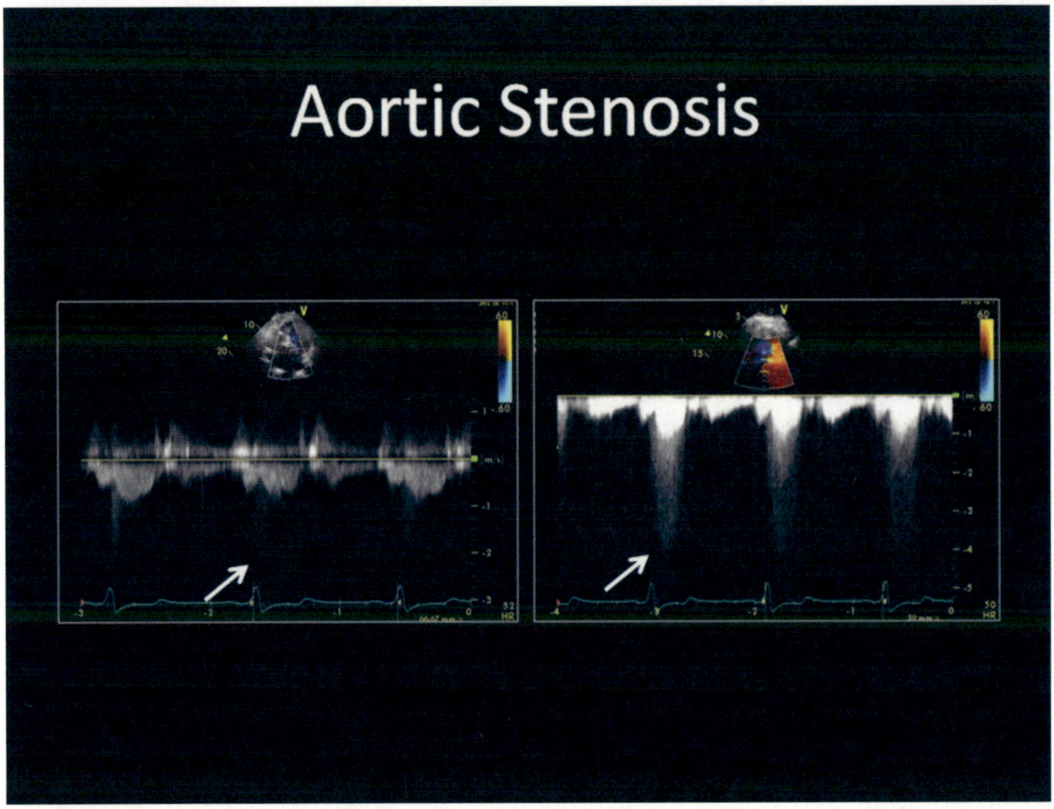

Fig. 5. Continuous wave spectral Doppler display of a patient with aortic stenosis. Left. Unenhanced image with weak tracing unable to confirm maximal gradient >30mmHg (arrow). Right. Contrast enhanced image (same patient as shown on the left) with optimal Doppler tracing confirming a maximal gradient > 70mmHg

Another interesting observation from this study, which these authors can confirm, was that the Doppler contrast augmentation effect lasted much longer than the LVO effect. This is a valuable property of contrast Doppler and by providing longer time window to capture the enhanced signals, the sonographer is able to complete the LVO portion of the 2D exam and then perform the enhanced Doppler exam afterwards. This phenomenon allows one to use a minimal amount of contrast for Doppler augmentation and does not require an additional contrast injection. In our experience, this latter spectral Doppler examination, performed after most of the contrast has 'washed out', retains the enhanced signal properties of the contrast agent while minimizing the potential for excess noise often created when the Doppler is used too soon.

Doppler parameter	Pathologic value	Clinical implication
Aortic Regurgitation PHT	< 200 ms	Elevated LVEDP
Aortic Stenosis	>4.0m/sec	Severe AS
Mitral Regurgitation (dP/dt)	<600mmHg/sec	Severe Systolic Dysfunction
PA Acceleration Time	< 90ms	Severely Elevated PASP
TR vti trace	> 25mmHg	Elevated PAMP

PHT, pressure half time; LVEDP, left ventricular end diastolic pressure; PASP, pulmonary artery systolic pressure; TR, tricuspid regurgitation; VTI, velocity time integral; PAMP, pulmonary artery mean pressure

Table 1.

Von Bibra et al used a saccharide based contrast agent and found a close correlation between the enhanced mitral spectral Doppler and TEE, thereby hinting an underestimation by the unenhanced TTE Doppler images. Their results echoed with findings of other investigators, emphasizing the role and utility of contrast in situations where the determination of MR severity is crucial (von Bibra H et al, 1995). Other investigators have demonstrated the role of contrast agents in patients with prosthetic mitral valves. In clinical situations of ambiguity or when discrepancies exist between different diagnostic modalities, adding contrast may be a simple technique to offer greater insight and clarification of valve patholophysiology (Donovan & Armstrong, 1996). Summarizing the limited published evidence, combined with our experiences, there is reasonable data to suggest that the use of contrast in cases where the spectral Doppler signals are low in intensity is warranted.

Aortic stenosis (AS) is a chronic progressive disease mainly affecting the elderly population. Assessment of the severity of AS is of crucial importance in the decision for timing of aortic valve replacement surgery. Evaluation of AS severity with TTE relies heavily on Doppler measurement of the transvalvular velocity, which in turn allows the estimation of the AV gradient and the calculation of aortic valve area (AVA) by use of the continuity equation (Otto CM, 2006). Alignment of the Doppler signal to the direction of blood flow is critical to obtain an accurate estimation of the jet velocity and gradients and hence the AVA. Underestimation is a valid concern when confronted with decision for surgery. Contrast has been shown to result in an improvement in the determination of the peak Doppler velocity AS profile, allowing a more accurate trans-aortic gradient estimation (Nakatani S et al, 1992). Importantly, in this study, the authors noted that patients with weak Doppler signals demonstrated improvements in their image profiles, but even those with adequate unenhanced Doppler signals were further improved by the use of contrast. As already demonstrated, contrast enhancement of the Doppler signal profile improves the ability to obtain the maximal velocity as well as the entire Doppler envelope trace. In AS, this portends to improvement in the estimation of the maximal and mean AV gradients. The normal protocol for obtaining maximal AS gradients requires the echo sonographer to utilize numerous ultrasound windows (usually > 3) in the hope of aligning the Doppler cursor with the actual AS flow. As the AV becomes diseased, the valve opening is altered and the blood flows in any number of directions from the LV to aorta. Therefore, it is uncommon that the optimal alignment can be predicted, as it is just as likely that the maximal velocity will be obtained in the right parasternal window as it will be in the apical

3, apical 5, subcostal, or suprasternal window. At times, there is a great variation in the maximal AS gradient from each of these windows. In our experience, the contrast enhanced Doppler signal is occasionally similar across multiple ultrasound windows. Whether this would portend to a quicker Doppler exam, by allowing the sonographer to limit the number of images acquired from multiple windows has yet to be proven.

4. Conclusion

Contrast agents have now been in use for more than five decades from their initial application by Gramiak and Shah in 1960s. The 2nd generation agents used today, are safe, have the ability to cross the pulmonary circulation, are inert and have higher acoustic properties to aid in the evaluation of a vast spectrum of clinical dilemmas. Because of recent post-marketing concerns raised by the FDA, there have been several important, large studies reported that demonstrate and confirm the safety of these agents (Borges AC et al, 2002; Piscaglia F et al, 2006; Raisinghani A et al, 2003). In this chapter, the role of these contrast agents in augmenting the spectral Doppler profile for both right and left sides of the heart and including both regurgitant and stenotic valve diseases was highlighted.

5. References

[1] Abdelmoneim SS, Bernier M, Scott CG et al. Safety of contrast agent use during stress echocardiography in patients with elevated right ventricular systolic pressure: a cohort study. *Circ Cardiovasc Imaging*. 2010 May; 3(3):240-8.

[2] Allen MR, Pellikka PA, Villarraga HR et al. Harmonic imaging: echocardiographic enhanced contrast intensity and duration. *Int J Card Imaging*.1999; 15:215-20.

[3] Beard JT, Byrd BF. Saline contrast enhancement of trivial Doppler tricuspid regurgitation signals for estimating pulmonary artery pressure. *Am J Cardiol*. 1988 Sep 1; 62(7):486-8.

[4] Borges AC, Walde T, Reibis RK et al. Does contrast echocardiography with Optison induce myocardial necrosis in humans? *J Am Soc Echocardiogr*. 2002; 15: 1080-6.

[5] Castello R, Pearson AC, Lenzen P et al. Evaluation of pulmonary venous flow by transesophageal echocardiography in subjects with a normal heart: comparison with transthoracic echocardiography. *J Am Coll Cardiol*. 1991 Jul; 18 (1):65-71.

[6] Donovan CL, Armstrong WF. Contrast enhancement of mitral regurgitation to estimate left ventricular systolic pressure. *Am Heart J*. 1996 Oct; 132(4):884-6.

[7] Enriquez-Sarano M, Miller FA Jr, Hayes SN et al. Effective mitral regurgitant orifice area: clinical use and pitfalls of the proximal isovelocity surface areamethod. *J Am Coll Cardiol*. 1995; 25:703-9.

[8] Feigenbaum H, Armstrong WF, Ryan T. (2009.12.30). Feigenbaum's Echocardiography. Lippincott Williams & Wilkins. Philadelphia, USA

[9] Gramiak R, Shah PM, Kramer DH. Ultrasound cardiography: contrast studies in anatomy and function. *Radiology*. 1969 Apr; 92(5):939-48.

[10] Hall SA, Brickner ME, Willett DL et al. Assessment of mitral regurgitation severity by Doppler color flow mapping of the vena contracta. *Circulation*.1997; 95: 636-42.

[11] Himelman RB, Stulbarg M, Kircher B, et al. Noninvasive evaluation of pulmonary artery pressure during exercise by saline-enhanced Doppler echocardiography in chronic pulmonary disease. *Circulation.* 1989 Apr; 79(4):863-71.

[12] Izumi C, Yoshida K, Akasaka T et al. Improved visualization of pulmonary venous flow Doppler signal by intravenous injection of sonicated albumin. 1996 Sep 1; 78 (5):598-600.

[13] Kitzman DW, Goldman ME, Gillam LD et al. Efficacy and safety of the novel ultrasound contrast agent perflutren (Definity) in patients with suboptimal baseline left ventricular echocardiographic images. *Am J Cardiol.* 2000; 86:669-74.

[14] Kornbluth M, Liang DH, Brown P et al. Contrast echocardiography is superior to tissue harmonics for assessment of left ventricular function in mechanically ventilated patients. *Am Heart J.* 2000 Aug; 140(2):291-6.

[15] Masuyama T, Kodama K, Kitabatake A, et al. Continuous-wave Doppler echocardiographic detection of pulmonary regurgitation and its application to noninvasive estimation of pulmonary artery pressure. *Circulation.* 1986 Sep; 74 (3):484-92.

[16] Williams MJ, McClements BM, Picard MH et al. Improvement of transthoracic pulmonary venous flow Doppler signal with intravenous injection of sonicated albumin. *JAm Coll Cardiol* 1995;26:1741-1746.

[17] Mulvagh SL, Rakowski H, Vannan MA et al. American Society of Echocardiography Consensus Statement on the Clinical Applications of Ultrasonic Contrast Agents in Echocardiography. *J Am Soc Echocardiogr.* 2008 Nov;21 (11):1179-201.

[18] Nakatani S, Imanishi T, Terasawa A et al. Clinical application of transpulmonary contrast-enhanced Doppler technique in the assessment of severity of aortic stenosis. *J Am Coll Cardiol.* 1992; 20:973-

[19] Otto CM. Valvular aortic stenosis: disease severity and timing of intervention. *J Am Coll Cardiol.* 2006 Jun 6; 47(11):2141-51.

[20] Piscaglia F, Bolondi L. Italian Society for Ultrasound in Medicine andBiology (SIUMB) Study Group on Ultrasound Contrast Agents. The safety of SonoVue in abdominal applications: retrospective analysis of 23188 investigations. *Ultrasound Med Biol.* 2006; 32: 1369-75.

[21] Pu M, Prior DL, Fan X et al. Calculation of mitral regurgitant orifice area with use of a simplified proximal convergence method: initial clinical application. *J Am Soc Echocardiogr.* 2001; 14:180-5.

[22] Raisinghani A, Wei KS, Crouse L et al. POINT Investigators. Myocardial contrast echocardiography (MCE) with triggered ultrasound does not cause premature ventricular complexes: evidence from PB127 MCE studies. *J Am Soc Echocardiogr.* 2003; 16: 1037-42.

[23] Rossvoll O, Hatle LK. Pulmonary venous flow velocities recorded by transthoracic Doppler ultrasound: relation to left ventricular diastolic pressures. *J Am Coll Cardiol.* 1993 Jun; 21 (7):1687-96.

[24] Shah PM, Raney AA. Tricuspid valve disease. *Curr Probl Cardiol.* 2008 Feb; 33(2):47-84.

[25] Tabata T, Thomas JD, Klein AL. Pulmonary venous flow by doppler echocardiography: revisited 12 years later. *J Am Coll Cardiol.* 2003 Apr 16; 41 (8):1243-50.

[26] Terasawa A , Miyatake K, Nakatani S et al. Enhancement of Doppler Flow Signals in the Left Heart Chambers by Intravenous Injection of Sonicated Albumin. *J Am Coll Cardiol.* 1993;21:737-42.
[27] van de Brink RB, Verheul HA, Hoedemaker G, et al. The value of Doppler echocardiography in the management of patients with valvular heart disease: Analysis of one year of clinical practice. *J Am Soc Echo*. 1991; 4: 109-20.
[28] von Bibra H, Sutherland G, Becher H et al. Clinical evaluation of left heart Doppler contrast enhancement by a saccharide-based transpulmonary contrast agent. The Levovist Cardiac Working Group. *J Am Coll Cardiol*. 1995 Feb; 25(2):500-8.

9

Factors Influencing Doppler Blood Flow and its Measurements

Tie-Sheng Cao and Li-Jun Yuan
Fourth Military Medical University
China

1. Introduction

Doppler ultrasound has become one of the most important imaging modalities for measuring hemodynamic changes in various clinical settings. The accuracy of these measurements is the preconditioning to the appropriate interpreting of clinical observations and to the reasonable therapeutic strategy-makings. In this chapter, we studied two major factors that influence Doppler blood flow and its measurements. One is the intrathoracic pressure changes and the other is cardiac motion.

2. Research done by other researchers and our contribution

Respiration, including spontaneous and resistant respiration, can cause intrathoracic pressure changes, which would lead to Doppler flow alterations due to heart-lung interactions. Although spontaneous respiration on hemodynamics in humans has been studied and its regularity has been proved, quantitative evaluation of resistant respiration and forced maneuvers on hemodynamics and the underlying mechanisms has not been fully elucidated. We started to investigate comprehensively the factors that influence Doppler flow and its measurements fifteen years ago, and found that the introthoracic pressure changes have great impact on Doppler blood flow and its measurements both in healthy subjects and patients with cardiopulmonary diseases. We comprehensively and quantitatively assessed the influence of spontaneous respiration and resistant respiration on cardiac transvalvular blood flow, superior vana caval and pulmonary venous blood flow in both healthy subjects and patients with pericardial effusion and chronic obstructive pulmonary diseases.

It is well known that blood flow velocity measured by Doppler ultrasound represents the net motion of the blood relative to the transducer. It is widely assumed that the measured velocity represents the actual flow. However, if the cardiac chamber or valvular annulus surrounding the blood has independent motion relative to the transducer, the flow we need to measure will be influenced by the motion of the heart and therefore will be the vector sum of the chamber or annulus velocity and blood flow velocity. For example, the pulsed Doppler flow velocity signal at the left ventricular outflow tract or through the aortic annulus is usually obtained from the apical five-chamber view. The blood moving away from the transducer during systole is ejected into the aortic root through the aortic annulus, while the annulus itself is moving towards the transducer at the same period of time. If we need to measure the left ventricular stroke volume, we need the velocity of the blood relative to the aortic annulus, not to the transducer. While, the blood flow velocity "observed" by the transducer is only the velocity of the blood relative to the transducer. Therefore, cardiac output has been underestimated by the approach of Doppler echocardiography due to the aortic annulus motion opposite to the flow direction. On the other hand, Doppler echocardiography overestimates aortic flow routinely by measuring the outer edge of the spectrum. So, the routine Doppler method of stroke volume measurement seems to be accurate because the two errors are in the opposite direction and cancel each other. Similar situations will be encountered for right ventricular outflow or inflow tracts or the Doppler measurements of flow velocity of valvular stenosis or regurgitations. We think this problem of Doppler echocardiography should be stressed and the method of the correction of these errors should be explored as it has been either unrecognized or ignored in the clinical practice.

We designed an in vitro model that allowed us to observe and independently control the motion of a chamber containing a liquid and the motion of the liquid itself. This model enabled to observe the effects of the movement of the chamber on the Doppler signal derived from the motion of the liquid. We tested the hypothesis that cardiac motion can alter the velocity of the Doppler signal generated by blood flow in the in vitro model. We measured cardiac motion with M-mode echocardiography in human subjects (in vivo model) and compared the data with the Doppler signal generated by cardiac motion.

The in vitro and in vivo models were used in their study to demonstrate that cardiac motion can influence the measured Doppler signal generated by blood flow and to investigate the influence of the motion of the heart on measured velocity. In the in vitro model, the velocity of the cornstarch-water slurry and the motion of the apparatus were varied independently to simulate cardiac motion and blood flow. This procedure allowed us to separate the two components of the measured velocities. By stopping the motion of the piston, they could observe the pure flow profile, which could be kept constant. Similarly, the flow through the apparatus could be stopped, allowing us to measure the motion of the apparatus. They illustrated the potential alterations in peak velocities as well as changes in the slope of the velocity curve (acceleration) and were able to cause apparent changes in cycle length. Although some of the relations between the motion of tubing and the flow of the slurry do not appear naturally on a recurring basis, they illustrate the capacity of certain changes in timing to alter apparent flow patterns. Intermittent changes in cardiac motion relative to flow could be caused by atrial or ventricular ectopic activity or respirations, resulting in changes in cardiac motion. Because such changes might not be synchronized with flow alterations, changes in both the slope and the height of the Doppler signal might occur. The velocity of cardiac motion also varies throughout the cardiac cycle and therefore may not affect events at different parts of the cycle similarly. In measurements utilizing slopes, such as mitral valve half-time or pulmonary acceleration time, changes in cardiac motion might cause a significant change in a Doppler-derived measurement.

Their experiments in vitro and in vivo provided important information about the interaction of cardiac motion and blood flow in the Doppler spectrum. The measured Doppler spectrum of blood flow velocity is modified by cardiac motion and could be corrected for more accurate measurement.

In reviewing the previous study, we noticed that it is important to find that the measured Doppler spectrum of blood flow velocity is modified by cardiac motion in the in vitro model. However, in the experiment of the in vitro model, the simulated blood, the cornstarch-water slurry, was carried by the simulated vessel and, thus, the velocity of the simulated blood would naturally be the vector sum of the two motions, the motion of the simulated blood itself and the motion of the vessel, i. e., there should be no difficult to understand that the transducer would record a modified velocity. In the echocardiographic laboratory examination, however, if we need, for example, to measure the left ventricular stroke volume, the transducer should be located at the apex of the heart and directed to the base to display the 5-chamber view. During systole, the aortic valve is open and therefore, the aortic root does not carry the blood to move in any direction, which is not like the in vitro model's condition. Is the previous in vitro experiment still valid to provide the important information? To further confirm the previous conclusion and to find out if the conclusion is valid in the Doppler echocardiographic examination, we designed the following experiments.

3. Methods

3.1 Methods of studying the influence of intrathoracic pressure changes on Doppler flow

3.1.1 Doppler Echocardiography

Echocardiography was performed in all adult subjects with left decubitus position and spontaneous respiration by Siemens Sequoia 512 (Mountain View, CA, USA) with a 2.5-4.0 MHz transducer. Electrocardiogram and respiratory tracing by a nasal thermo-sensitive transducer (E99H450, fittings to Sequoia 512) were recorded simultaneously with echocardiograms. The protocol was approved by the Human Subjects Ethics Committee of the Fourth Military Medical University, and each subject provided an informed written consent.

The Doppler flow spectra across the four cardiac valves were recorded by pulsed Doppler echocardiography. The sample volume was put at the tips of mitral and tricuspid valves and 1 cm above the aortic and pulmonary valve. The superior vena cave (SVC) blood flow spectra were recorded by placing the transducer in the right supraclavicular region. The right-upper pulmonary venous flow was studied by pulsed Doppler from the apical four-chamber view, and the sample volume for Doppler examination was placed 0.5-1.0 cm into the right-upper pulmonary vein proximal to where it enters the left atrium and at an angle as parallel as possible to the direction of the blood flow.

3.1.2 Quantification of intrathoracic pressure

In order to quantify the influence of intrathoracic pressure on Doppler flow measurements, we developed an instrument that could quantify intrathoracic pressures. The device for quantification of intrathoracic pressure was refit by a watch sphygmomanometer, a mask and tubes. The examinees were told to press the mask tight against their nose and mouth, making the oral cavity and the thorax a closed system. Then, ask the examinees to inspire or expire through the mask of the device with their mouth open to generate negative or positive intrathoracic pressure changes. These pressure changes could be quantified and read directly from the attached watch sphygmomanometer.

3.2 Methods for studying the effect of cardiac motion on Doppler flow

We designed an in vitro model that allowed us to observe if the motion of the simulated blood vessel or heart chamber may modulate the Doppler spectrum of the motion of the simulated blood in it to further confirm the previous study. To test the hypothesis that cardiac motion can alter the velocity of the Doppler signal generated by blood flow and that the motion of the vessel would also influence the resultant flow velocity measurement, we used combined motion of the simulated blood vessel and the simulated blood flow. Using the measurement of left ventricular stroke volume as an example, we analyzed the error generated in the routine Doppler echocardiographic examination and proposed some approaches to correct it. We, then, discussed the theoretical meaning of the study.

3.2.1 Echocardiographic equipment

An Acuson Sequoia 256 ultrasound system with a 5- or 3-MHz transducer was used for the in vitro model experiments. Images were recorded on the hard disc in the equipment. Machine factors were adjusted as shows in the screen. It reads as follows: the pulsed Doppler transmit power was set at <100; the log compress was set at 35 dB; the length of the gate was 6.0mm; the width of the gate or the focus was 3mm. For the in vitro apparatus, the depth of the pulsed Doppler gate was 55mm, and the gate was placed within the middle of the straight portion of the tubing, away from the walls.

3.2.2 In vitro model

The in vitro model was designed to independently control the flow of simulated blood through a chamber and the motion of the chamber relative to the Doppler beam (Figure 1 and 2). A 220-cm length of silicon rubber tubing with an inner diameter of 6mm was connected to a variable pulse rate and flow velocity perfusion pump (Longer Pump YZ1515X). A 5% (5g Fiber/100ml tap water, equate Fiber Therapy, original texture.) fiber-water slurry was driven by the pulsatile pump through the tubing to simulate the blood flow within the vessel or heart chamber. Both the velocity of flow and the frequency could be independently controlled along a continuum. The flow rate for pulsatile flow through the pump was varied from 100 to 300ml/min, corresponding to average linear velocities of 8 to 25cm/s. A 6-cm section of the silicon tubing was fixed to a rigid plastic board (Figure 1b), and the board was cyclically moved by a specially designed machine (TD-4 cardiac motion simulator) to simulate the heart base motion. The tubing attached to the board was aligned with the echocardiographic transducer placed above it, and the motion of the board was parallel to the Doppler ultrasound beam as well. This eliminated possible artifacts from beam angulation. The pulsed Doppler gate was within the tubing, away from the wall and well above the curved portion of the tubing. The Doppler beam was parallel to the motion of the simulated blood and the tubing. The plastic board was coupled by means of gears, rubber bands and connectors to TD-4 cardiac motion simulator with a variable rate control. The board could be cyclically moved up and down to mimic the motion of cardiac base. Both the rate and the excursion of the board could be controlled and varied independently of the flow within the tubing. The motion of the board could be continuously varied over a range of velocities from 0.3 to 60cm/s, and its maximal excursion for these series of experiments was 1 to 2cm. This is comparable to the motion of cardiac base in humans (Strunk et al., 1976). The tubing and board were placed within a water bath, with the echocardiographic transducer above the vertical portion of the tubing.

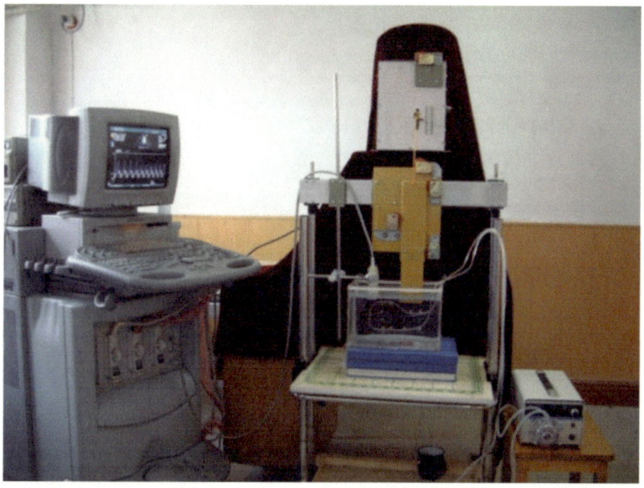

Fig. 1a. Photo of the whole set of the in vitro model experiment. From the right to the left of the photo the whole set is displayed. Right: the perfusion pump which drives the simulated blood in the tubing; Middle (from top to the bottom): the top is the TD-4 cardiac motion simulator (specially designed and home-made) that moves the plastic board up and down; the middle is the gears and connectors that connects the plastic board below; the bottom is the water tank with the plastic board in it. The tubing with 5% fiber-water slurry, the simulated blood, is fixed on the plastic board that is connected with the connector above. The plastic board with the tubing may move up and down freely by the simulator.
The echo transducer is separately fixed on the frame of the setup; Left: Ultrasound machine, Sequoia 256

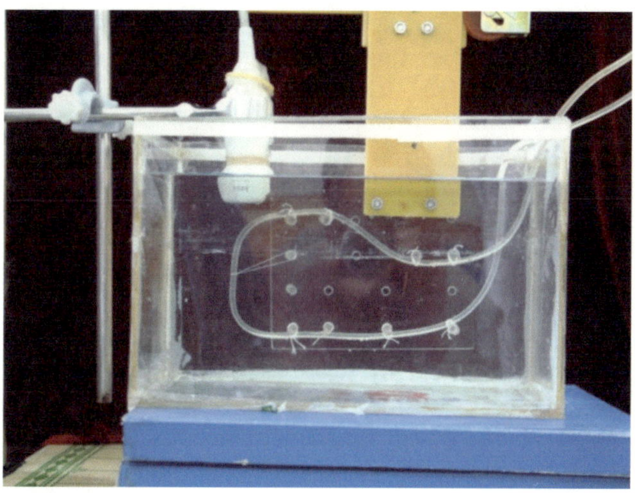

Fig. 1b. Photo of the plastic board. The board carries the tubing which should have a straight and vertical part outside the board

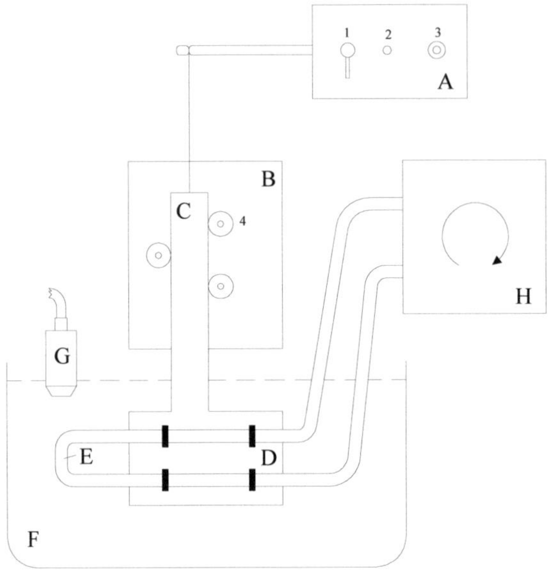

Fig. 2. Sketch of the in vitro model. A, the cardiac motion simulator; B, the connector with the gears; C, the connection of the connector with the plastic board; D, the plastic board that carries the tubing; E, the tubing with the fiber-water slurry in it; F, the water tank; G, the echocardiographic transducer

4. Results

4.1 Influence of the intrathoracic pressure changes on Doppler flow

4.1.1 Influence of spontaneous respiration on Doppler flow measurements in healthy subjects

4.1.1.1 Four cardiac valves

The transmitral and aortic Doppler flow velocities increased significantly on expiration compared on inspiration, while the tricuspid and pulmonary Doppler flow velocities increased significantly on inspiration compared on expiration (Figure 3-6, Table 1). The averaged respiratory variation index (RVI), which was calculated as the [(average velocity on expiration-the average velocity on inspiration)/average velocity on expiration] for mitral valve, aortic valve and pulmonary vein, and [(average velocity on inspiration-the average velocity on expiration)/average velocity on inspiration] for the four cardiac valves were shown in table 1.

	MV	AV	TV	PV
Inspiration	76.6±15.5	104.2±13.7	62.2±17.2	89.8±15.8
Expiration	83.8±17.7	109.4±14.1	52.8±14.1	84.8±15.0
RVI	8.4±3.7%	4. 7±2.0%	16.4±5.7%	5.7±2.6%

Note: MV, mitral valve; AV, aortic valve; TV, tricuspid valve; PV, pulmonary valve.

Table 1. Doppler flow velocities across the cardiac valves during expiration and inspiration and the respiratory variation index

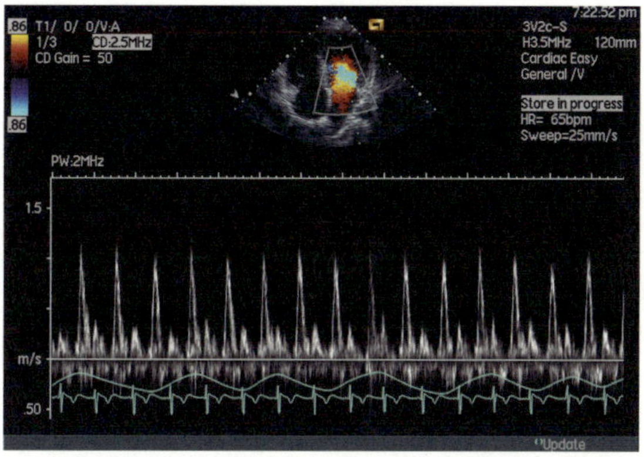

Fig. 3. The velocity across the mitral valve is decreased during inspiration and increased during expiration with RVI 8.4%. From top to the bottom are: color Doppler imaging, Doppler wave, respiratory wave (upward, inspiration; downward, expiration), and electrocardiogram

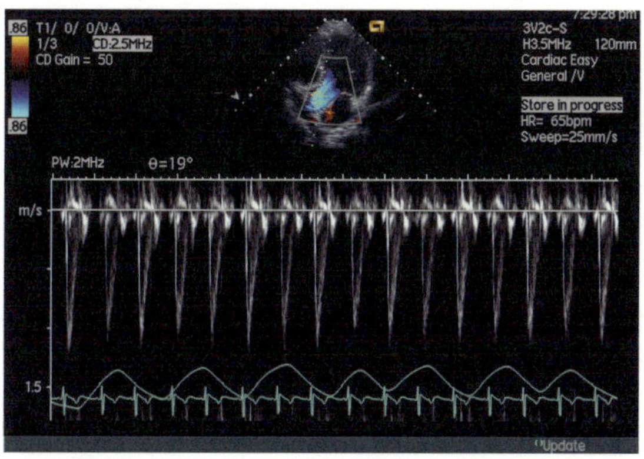

Fig. 4. The velocity across the aortic valve is decreased during inspiration and increased during expiration with RVI 4.7%

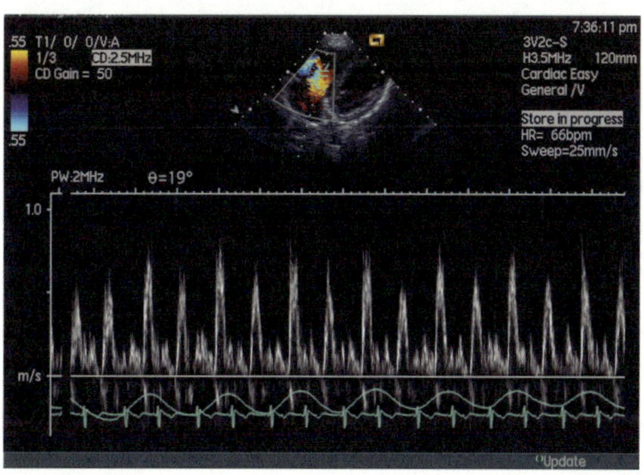

Fig. 5. The velocity across the tricuspid valve is increased during inspiration and decreased during expiration with RVI 16.4%

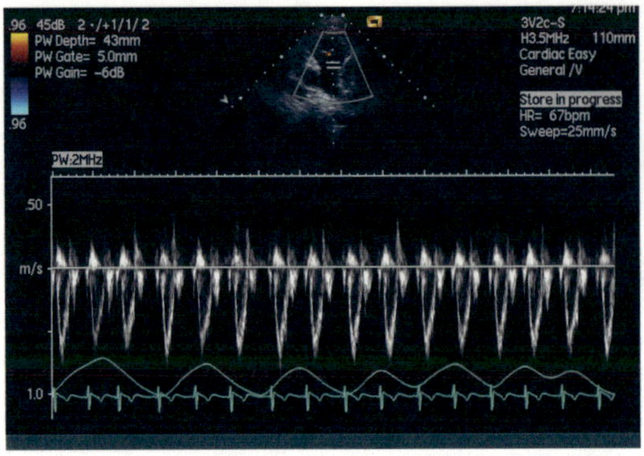

Fig. 6. The velocity across the pulmonary valve is increased during inspiration and decreased during expiration with RVI 5.7%

4.1.1.2 Pulmonary veins

The systolic peak flow velocity (PVs) and its integral (PV VTIs) of the pulmonary vein did not vary dramatically between inspiration and expiration; however, the diastolic peak flow velocity (PVd) and its integral (PV VTId) increased remarkably from inspiration to expiration, resulting in significantly decreased PVs/PVd and PV VTIs/PV VTId from inspiration to expiration.

4.1.1.3 Superior and inferior vena cava (SVC and IVC)

Both the systolic and diastolic peak flow velocities of SVC and IVC significantly increased from inspiration to expiration, while the reversed flow velocity during systole and diastole showed no significant difference between inspiration and expiration.

4.1.2 Influence of resistant respiration on cardiac valvular Doppler flow measurements in healthy subjects

There was no significant difference in RVIs between the spontaneous respiration and with the intrathoracic pressure change of -4mmHg, while significant difference in RVIs were found between the spontaneous respiration and with the intrathoracic pressure change of -8mmHg and -12mmHg, respectively (Figure 7-10, $p<0.01$).

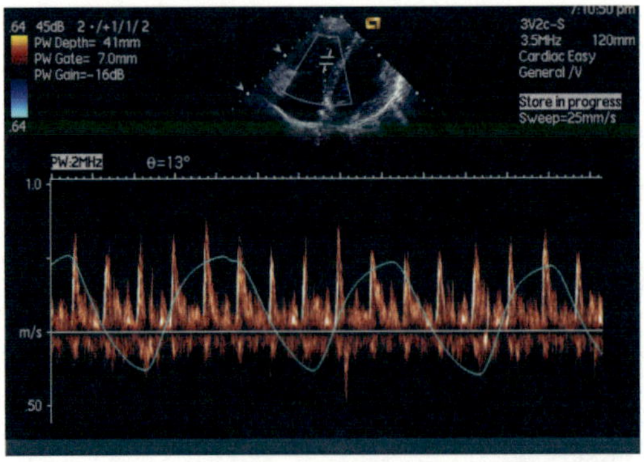

Fig. 7. Effects of spontaneous respiration on tricuspid flow. The velocity across the tricuspid valve is increased during inspiration and decreased during expiration with RVI 10.1%. From top to the bottom are: color Doppler imaging, Doppler wave, respiratory wave (upward, inspiration; downward, expiration), and electrocardiogram

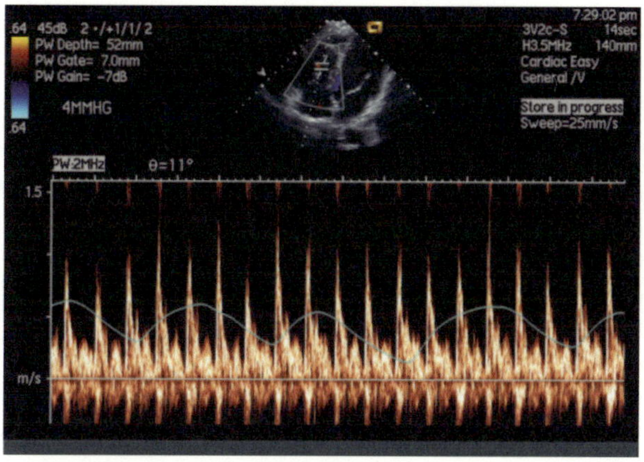

Fig. 8. Doppler spectra across the tricuspid valve with the intrathoracic pressure decrease of 4mmHg in the same subject as in figure 1. RVI is 11.35 %

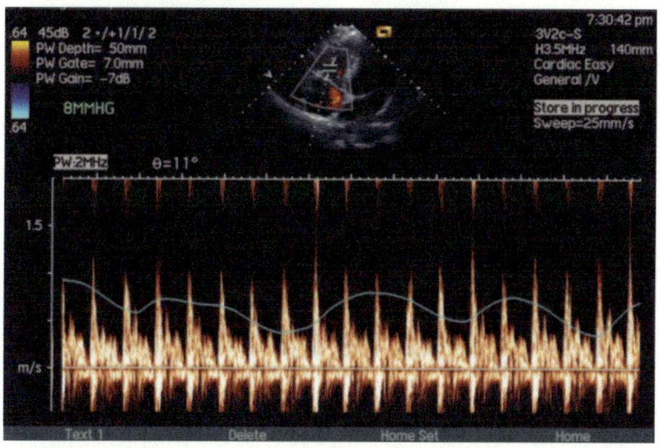

Fig. 9. Doppler spectra across the tricuspid valve with the intrathoracic pressure decrease of 8mmHg in the same subject as in figure 1. RVI is 19.0%

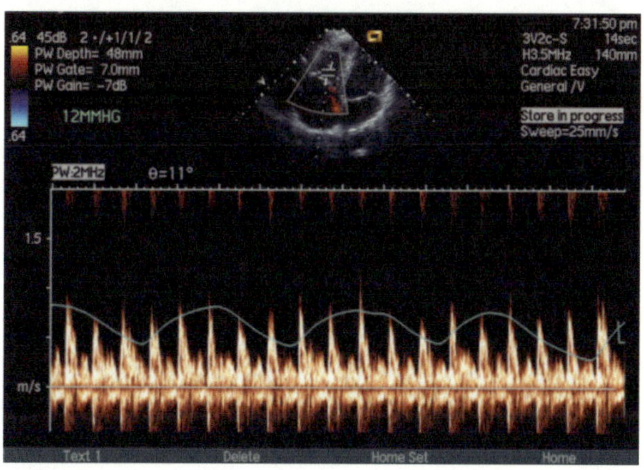

Fig. 10. Doppler spectra across the tricuspid valve with the intrathoracic pressure decrease of 12mmHg in the same subject as in figure 1. RVI is 21.3%

4.1.3 Influence of spontaneous respiration on Doppler flow measurements in patients with pericardial effusion

4.1.3.1 Four cardiac valves

In patients with pericardial effusion (PE), The RVI of the velocities across the mitral and the aortic valves increased significantly in patients with PE compared with normal subjects (Figure 11-14, Table 2).

Groups	MV	AV	TV	PV
Control	9.71±3.39	4.67±1.79	14.82±3.70	5.86±2.55
PE	14.57±7.89*	11.61±4.96**	24.97±6.19**	23.93±10.12**

Notes: PE, Pericardial effusion. *Compared to normal, $p<0.05$; **Compared to normal, $p<0.001$.

Table 2. Comparison of RVI between patients with PE and normal subjects

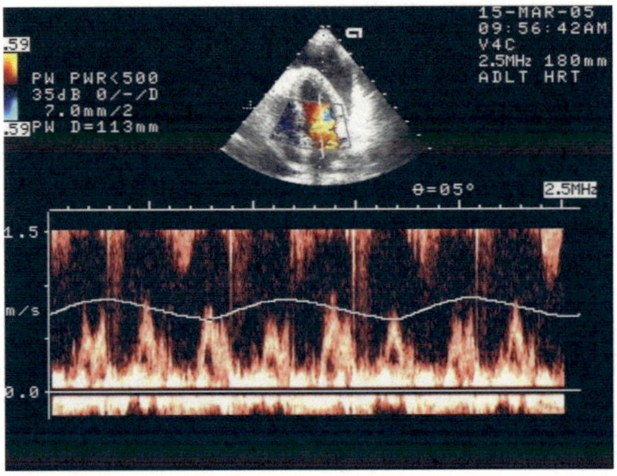

Fig. 11. RVI of the Doppler flow velocity across the mitral valve is significantly increased in a patient with large amount of pericardial effusion compared to normal subject shown in figure 1 (29.8% vs. 8.4%)

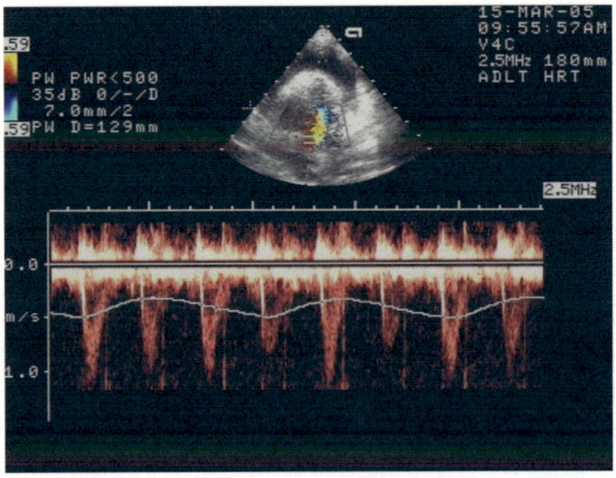

Fig. 12. RVI of the Doppler flow velocity across the aortic valve is significantly increased in a patient with large amount of pericardial effusion compared to normal subject shown in figure 2 (33.3% vs. 4.7%)

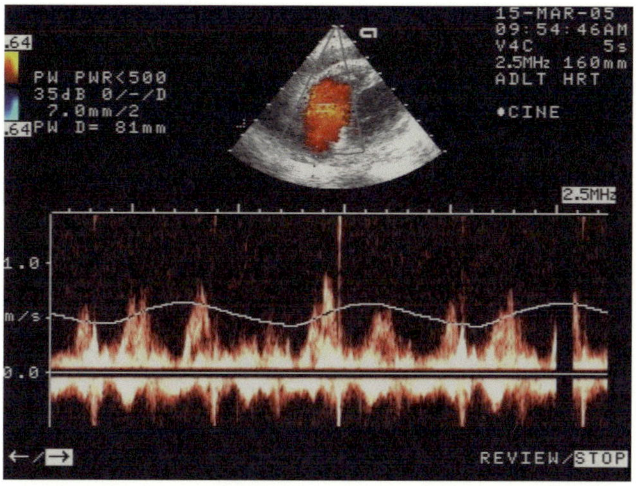

Fig. 13. RVI of the Doppler flow velocity across the tricuspid valve is significantly increased in a patient with large amount of pericardial effusion compared to normal subject shown in figure 3 (48.9% vs.16.4%)

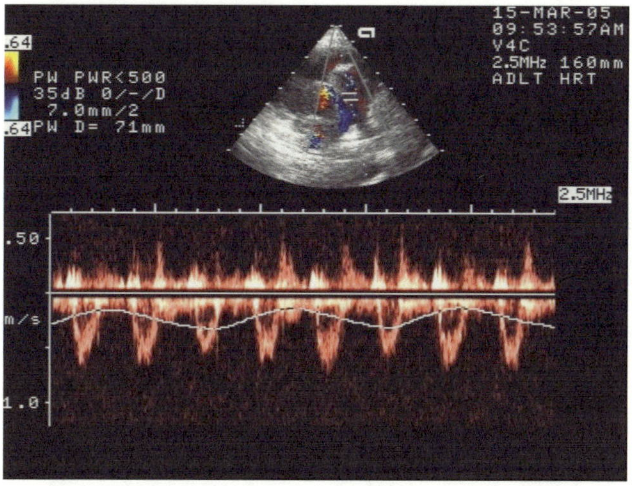

Fig. 14. RVI of the Doppler flow velocity across the pulmonary valve is significantly increased in a patient with large amount of pericardial effusion compared to normal subject shown in figure 4 (27.7% vs. 5.7%)

4.1.3.2 Inferior vena cava (IVC)

In patients with pericardial effusion, RVI of the systolic and diastolic peak flow velocities of IVC significantly increased compared to normal subjects ($p<0.001$).

4.1.4 Influence of spontaneous respiration on Doppler flow measurements in patients with chronic obstructive pulmonary disease (COPD)

RVI of the four cardiac valves in COPD patients were significantly higher than that in normal subjects (Figure 15-18; Table 3)

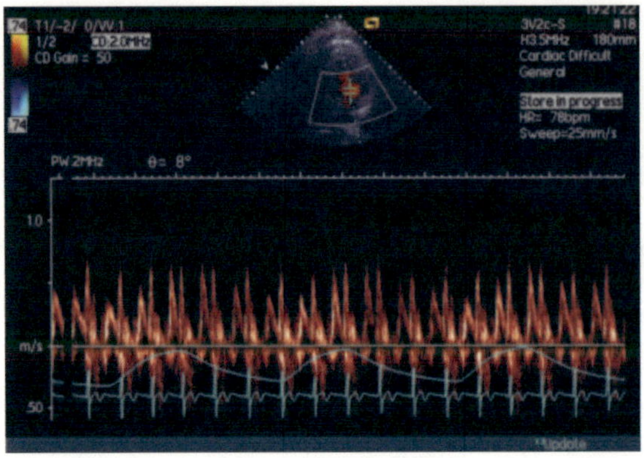

Fig. 15. RVI of the Doppler flow velocity across the mitral valve is significantly increased in a patient with obstructive pulmonary disease compared to normal subject shown in figure 1 (14.27% vs. 8.4%)

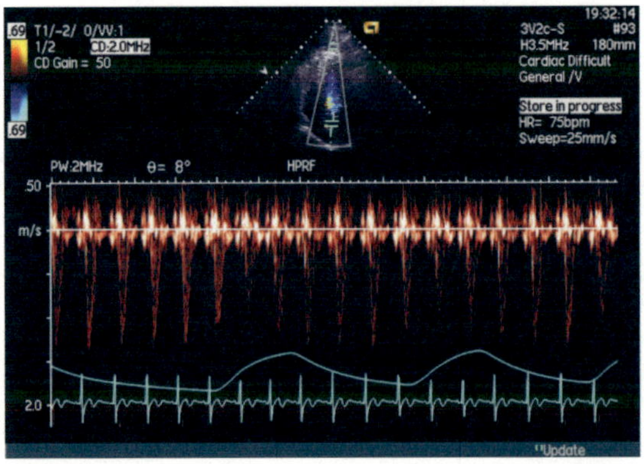

Fig. 16. RVI of the Doppler flow velocity across the aortic valve is significantly increased in a patient with obstructive pulmonary disease compared to normal subject shown in figure 1 (11.6% vs. 4.7%)

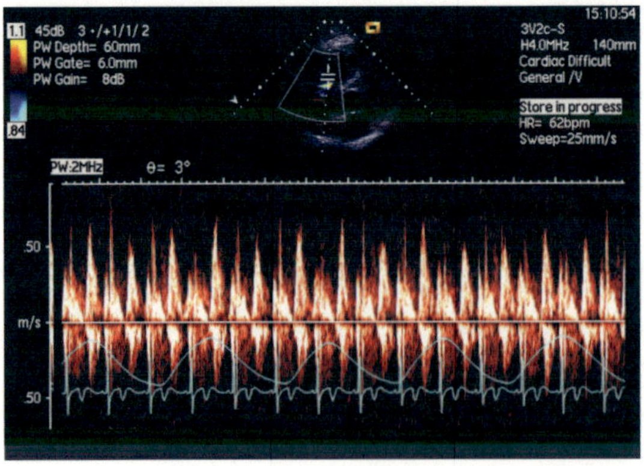

Fig. 17. RVI of the Doppler flow velocity across the tricuspid valve is significantly increased in a patient with obstructive pulmonary disease compared to normal subject shown in figure 1 (27.7% vs.16.4%)

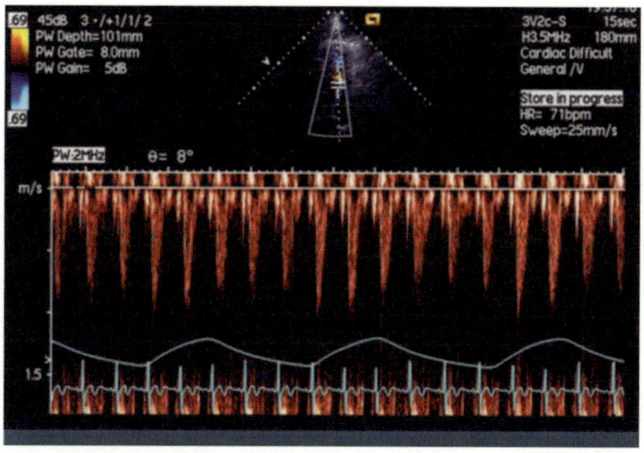

Fig. 18. RVI of the Doppler flow velocity across the pulmonary valve is significantly increased in a patient with obstructive pulmonary disease compared to normal subject shown in figure 1 (16.8% vs.5.7%)

Groups	MV	AV	TV	PV
Control	10.5±8.7	4. 7±1.8	14.9±6.3	8.6±2.3
COPD	16.3±8.7*	11.6±5.0**	27.7±8.4**	13.5±5.0**

Notes: COPD, Chronic obstructive pulmonary disease. *Compared to normal, p<0.05; **Compared to normal, p<0.001.

Table 3. Comparison of RVI between patients with COPD and normal subjects

With the whole set of the in vitro model devices, the Doppler spectra were recorded in series. Measurements of the velocity and amplitude of the tubing in the in vitro apparatus was either by the M-mode echocardiography or directly read from the Doppler blood flow velocity waveforms. The distance the tubing moved was determined by measuring the amplitude of the M-mode tracing of the tubing. It was compared with direct measurements of the distance that the apparatus moved. The sloped of the M-mode measurements represents the velocity of the tubing. We compared the M-mode measurements with the Doppler velocities obtained with the apparatus maintained at a constant speed.

4.2 Effect of cardiac motion on Doppler flow

Figures 19 to 21 demonstrate the Doppler signals derived from the motion of the silicon tubing, the motion of the fiber-water slurry within the tubing during peristaltic pumping and their combined motions. The motion of the tubing was parallel to the flow of the slurry within the tube. Figure 19 shows Doppler spectrum of the motion of the tubing being moved by TD-4 cardiac motion simulator while the fluid is not being pumped. The sample volume of the Doppler ultrasound is in the center of the tubing in figure 19. However, we noticed that we may record similar spectrum with the sample volume located anywhere outside the tubing, but close to it or to the plastic board. The apparent Doppler signal is a sinusoidal pattern with a maximal velocity of 15 cm/s and occurs regularly with a frequency of about 2 Hz. Figure 20 demonstrates a typical pulsed Doppler recording generated by the pulsatile motion of the fluid alone while the tubing is stationary. The maximal velocity is approximately 45 cm/s and occurs regularly with a frequency of about 4 Hz.

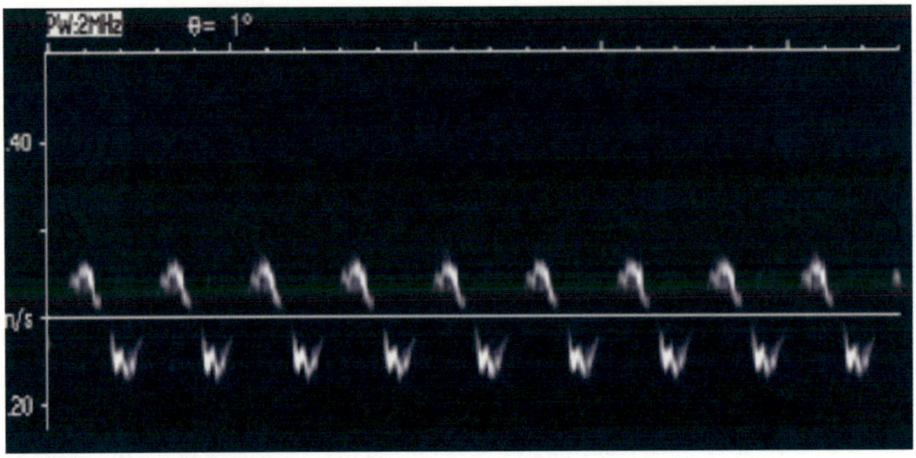

Fig. 19. Doppler signal derived from only the motion of the tubing. The fiber-water slurry is within the tubing but is not being pumped. The Doppler signal is generated entirely by the motion of the tubing, reflected by the fiber-water slurry

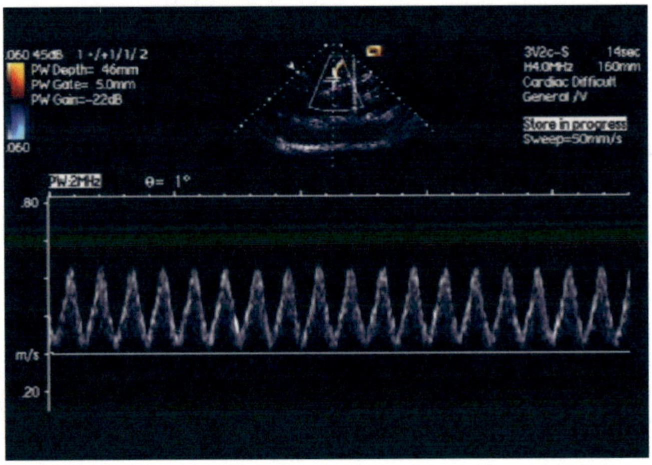

Fig. 20. Doppler signal derived from the pulsatile pumping of the simulated blood, the fiber-water slurry, while the tubing remains stationary

The complexity of the interaction between the motion of the tubing and the simulated blood is demonstrated in Figures 21, where the frequencies of the two motions are varied relative to each other. Flow of the simulated blood and motion of the tubing were controlled independently to create synchronized and desynchronized motion combination. We have recorded different combinations of the synchronized motions. But to make our description brief, we only use the desynchronized motion. The desynchronized motion actually covered the waveforms of all the motion combinations. In Figure 21, the frequency of the pulse rate of the peristaltic flow was slower than the motion of the tubing and is therefore slightly dissociated. This resulted in a continually varying alternant pattern of the peak amplitudes of the Doppler signals. The resultant waves change not only in amplitude (velocity), but also in apparent slope (acceleration and deceleration).

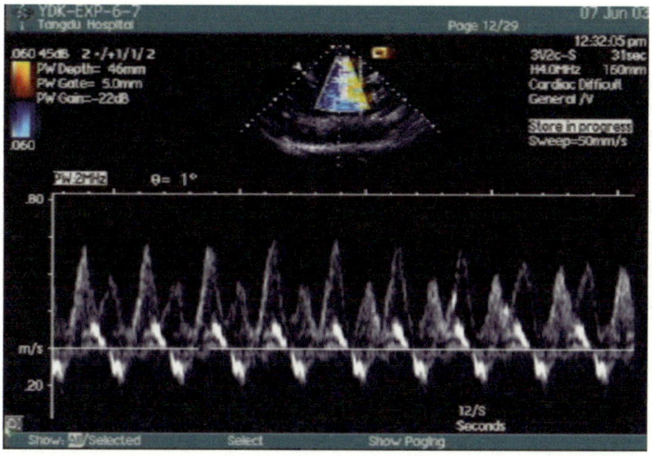

Fig. 21. Doppler signals generated by fluid and tubing motions. The frequency of the motion of the tubing and the frequency of the peristaltic pump were varied. The frequencies of two motions were very close, but desynchronized. The relative magnitude of the measured signals during the cycle varies even though the actual frequencies and velocities of motion and flow were constant. The two motions may have various phase combinations, yielding different modified Doppler flow velocity spectra

The Doppler signals of Figure 21 demonstrate the combined effect of motion of the tubing and flow through it. Although the actual velocity of the fluid through the tubing has not changed, its measured velocity has been altered by the motion of the tubing.

When the peak velocities are in phase (the ninth wave of the flow waveforms counted from the left side), the maximal velocities of both signals are additive, resulting in an increase in the measured velocity of the simulated blood. The maximal velocity of the wave is about 60 cm/s that equals to the algebraic sum of the two maximal velocities, 45 cm/s + 15 cm/s.

When the peak velocities are out of phase (the eighth wave of the flow waveforms counted from the left side in figure 21), they negate each other. The measured velocity is thus the vector sum of the two velocities. The maximal velocities of both signals are subtractive, resulting in a decrease in the measured velocity of the simulated blood. The maximal velocity of the wave is about 30 cm/s that equals to the subtraction of the two maximal velocities, 45 cm/s - 15 cm/s. Although flow through the tubing remains constant throughout, the desynchronized motion of the tubing (relative to the frequency of the pulsatile pump) results in an apparent twofold difference in velocity (30 to 60 cm/s) between adjacent peaks.

The waves of 16th and 17th in figure 21 (counted from left side of the figure) demonstrates the Doppler flow pattern when the frequency of the motion of the tubing and the pulsatile flow are out of phase but are integral multiples of each other. When the flow and movement of the tubing are at similar frequency but out of phase, the observed relationship may have this pattern. Although the flow of the simulated blood is unchanged, the velocity patterns are quite different. These patterns were achieved merely by changing the degree of phase synchronization of the motion of the tubing relative to the simulated blood. The resultant Doppler spectrum of the combined motion is the algebraic sum of their Doppler signals, resulting in apparent changes in maximal velocity as well as slope of the velocity curve. There are different combinations of the two motions in figure 21.

5. Discussion

The present study shows that both spontaneous and resistant respiration could have great impact on the Doppler flow velocity measurements, and this impact may be augmented in some diseased states, including pericardial effusion and chronic obstructive pulmonary diseases. The results of these experiments revealed the influence of intrathoracic pressure changes on Doppler blood flow and furthered the understanding of the mechanism of respiration-driven hemodynamics or heart-lung mechanical interactions that have remained controversial for over a century.

Similar findings of spontaneous respiration effects on Doppler flow velocities across the mitral and tricuspid valves in adults were reported previously (Dabestani et al., 1988). Some other studies investigated the influence of respiration on Doppler flow velocities across the mitral and tricuspid valves in children aged from 3 to 12.5 and from 1.5 to 11, respectively, and found that the early peak flow velocity across the mitral valve decreased 7% and 8% (Alehan, et al., 1996; Riggs, et al., 1989), which are similar to those in the adults shown in the present study.

The present study showed that the diastolic peak flow velocity and its integral increased remarkably from inspiration to expiration, resulting in significantly decreased PVs/PVd and PV VTIs/PV VTId from inspiration to expiration. The similar respiratory effects on the pulmonary venous flow were also demonstrated in one study using transesophageal pulsed Doppler echocardiography. In addition, this study showed that compared to the spontaneous respiration, Valsalva maneuver has greater impacts on the pulmonary venous flow (Meijburg et al., 1992). These effects should be considered when the pulmonary venous Doppler variables are applied for clinical purposes, and it would be of importance if considering the respiratory variation of the pulmonary venous flow when adopting PVs/PVd to identify pseudonormal left ventricular function.

In the condition of resistant respiration in normal subjects or in patients with chronic obstructive pulmonary diseases, in which the intrathoracic pressure changes are increased as in the resistant respiration, the impacts of respiration on Doppler flow measurements are much greater than that in normal subjects. Thus, the respiratory variation index may be an alternative parameter for assessing the severity and the therapeutic effect of COPD in clinic. This should be also applied in patients with pericardial effusion and the respiratory variation index of these Doppler flow velocities may better reflect the severity of pericardial effusion combined with the quantity of the fluid collection.

It has long been known that the interventricular septal shift that periodically occurs in the short-axis of the right ventricle and left ventricle is the key point of respiration-driven hemodynamics (Masuyama et al., 1986; Miller et al., 2006; Mitchell et al., 2005; Neumann et al., 2005). However, the mechanism of the septal shift has remained controversial.

In spite of its complexity, the circulatory system can be regarded hydromechanically as two enclosed fluid systems which are connected sequentially. One is the fully-intrathoracic fluid system, which includes the left ventricle, left atrium and pulmonary veins, and the other one is the partially-intrathoracic fluid system, which includes the right ventricle, right atrium and the vena cavae. Based on Pascal's law, the intrathoracic pressure changes during respiration may be transmitted without loss to all areas within the chest, including the fully-intrathoracic system. On the contrary, the intrathoracic pressure changes affect only the intrathoracic part, i.e., the right ventricle and atrium of the partially-intrathoracic system. With inspiration, the right ventricular pressure decrease will be mostly compensated by venous return from the peripheral veins. Thus, the pressure difference occurs between the two sides of the interventricular and atrial septa would push the septa to move toward the left ventricle and left atrium on inspiration, and vice versa. So the filling of the left ventricle and left atrium is impeded, and consequently the blood flow velocities across the mitral and aortic valves decrease on inspiration compared to those on expiration. In the condition of chronic obstructive pulmonary disease, the intrathoracic pressure changes is greater compared to normal subjects, thus, the respiratory variation of the cardiac blood flow velocities is increased. For the pericardial effusion where the pericardial pressure usually increases, the pressure difference between the two sides of the interventricular and atrial septa is exaggerated, and thus causes greater respiratory variation of these Doppler parameters.

The motion of blood cells within the heart or great vessels consists of the propulsion of blood cells driven by the contraction of the heart and the motion of blood cells as a component of the chamber, which is moving cyclically. In the past, the "flow" signal generated by cardiac motion was neglected.

The motion of the base of the heart has been observed by many investigators (Isaaz et al., 1993). Atrioventricular and semilunar valvular annuli and the fibrous framework in the adjacent tissues should have similar patterns of motion because they move together as part of the base of the heart (Ormiston et al., 1993). The blood flowing through the chambers or the great vessels will have independent motion relative to the transducer. What the transducer observes, for example, in the apical five-chamber view, is motion of the annuli toward the transducer during systole while blood is flowing in the opposite direction from the aorta. We mimic this with our apparatus. By positioning the tubing and motion of the board along the ultrasound beam of the transducer, we were able to eliminate problems of angle correction from our calculations. The impact of the twisting motion that occurs in normal hearts was not included in our in vitro analysis. Although the motion of the heart is complex, the ultrasound transducer observes only one-dimensional signals in both Doppler and M-mode studies.

Even though the Doppler sample volume had a focus of 3 mm within the central portion or bore of the tubing, we believe that the signals generated by the motion of the tubing are caused primarily by reflection of the ultrasound beam off the walls of the tubing and are a result of beam width. Some of this signal may also be generated by the fiber particles close to the wall, which move with the tubing as it accelerates. We placed the Doppler sample volume outside the tubing, in the water bath itself, and outside the cardiac chamber, within muscle (data not shown), and we were still able to record the Doppler signals, although they were much weaker. Whether the source of the signal is reflectors adjacent to the wall of the chamber, the chamber itself or beam width artifact, these signals alter the measured signal generated by blood flow, and the direction and timing of the alteration correlate with the motion of the chamber.

The measured Doppler spectrum of blood flow velocity in clinical echocardiography always has the built-in error caused by cardiac motion. The resultant spectrum is different from the pure spectrum, not only in the amplitude of the peak velocity but also in the slope of the measured velocity. Thus, cardiac motion can alter the velocity signals used to measure hemodynamic variables. In mitral inflow, for example, the maximal velocity, the half-time and the relation between the E and A waves could be altered by movement of the annulus. Because the direction and the velocity of the motion of the annulus vary throughout the cardiac cycle, the slopes of the E and A waves and their relative heights might not be affected equally. This observation may in part explain the difficulty in utilizing mitral inflow to analyze diastolic events (Shapiro et al., 1991). The changes seen in diastolic filling that are attributed to changes in compliance and relaxation might be overshadowed by the changes due to cardiac motion. This might further obscure the already difficult to understand effects of diastolic relaxation on the Doppler signal. Measurements of mitral valve area might also be inaccurate because of changes in slope caused by cardiac motion. Another example of problems that can be created by not considering the effect of cardiac motion on Doppler measurements is the use of the pulmonary artery flow acceleration time to diagnose pulmonary hypertension. Cardiac motion could alter the slope and therefore the acceleration time.

In this and our previous study, the in vitro models demonstrated an important phenomenon: the measured Doppler spectrum of blood flow velocity in clinical echocardiography has been modulated by the cardiac motion. The resultant spectrum is different from the pure spectrum. This may be easily understood as both the in vitro models used the tubing that carried the simulated blood. When the tubing is moving with a moving simulated blood in it, the velocity of the tubing motion is naturally added to the velocity of the blood. However, the clinical situation is different. In the Doppler echocardiographic settings, the heart chamber or the great vessels do not carry the blood moving. For example, the pulsed Doppler flow velocity signal at the left ventricular outflow tract or through the aortic annulus is usually obtained from the apical five-chamber view. The blood moving away from the transducer during systole is ejected into the aortic root through the aortic annulus, while the aortic valve is open and, thus, it does not carry the blood moving which is different from the situation of the in vitro models. So, it is hard to explain and compare the two situations. However, based on the theoretical analysis and our this study, we understood that when the blood is ejected into the aortic root in systole, the aortic annulus itself is moving towards the transducer at the same period of time. Now we may explain that the two motions in the opposite direction should be added. That means If we need to measure the left ventricular stroke volume, we need the velocity of the blood relative to the aortic annulus and that is the vector sum of the two velocities, or we may explain that the algebraic sum of the velocity of the aortic blood flow away from the transducer and the velocity of the aortic annulus towards the transducer is the net flow velocity of the blood relative to the annulus.

The measured Doppler spectrum of blood flow velocity in clinical echocardiography always has the built-in error caused by cardiac motion. We believe, however, that one could partially correct for the error generated by cardiac motion by using the M-mode recording to measure cardiac motion or by measuring the Doppler signal derived from the cardiac motion and using one of these to correct the measured Doppler velocity signal or we can use Doppler tissue imaging modality attached to some ultrasound equipments to measure the velocity of the adjacent annulus or wall and correct the error. These methods of correction may be useful, but they are time-consuming and not convenient in the clinical echocardiographic practice. New, simple and convenient methods need to be explored.

With the development of Doppler tissue imaging (DTI), the direct measurement of the tissue velocity becomes available (Isaaz et al., 2000). Using DTI, the velocity measurements of the cardiac chamber walls or valvular annuli become convenient and simple. We are now on the work of this research and hope get the results soon. As mentioned above, the routine

Doppler method of hemodynamic data analysis, for example, the stroke volume measurement seems to be accurate because the two errors are in the opposite direction and cancel each other. In addition to correct the errors of the Doppler spectra caused by cardiac motion, we need to explore new modality of tissue velocity measurement. The use of the outer edge of Doppler spectrum as the velocity will overestimate the value and to obtain accurate blood flow velocity measurement, we need to explore a method to obtain the average special velocity of the blood cells in the measured cross-section of the vessel at any moment and then we may have an accurate flow velocity curve. To correct these errors, there is much to be done.

6. Conclusion

Intrathoracic pressure change is one of the factors that influence Doppler blood flow and its measurements. These effects should be considered when applying these parameters for clinical purposes. In addition, the respiratory variation index may be an alternative parameter for assessing the respiratory-related hemodynamic changes both in normal condition and in patients. The measured Doppler spectrum of blood flow velocity in clinical echocardiography always has the built-in error caused by cardiac motion. The resultant spectrum is different from the pure spectrum, not only in the amplitude of the peak velocity but also in the slope of the measured velocity. In addition to correct the errors of the Doppler spectra caused by cardiac motion, we need to explore new modality of tissue velocity measurement.

7. References

Alehan FK., Ozkutlu S., Alehan D (1996). Effects of respiration on left ventricular diastolic function in healthy children. *Eur Heart J,* Vol 17, No.3, pp. 453-456.

Dabestani A., Takenaka D., Allen B., et al (1988). Effects of spontaneous respiration on diastolic left ventricular filling assessed by pulsed Doppler echocardiography. *Am J Cardiol,* Vol 61, No.15, pp. 1356-1358.

Isaaz K., Munoz L., Lee E., et al (1993). Quantitation of the cardiac base motion in normal man by Doppler echocardiography. J Am Soc Echo, Vol 6, No. 2, pp. 166 –176.

Isaaz K (2000). What are we actually measuring by Doppler tissue imaging? J Am Coll Cardiol, Vol 36, No. 3, pp. 897–899.

Masuyama T., Uematsu M., Sato H., et al (1986). Pulmonary arterial end-diastolic pressure noninvasively estimated by continuous wave Doppler echocardiography. *J Cardiogr,* Vol 16, No. 3, pp. 669-675.

Meijburg HW., Visser CA., Westerhof PW, et al (1992). Normal pulmonary venous flow characteristics as assessed by transesophageal pulsed Doppler echocardiography. *J Am Soc Echocardiogr,* Vol 5, No. 6, pp. 588–597.

Miller JD., Smith CA., Hemauer SJ, et al (2006). The effects of inspiratory intrathoracic pressure production on the cardiovascular response to submaximal exercise in health and chronic heart failure. *Am J Physiol Heart Circ Physiol.* Vol 292, No.1, pp. H580-592.

Mitchell JR., Sas R., Zuege DJ., et al (2005). Ventricular interaction during mechanical ventilation in closed-chest anesthetized dogs. *Can J Cardiol,* Vol 21, No. 1, pp. 73-81.

Neumann P., Schubert A., Heuer J (2005). Hemodynamic effects of spontaneous breathing in the post-operative period. *Acta Anaesthesiol Scand*, Vol 49, No. 10, pp. 1443-1448.

Ormiston JA., Shah PM., Tei C., et al (1981). Size and motion of the mitral valve annulus in man-A two-dimensional echocardiographic method and findings in normal subjects. Circulation, Vol 64, No. 1, pp. 113-120.

Riggs TW., Snider AR (1989). Respiratory influence on right and left ventricular diastolic function in normal children. *Am J Cardiol*, Vol 63, No. 12, pp. 858-861.

Shapiro SM., Bersohn MM., Laks MM (1991). In search of the Holy Grail: the study of diastolic ventricular function by use of Doppler echocardiography. J Am Coll Cardiol,Vol 17, No.7, pp. 1145-1147.

Strunk BL, Fitzgerald JW, Lipton M, et al (1976). The posterior aortic wall echocardiogram: its relationship to left atrial volume change. Circulation, Vol 54, No.5,pp. 774-750.

10

The Importance of Doppler-echocardiography in the Assessment of the Athlete's Heart

Gábor Pavlik and Zsuzsanna Kneffel
Department of Health Sciences and Sports Medicine, Faculty of Physical Education and Sports Sciences, Semmelweis University
Hungary

1. Introduction

Summarizing observations of several authors characteristics of the athlete's heart can be divided into three groups:

- morphological characteristics, among which the most important modification of athlete's heart is a marked left ventricular (LV) hypertrophy,
- functional characteristics, which could mean better systolic and diastolic function and
- regulatory characteristics, a higher parasympathetic and a lower sympathetic activity at rest, resulting mostly in a lower heart rate, lower cardiac output, circumferential shortening velocity (*Pavlik et al. 2010*).

In the general medical practice LV hypertrophy is considered as a risk factor caused by some diseases as hypertension, obesity, cardiomyopathy, etc. To separate pathological and physiological hypertrophy the most important factors are functional and regulatory characteristics of the heart which can be mostly detected by Doppler-echocardiography.

2. The importance of Doppler-echocardiography in the distinguishing between physiologic and pathological left ventricular hypertrophy

2.1 Flow velocities

With the help of Doppler echocardiography the flow velocities and the time durations of different intervals can be estimated. The ratio between the early and late peak velocities (E/A) is linearly proportional to the diastolic function, i.e. to the ventricular distensibility. Data of different authors are in accordance that against the LV hypertrophy, E/A quotient does not decrease in athletes. Whether it is higher in athletes, or there is no difference between athletic and non-athletic groups, data are discordant. Based on different data and on our own investigations it seems that in young age, when diastolic function is perfect also in non-athletic subjects, regular physical training does not cause a marked improvement. If there is any, it is manifested in the male endurance athletes. It seems to be more probable; however, that regular physical activity attenuates the age-associated impairment of the diastolic function. A collection of data is shown in the Table 1.

AUTHORS	STUDY	RESULT
Shapiro, Smith 1983	different athletes	=
Granger et al. 1985	different athletes	=
Fagard et al. 1987	cycle racers	=
Missault et al. 1993	cycle racers	=
Pearson et al. 1986	weight lifters	=
Pavlik et al. 2001	children athletes	=
Pavlik et al. 1999a	women athletes	=
Vinereanu et al. 2001	power athletes	=
D'Andrea et al. 2007	power athletes	=
Perseghin et al. 2007.	different athletes	=
Teske et al. 2009.	different athletes	=
Matsuda et al. 1983	different athletes	+
Colan et al. 1985	different athletes	+
Douglas et al. 1986	triathlonists	+
Möckel et al. 1992	triathlonists	+
Finkelhor et al. 1986.	endurance athletes	+
Pavlik et al. 2001	different athletes	+
Vinereanu et al. 2001	runners	+
Rodrigues et al. 2006	6 months training	+
D'Andrea et al. 2007	endurance athletes	+
Spurgeon et al.1983	animal experiments	+
Starnes et al. 1983	animal experiments	+
Tate et al. 1990	animal experiments	+
Gwathmey et al. 1990	animal experiments	+
Schulman et al. 1992	older humans	=
Fleg et al. 1995	older humans	=
Sadaniantz et al. 1996	1 yr training in older humans	=
Baldi et al. 2003.	older humans	=
Teske et al. 2009.	older humans	=
Takemoto et al. 1992	older humans	+
Douglas, O'Toole 1992	older humans	+
Levy et al. 1993	6 months training in older humans	+
Pavlik et al. 2001	older humans	+
Galetta et al. 2004	older humans	+
Limongelli et al. 2006	older soccer players	+
Prasad et al. 2007	older humans	+

Table 1. Effect of regular physical training on the E/A quotient in different studies.
= : physically trained hearts and non-trained hearts show similar values, + : physically trained hearts demonstrates an increased quotient

In our studies altogether 3076 subjects of different ages have been investigated since 1994 until now. The number of males was 1896 (non-athletic: 243, physically trained: 1653), number of females was 1180 (non-athletic 290, physically trained: 890). Results are shown in the Figure 1.

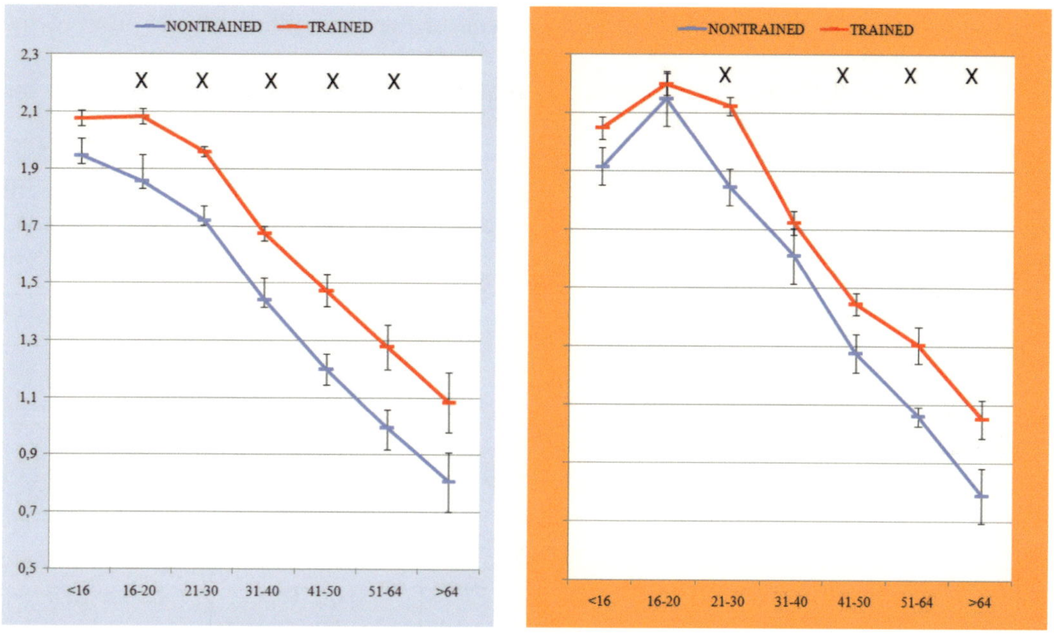

Fig. 1. The E/A quotient in the function of age in athletic (red lines) and non-athletic (blue lines) males (left graph) and females (right graph) (mean ± s.e.m.). x: significant difference ($p < 0.05$)

Results are quite similar to those published in our older studies (*Pavlik et al. 1999a, 1999b, 2001*). In the younger groups LV distensibility is very good also in the non-athletic subjects; regular physical training does not induce a further improvement. In the adult and older groups E/A of the athletic groups is markedly higher than that of non-athletic groups.

In the evaluation of E/A it is disturbing that the quotient is inversely related to the heart rate: the higher is the heart rate, the lower is the E/A. The bradycardia of the athlete's heart is well known, sometimes it is very difficult to establish: the higher E/A of some athletic groups is a consequence of their lower heart rate, or it is an independent effect of the regular physical training. In our recent analysis heart rate dependent equations of the E/A quotient were compared between athletic and non-athletic subjects in different ages. It seems that in young subjects differences can be attributed to the frequency differences, while in older subjects the higher E/A is an independent effect of regular physical activity (*Kneffel et al. 2011*).

2.2 Cardiac cycle intervals

Bradycardia of the athlete's heart results significantly longer duration of the cardiac cycle in athletes than in non-athletes, there are, however, very few reports about the training induced modifications of the different phases of the cardiac cycle. Doppler echocardiographic investigations help to reveal differences between the modifications of the different phases and sub phases. In our previous study (*Pavlik et al. 1999b*) in 221 male athletes and non athletes we made two main establishments.

1. There is one period, which is definitely increased in the athletes: it is the E-A period, i.e. the period of diastasis extending from the end of the early filling till the onset of the atrial systole.
2. The lengths of the two main cardiac phases are also different: the proportion of the systole is decreased in the athlete's heart.

Our further investigations confirmed the above mentioned establishments. Our data since 1994 until now are summarized in the Table 2 and 3. In this analysis data of different athletes were collected to common groups, in the tables data of 19-35 yr. old 846 males (62 non-athletes and 784 athletes) and 561 females (84 non-athletes and 477 athletes) are demonstrated.

Interval	Non-athletes		Athletes	
	Abs. (ms)	Rel. (%)	Abs. (ms)	Rel. (%)
ICT	41.2 ± 13.2	4.62 ± 1.58	**46.4 ± 19.7**	4.31 ±1.78
AOAT	91.5 ± 18.6	10.37 ± 2.21	93.6 ± 16.5	**8.81 ± 1.75**
AODT	190.6 ± 20.4	21.28 ± 2.81	**205.7 ± 24.6**	**19.1 ± 2.69**
SYSTOLE	323.6 ± 30.0	36.28 ± 4.45	**345.5 ± 36.8**	**32.25 ± 4.22**
IVRT	77.9 ± 20.5	8.95 ± 2.55	**88.4 ± 21.6!**	**8.29 ± 2.11**
EACC	87.6 ± 14.3	9.81 ± 1.69	**95.7 ± 16.3**	**8.94 ± 1.72**
EDT	147.4 ± 42.0	16.06 ± 3.81	155.5 ± 34.6	**14.36 ± 3.18**
E-A	108.6 ± 82.3	11.30 ± 7.48	**233.5 ± 136.7**	**20.27 ± 9.50**
A	157.4 ± 36.1	17.60 ± 4.00	**169.6 ± 39.2**	**15.90 ± 4.06**
DIASTOLE	579.0 ± 109.9	64.2	**742.0 ± 154.1**	68.2
TOTAL	902 ± 121.4		**1087.5 ± 121.4**	

Table 2. Absolute and relative time durations of the cardiac cycle (mean ± s.d.) in 19-35 yr. old men. ICT: isovolumetric contraction time, AOAT: acceleratory phase of the aortic flow, AODT: deceleratory phase of the aortic flow (=decreased ejection), IVRT: isovolumetric relaxation time, EACC: acceleratory phase of the early transmitral flow (E), EDT: deceleratory phase of the early transmitral flow (E), E-A: a period from the end of the early transmitral flow (E) to the beginning of the atrial systole (A) (diastasis), A: atrial systole. Bold numbers: significant difference from the control values, where $p < 0.05$

Interval	Non-athletes		Athletes	
	Abs. (ms)	Rel. (%)	Abs. (ms)	Rel. (%)
ICT	38.2 ± 11.9	4.46 ± 1.58	**43.7 ± 16.2**	4.19 ±1.57
AOAT	87.6 ± 16.6	10.30 ± 2.22	**92.0 ± 15.9**	**8.92 ± 1.95**
AODT	198.3 ± 21.9	23.00 ± 3.20	**214.6 ± 22.2**	**20.5 ± 2.99**
SYSTOLE	325.9 ± 27.6	37.76 ± 4.98	**350.4 ± 30.8**	**33.61 ± 4.53**
IVRT	77.4 ± 18.5	9.18 ± 2.02	**85.8 ± 19.5**	**8.23 ± 2.01**
EACC	83.7 ± 14.7	9.65 ± 1.71	**91.6 ± 13.0**	**8.82 ± 1.70**
EDT	135.8 ± 30.6	15.18 ± 2.98	**155.0 ± 32.5**	14.69 ± 3.06
E-A	81.2 ± 73.8	8.58 ± 6.81	**207.4 ± 138.8**	**18.12 ± 9.85**
A	171.7 ± 42.9	19.65 ± 4.09	172.9 ± 39.9	**16.54 ± 4.04**
DIASTOLE	549.6 ± 111.1	62.8	**712.9 ± 161.4**	67.1
TOTAL	875.5 ± 117.9		**1062.5 ± 176.7**	

Table 3. Absolute and relative time durations of the cardiac cycle (mean ± s.d.) in 19-35 yr. old women. ICT: isovolumetric contraction time, AOAT: acceleratory phase of the aortic flow, AODT: deceleratory phase of the aortic flow (=decreased ejection), IVRT: isovolumetric relaxation time, EACC: acceleratory phase of the early transmitral flow (E), EDT: deceleratory phase of the early transmitral flow (E), E-A: a period from the end of the early transmitral flow (E) to the beginning of the atrial systole (A) (diastasis), A: atrial systole. Bold numbers: significant difference from the control values, where $p < 0.05$

It is quite obvious that due to training bradycardia, the cardiac cycle of the athletes is longer. The contribution of the different phases can be seen on the tables. There is a basic difference in the elongation of the systole and of the diastole: systole is slightly (6.8 % in males, 7.5 % in females) longer in athletes, while the difference in the diastole is very definite (28.2 % and 29.7 % respectively).

The absolute duration of most of the subphases are a little longer in athletes. This increase can be attributed due to the resting bradycardia, but it is not proportional to the elongation of the whole cardiac cycle, the relative durations are decreased. There is only one period which shows a definite increase in absolute as well as in relative duration: E-A, i.e. the period from the end of the early phase to the beginning of late filling, when flow velocity is minimal or zero. This phase seems to be the most sensitive to the exercise training.

If we investigate the stability or variability of the different periods of the cardiac cycle, the ratio of the standard deviations to the mean absolute values can be calculated. Results are indicated in Table 4.

	Males		Females	
Period	non-athletes	athletes	non-athletes	athletes
ICT	32.0	42.5	31.1	37.1
AOAT	20.3	17.6	18.9	17.3
AODT	10.7	11.6	11.0	10.3
SYSTOLE	9.3	10.7	8.5	8.8
IVRT	26.3	24.4	23.9	22.7
EACC	16.3	17.0	17.6	14.2
EDT	28.5	22.3	22.5	21.0
E-A	75.8	58.5	90.9	66.9
A	22.9	23.1	25.0	23.1
DIASTOLE	19.0	20.8	20.2	22.6
TOTAL	13.5	11,2	13.5	16.6

Table 4. Ratio of the standard deviation to the mean value of different periods of the cardiac cycle in male and female subjects (s.d./mean)

Systole is more stable than diastole. Among the sub phases of the cardiac cycle in which an active flow is occurring are the most stable: AOAT, AODT, EACC, EDT. It is outstanding that the phase from the end of E to the beginning of A (E-A period) is very variable: its coefficient of variation is much higher than those of other periods.

The stability of systole is quite obvious: the pumping function, the ejection of the blood needs a rapid, abrupt contraction in any case, so it cannot be much longer even in case of the bradycardia of the athletic heart. All that means that training bradycardia arises from the elongation of diastole, which means a more economic cardiac function: longer relaxation time, more time for recovery and, as coronary circulation is free only during diastole, better coronary circulation.

Considering all cardiac phases, the greatest variability was seen in the period occurring between the end of the E and the beginning of the A phase, i.e. during which transmitral flow is practically minimal: the period of diastasis. This period is the most variable among all of the periods; the s.d./mean ratio of the absolute length is above 50 % in both groups. Thus, it seems that this is the period that can be modified to the greatest extent; training bradycardia seems to develop through elongation of this period.

Periods of the cardiac cycle seem to provide further data on the function and regulation of the athletic heart. Some data and some indices may widen the arsenal of the different signs characterising of the athlete's heart. Our data indicate that the E-A period, namely the diastasis period of the diastolic filling is the most characteristic of the physically trained heart.

3. Tissue Doppler echocardiography

During the last two decades the used of the methods has been richer with the Tissue Doppler Imaging (TDI) technique. The main advantage of this method is that it offers direct measurements of local myocardial movements and velocities, it is less dependent on hemodynamic conditions and it makes also possible to establish wall movements at different segments of the heart. These advantages are used mostly in clinical cardiology for detailed investigations of some cardiac diseases or damages. The method has been introduced to the sports medicine as well. Several authors compared cardiac morphology, traditional Doppler and TDI indices of athletes to those of non-athletic healthy subjects and some cardiac patients (*Caso et al. 2000, Vinereanu et al. 2001, Baldi et al. 2003, Galetta et al. 2004, Kasikcioglu et al. 2006, Rodrigues et al. 2006, D'Andrea 2007, Prasad et al. 2007, Caselli et al. 2009*). An extensive review has been published recently (*Krieg et al. 2007*).

The main advantages of the TDI vs. traditional Doppler investigations in the sports medicine can be summarized as follows:

1. TDI results are less dependent on the heart rate than the traditional transmitral Doppler investigation findings (*Caso et al. 2000, Baldi et al. 2003*),
2. it offers a new index: ratio of the blood flow to tissue movement velocity (E/E′) is inversely related to the LV filling pressure and hence, it is postulated to be lower in athletes (*Baldi et al. 2003, Kasikcioglu et al. 2006*),
3. it is not excluded that an enhanced systolic wall movement velocity (S′) might show a better dynamic systolic function of the athletes heart (*Baldi et al. 2003, Rodrigues et al. 2006, D'Andrea 2007*).

During the last years we also made some investigations with TDI, our results are presented in the focus of the above mentioned three points.

1. Correlation coefficients between heart rate and the transmitral E/A and TDI determined E′/A′ quotients were established in 19-35 yr old males and females (Table 5 and 6).

Heart rate / E/A	N	r	p
Transmitral E/A	144	**-0.305**	**< 0.001**
Mitr. med. E′/A′	144	-0.090	> 0.2
Mitr. lat. E′/A′	144	-0.080	> 0.3
Tric. med. E′/A′	144	-0.068	> 0.4
Tric. lat. E′/A′	144	-0.130	> 0.1

Table 5. Correlation coefficients between heart rate and E/A quotients in 19-35 yr old males. E: early phase of the diastolic filling, A: late (atrial) phase of the diastolic filling, E′, A′: TDI determined velocities

Heart rate / E/A	N	r	p
Transmitral E/A	44	**-0.366**	**< 0.02**
Mitr. med. E'/A'	44	**-0.517**	**< 0.001**
Mitr. lat. E'/A'	44	-0.181	> 0.2
Tric. med. E'/A'	44	-0.090	> 0.5
Tric. lat. E'/A'	44	-0.002	> 0.9

Table 6. Correlation coefficients between heart rate and E/A quotients in 19-35 yr old females
E: early phase of the diastolic filling, A: late (atrial) phase of the diastolic filling, E', A': TDI determined velocities

Results indicate that the disturbing effect of the heart rate is really stronger in case of the E/A, both in males and in females significant correlations were found. Relationship is much poorer with E'/A' values: it was only the mitral medial wall movement which correlated significantly with heart rate in women, the other r values were negative but not significant.

2. E/A, TDI determined E'/A', E/E' and S' values are indicated in the Table 7.

	Males		Females	
	Non athletes	Athletes	Non athletes	Athletes
E/A	**1.63 ± 0.34**	**1.93 ± 0.40**	**1.88 ± 0.55**	**2.08 ± 0.55**
Mitr. med. E'/A'	**1.56 ± 0.49**	**1.88 ± 0.62**	**1.54 ± 0.39**	**2.01 ± 0.60**
Mitr. med. E/E'	6.99 ± 1.27	7.48 ± 1.50	7.58 ± 1.12	7.77 ± 1.47
Mitr. med. S'	0.088 ± 0.013	0.088 ± 0.015	0.088 ± 0.015	0.084 ± 0.013
Mitr. lat. E'/A'	2.56 ± 0.59	2.69 ± 0.97	2.26 ± 0.68	2.43 ± 0.93
Mitr. lat. E/E'	5.76 ± 1.98	5.07 ± 2.07	6.30 ± 1.71	5.62 ± 1.47
Mitr. lat. S'	0.11 ± 0.030	0.12 ± 0.033	0.10 ± 0.015	0.12 ± 0.024
Tric. med. E'/A'	1.94 ± 0.21	2.01 ± 1.05	2.09 ± 1.06	2.05 ± 0.62
Tric. med. S'	0.094 ± 0.014	0.098 ± 0.026	0.088 ± 0.012	0.091 ± 0.013
Tric. lat. E'/A'	1.59 ± 0.86	1.65 ± 0.67	1.50 ± 0.36	1.94 ± 0.66
Tric. lat. S'	0.137 ± 0.022	0.140 ± 0.029	0.127 ± 0.021	0.131 ± 0.023

Table 7. Transmitral and TDI determined velocities and indices in 19-35 yr old male and females
E: early phase of the diastolic filling, A: late (atrial) phase of the diastolic filling, E', A': TDI determined velocities. S' systolic velocity. Bold numbers: significant difference from the control values where, $p < 0.05$

Significant differences were seen only in the E/A values and in the TDI measurements of the medial part of the mitral valve (med. E'/A'). If we examine other parameters in which differences were suggested by other authors, only some small, non-significant differences were seen. It is possible that by a refined selection restricted to top-level endurance athletes more significant differences could be found.

4. Conclusion

Doppler echocardiography is a very important method in distinguishing physiologic hypertrophy from the pathologic one.

In this respect the most important point is the LV diastolic function. Commonly, the increase of the LV wall thickness and the LV muscle mass is associated with a decreased distensibility, an impaired diastolic function. In the athlete's heart despite of the LV hypertrophy an improved diastolic function can be detected either by transmitral or by TDI echocardiography.

Doppler echocardiography is also suitable to establish changes in the duration of the phases of the cardiac cycles. Training bradycardia results in a much more marked elongation of diastole than systole. Among the sub phases the E-A period i.e. the final phase of the diastole changes the most consequently, in the athlete's heart in will be longer.

5. References

[1] Baldi, J.C.; McFarlaine, K.; Oxenham, H.C; Whalley, G.A.; Walsh, H.J.; Doughty, R.N. (2003). Left ventricular diastolic filling and systolic function of young and older trained and untrained men. *Journal of Applied Physiology*, Vol.95, No.6, (December 2003), pp. 2570-2575, ISSN 8750-7587

[2] Caselli, L.; Galanti, G.; Padeletti, L.; Nieri, M.; Cecchi, F.; Cipollini, F.; Baldi, M.; Perrotta, L.; Vignini, S.; Michelucci, A. (2009). Diagnostic accuracy to extended-length electrocardiogram in differentiating between athlete's heart and hypertrophic cardiomyopathy. *Journal of Electrocardiology*, Vol.42, No.6, (July 2009) pp. 636-641, ISSN 1532-8430

[3] Caso, P.; D'Andrea, A; Galderisi, M; Liccardo, B; Severino, S; De Simone, L.; Izzo, A; D'Andrea, L.; Minnini, N. (2000). Pulsed Doppler tissue imaging in endurance athletes: relation between left ventricular preload and myocardial regional diastolic function. *American Journal of Cardiology*, Vol.85, No.9, (May 2000) pp. 1131-1136, ISSN 0002-9149

[4] Colan, S.D.; Sanders, S.P.; MacPherson, D.; Borow, K. (1985). Left ventricular diastolic function in elite athletes with physiologic cardiac hypertrophy. *Journal of American College of Cardiology*, Vol.6, No.3, (September 1985), pp. 545-549, ISSN 0735-1097

[5] D'Andrea, A.; Caso, P.; Scarafile, R.; Salerno, G.; De Corato, G.; Mita, C.; Di Salvo, G.; Allocca, F.; Colonna, D.; Caprile, M.; Ascione, L.; Cuomo, S.; Calabró, R. (2007). Biventricular myocardial adaptation to different training protocols in competitive master athletes. *International Journal of Cardiology*, Vol.115, No.3, (February 2007), pp. 342-349, ISSN 1874-1754

[6] Douglas, P.S.; O'Toole, M.L.; Hiller, D.B.; Reichek, N. (1986). Left ventricular structure and function by echocardiography in ultraendurance athletes. *American Journal of Cardiology*, Vol.58, No.9, (October 1986), pp. 805-809, ISSN 0002-9149

[7] Douglas, P.S.; & O'Toole, M. (1992). Ageing and physical activity determine cardiac structure and function in the older athlete. *Journal of Applied Physiology,* Vol.72, No.5, (May 1992), pp. 1969-1973, ISSN 8750-7587

[8] Fagard, R.H.; van den Broeke, C.; Bielen, E.; Vanhees, L.; Amery, A. (1987). Assessment of stiffness of the hypertrophied left ventricle of bicyclists using left ventricular inflow Doppler velocitometry. *Journal of American College of Cardiology,* Vol.9, No.6, (June 1987), pp. 1250-1254, ISSN 0735-1097

[9] Finkelhor, R.S.; Hanak, L.J.; Behler, R.C. (1986). Left ventricular filling in endurance-trained subjects *Journal of American College of Cardiology,* Vol.8, No.8, (August 1986), pp. 289-293, ISSN 0735-1097

[10] Fleg, J.L.; Shapiro, E.P.; O'Connor, F.; Taube, J.; Goldberg, A.P.; Lakatta, E.G. (1995). Left ventricular diastolic filling performance in older male athletes. *Journal of the American Medical Association,* Vol.273, No.17, (May 1995), pp. 1371-1375, ISSN 0077-8923,

[11] Galetta, F.; Franzoni, F.; Femia, F.R.; Bartolomucci, F.; Carpi, A.; Santoro, G. (2004). Left ventricular diastolic function and carotid artery wall in elderly athletes and sedentary controls. *Biomedichine & Pharmacotherapy,* Vol. 58, No.8, (October 2004), pp. 437-442, ISSN 0753-3322

[12] Granger, C.B.; Karimeddini, M.K.; Smith, V.E.; Shapiro, H.R.; Katz, A.M.; Riba, A.L. (1985). Rapid ventricular filling in left ventricular hypertrophy: I. Physiologic hypertrophy. *Journal of American College of Cardiology,* Vol.5, No.4, (April 1985), pp. 862-868, ISSN 0735-1097

[13] Gwathmey, J.K.; Slawsky, M.T.; Perreault, C.L.; Briggs, G.M.; Morgan, J.P.; Wei, J.Y. (1990). Effect of exercise conditioning on excitation-contraction coupling in aged rats. *Journal of Applied Physiology,* Vol.69, No. 4, (October 1990), pp. 1366-1371, ISSN 8750-7587

[14] Kasikcioglu, H.A.; Kasikcioglu, E.; Oflaz, H.; Unal, S.; Topcu, B.; Tartan. Z.; Arslan. A.; Cam, N.; Kayserilioglu, A. (2006). Discrimination between physiologic and pathologic left ventricular dilatation. *International Journal of Cardiology,* Vol.109, No.2, (May 2006) pp. 288-290, ISSN 1874-1754

[15]Kneffel, Zs.; Varga-Pintér, B.; Tóth, M.; Major, Zs.; Pavlik, G. (2011) Relationship between the heart rate and E/A ratio in athletic and non-athletic males. *Acta Physiologica Hungarica,* In Press, ISSN 1588-2683

[16] Krieg, A.; Scharhag, J.; Kindermann, W.; Urhausen, A. (2007). Cardiac tissue Doppler imaging in sports medicine. *Sports Medicine,* Vol.37, No.1, (2007), pp. 15-30, ISSN 0112-1642

[17] Levy, W.C.; Cerqueira, M.D.; Abrass, I.B.; Schwartz R.S. ; Stratton J.R. (1993). Endurance exercise training augments diastolic filling at rest and during exercise in healthy young and older men. *Circulation,* Vol.88, (1993), pp. 116-126, ISSN 0009-7322

[18] Limongelli, G.; Verrengia, M.; Pacileo, G.; Da Ponte, A.; Brancaccio, P.; Canonico, R.; D'Andrea, A.; Sarubbi, B.; Cerasuolo, F.; Calabró, R.; Limongelli, F.M. (2006). Left ventricular hypertrophy in Caucasian master athletes: differences with hypertension and hypertrophic cardiomyopathy. *International Journal of Cardiology,* Vol.111, No.1, (July 2006), pp. 113-119, ISSN 1874-1754

[19] Matsuda, M.; Sugishita, Y.; Koseki, S.; Ito, I.; Akatsuka, T.; Takamtso, K. (1983). Effect of exercise on left ventricular diastolic filling in athletes and non-athletes. *Journal of Applied Physiology,* Vol.55, No.2, (August 1983), pp. 323-328, ISSN 8750-7587

[20] Missault, L.; Duprez, D.; Jordaens, L.; Buyzere, M.de.; Bonny, K.; Adang, L.; Clement, D. (1993). Cardiac anatomy and diastolic filling in professional road cyclists. *European Journal of Applied Physiology,* Vol.66, No.5, (1993), pp. 405-408, ISSN 1439-6319

[21] Möckel, M.; Störk, T.; Müller, R.; Eichstadt, H.; Hochrein, H. (1992). Left ventricular diastolic function in triathletes and untrained subjects: A stress Doppler-echo study. *Perfusion,* Vol.5, (1992), pp. 69-74,

[22] Pavlik, G.; Olexó, Zs.; Bánhegyi, A.; Sidó, Z.; Frenkl, R. (1999a). Gender differences in the echocardiographic characteristics of the athletic heart. *Acta Physiologica Hungarica,* Vol.86, No.3-4 (October 1999), pp. 273-278, ISSN 1588-2683

[23] Pavlik, G.; Olexó, Zs.; Osváth, P.; Sidó, Z; Frenkl, R. (2001). Echocardiographic characteristics of male athletes of different age. *British Journal of Sports Medicine,* Vol.35, No.2, (April 2001), pp. 95-99, ISSN 1473-0480

[24] Pavlik, G.; Olexó, Zs.; Sidó, Z; Frenkl, R. (1999b). Doppler-echocardiographic examinations in the assessment of the athletic heart. *Acta Physiologica Hungarica,* Vol.86, No.1, (1999), pp. 7-22, ISSN 1588-2683

[25] Pavlik, G.; Major, Zs.; Varga-Pintér, B.; Jeserich, M.; Kneffel, Zs. (2010). The athlete's heart. *Acta Physiologica Hungarica,* Vol.97, No. 4, (December 2010), pp. 337-353, ISSN 1588-2683

[26] Pearson, A.C.; Schiff, M.; Mrosek, D.; Labovitz, A.J.; Williams, G.A. (1986). Left ventricular diastolic function in weight lifters. *American Journal of Cardiology,* Vol.58, No.13. (December 1986), pp. 1254-1259, ISSN 0002-9149

[27] Perseghin, G,; De, Cobelli, F.; Esposito, A.; Lattuada, G.; Terruzzi, I.; La, Torre, A.; Belloni, E.; Canu, T; Scifo, P.; Del, Maschio, A.; Luzi, L.; Alberti G. (2007). Effect of the sporting discipline on the right and left ventricular morphology and function of elite male track runners: A magnetic resonance imaging and phosphorus 31 spectroscopy study. *American Heart Journal,* Vol.154, No.5, (November 2007), pp. 937-942, ISSN 0002-8703

[28] Prasad, A.; Popovic, ZB.; Arbab-Zadeh, A.; Fu, Q.; Palmer, D.; Dijk, E.; Greenberg, N.L.; Garcia, M.J.; Thomas, J.D.; Levine, B.D. (2007). The effects of aging and physical activity on Doppler measures of diastolic function. *American Journal of Cardiology,* Vol.99, No.12, (June 2007), pp. 1629-1636, ISSN 0002-9149

[29] Rodrigues, A.C.T.; Melo, Costa, J.; Alves, G.B.; Silva, F.; Picard, M.H.; Andrade, J.L.; Mathias, W.; Negrão, C.E. (2006). Left ventricular function after exercise training in young men. *American Journal of Cardiology,* Vol.97, No.7, (April 2006), pp. 1089-1092, ISSN 0002-9149

[30] Sadaniantz, A.; Yurgalevitch, S.; Zmuda, J.M.; Thompson, P.D. (1996). One year of exercise training does not alter resting left ventricular systolic or diastolic function. *Medicine and Science in Sports and Exercise,* Vol.28, No. 11, (November 1996), pp. 1345-1350, ISSN 0195-9131

[31] Schulman, S.P.; Lakatta, E.G.; Fleg, J.L.; Lakatta, L.; Becker, L.C;, Gerstenblith, G. (1992). Age-related decline in left ventricular filling at rest and exercise. *American Journal of Physiology,* Vol.263, No. 6, (December 1992), pp. H1932-H1938, ISSN 0363-6127

[32] Shapiro, L.M. & Smith, R.G. (1983). Effect of training on left ventricular structure and function: an echocardiographic study. *British Heart Journal,* Vol.50, No.6, (November 1983) pp. 534-539, ISSN 0007-0769

[33] Spurgeon, H.A.; Steinbach, M.F.; Lakatta, E.G. (1983). Chronic exercise prevents characteristic age-related changes in rat cardiac contraction. *American Journal of Physiology*, Vol.244, No.4, (April 1983) pp. H513-H518, ISSN 0363-6127

[34] Starnes, J.W.; Beyer, R.E.; Edington, D.W. (1983). Myocardial adaptations to endurance in aged rats. *American Journal of Physiology*, Vol.245, No.4, (October 1983), pp. H560-H566, ISSN 0363-6127

[35] Takemoto, K.A.; Bernstein, L.; Lopez, J.F.; Marshak, D.; Rahimtoola, S.H.; Chandraratna, P.A.N. (1992). Abnormalities of diastolic filling of the left ventricle associated with ageing are less pronounced in exercise trained individuals. *American Heart Journal,* Vol.124, No.1, (July 1992), pp. 143-148, ISSN 0002-8703

[36] Tate, C.A.; Taffet, G.E.; Hudson, E.K.; Blaylock, S.L.; McBride, R.P.; Michael, L.H. (1990). Enhanced calcium uptake of cardiac sarcoplasmatic reticulum in exercise-induced old rats. *American Journal of Physiology*, Vol.258, No.2, (February 1990), pp. H431-H435, ISSN 0363-6127

[37] Teske, A.J.; Prakken, N.H.; De, Boeck, B.W.L.; Velthuis, B.K.; Doevendans, P.A.; Crame,r M.J.M. (2009). Effect of long term and intensive endurance training in athletes on the age related decline in left and right ventricular diastolic function as assessed by Doppler echocardiography. *American Journal of Cardiology,* Vol.104, No.8, (October 2009), pp. 1145-1151, ISSN 0002-9149

[38] Vinereanu, D.; Florescu, N.; Sculthorpe, N.; Tweddel, A.C.; Stephens, M.R.; Fraser, A.G. (2001). Differentiation between pathologic and physiologic left ventricular hypertrophy by tissue Doppler assessment of long-axis function in patients with hypertrophic cardiomyopathy or systemic hypertension and in athletes. *American Journal of Cardiology,* Vol.88, No.1, (July 2009), pp. 53-58, ISSN 0002-9149

11

Cardiopulmonary Disease in the Liver Transplant Patient: The Role of Doppler Echocardiography

Michael Ramsay
Baylor University Medical Center
USA

1. Introduction

End-stage liver disease and in particular cirrhosis of the liver may have a deleterious effect on all major organ systems. A significant cause of this effect is endothelial cell dysfunction. This dysfunction may be the result of the excessive shear force on the blood vessel wall caused by the typical high flow circulation that is seen in many cirrhotic patients. Inflammatory and vasoactive molecules that are either not cleared by the liver or are released by the diseased liver may also play a significant role in causing this endothelial dysfunction. It is well known that cardiac failure may cause liver dysfunction and damage, also the reverse is true. Cirrhosis of the liver may cause cardiac dysfunction. In fact if closely examined beta-receptor down-regulation may be present in every cirrhotic patient. Because the splanchnic arteriolar vasodilatation and overall reduction in systemic vascular resistance results in an increased cardiac output in the typical cirrhotic patient, a false sense of dynamic cardiac function may be engendered. Clinically significant cirrhotic cardiomyopathy may be present and not recognized.

The effect of liver cirrhosis on the pulmonary vascular endothelium may result in arteriolar vasodilatation and the creation of pulmonary vascular shunts causing hypoxia. This is termed hepatopulmonary syndrome (HPS). If vascular remodeling with proliferation of vascular smooth muscle cells and medial hyperplasia occurs resulting in an increased resistance to blood flow, this causes pulmonary hypertension and right ventricular dysfunction. If this is associated with portal hypertension it is termed portopulmonary hypertension (POPH).

The patient with cirrhosis of the liver presenting for liver transplantation requires careful evaluation preoperatively and intense monitoring perioperatively. The role of the Doppler echocardiogram has now become an essential tool for the successful management of these patients.

2. Cirrhotic cardiomyopathy

Typically the cardiovascular changes observed in the patient with liver cirrhosis are that of a hyperdynamic circulation. This is clearly manifested by a very increased cardiac output and a reduced systemic vascular resistance. The peripheral arterial vasodilatation, especially in the splachnic bed, is caused by an excessive release of endothelial derived nitric oxide, carbon monoxide and endogenous cannabinoids. (Woitas et al, 1997). In the cirrhotic liver there is an increased hepatic sinusoidal resistance to blood flow due to impaired endothelial nitric oxide production and the fibrotic changes that develop. This results in portal hypertension.

Despite the high resting cardiac output there is a blunted cardiac ventricular contractile response to stress. Cirrhotic cardiomyopathy that was initially thought to only occur in alcoholic cirrhosis or conditions causing iron overload can now be demonstrated in nearly all patients with severe liver cirrhosis. (Lee, 1989). This is well masked in most patients by the reduction in afterload caused by the low systemic vascular resistance. And it may be revealed during times of stress such as liver transplantation or when there is a sudden shunting of venous return to the heart by the performance of a transjugular intrahepatic portosytemic shunt stent placement procedure. (Van der Linden et al, 1996)

Cirrhotic cardiomyopathy is defined as chronic cardiac dysfunction in patients with cirrhosis, and is demonstrated by a reduced contractile response to stress, altered diastolic relaxation, down regulation of beta-adrenergic receptors and electrophysiological changes without other known causes of cardiac disease. This is a high output cardiomyopathy that may result in cardiac failure and pulmonary hypertension when an acute rise in cardiac output occurs such as at reperfusion of a new liver graft. (Ramsay, 2007)

The examination of cardiac function by echocardiography may initially be interpreted as normal cardiac function because of the significant reduction in afterload caused by the low systemic vascular resistance. However on closer examination both systolic and diastolic dysfunction may be demonstrated. The diagnostic features are: an E/A ratio < 1, a prolonged deceleration time > 200ms, a prolonged isovolumetric relaxation time > 80ms, enlarged left atrium, overall decreased pattern of contractility, decreased wall motion, increased wall thickness, resting ejection fraction < 55%, ratio of pre-ejection period to LV ejection time is prolonged > 0.44s (rate corrected). (Zardi et al. 2010). Therefore the clinician has to perform a precise echocardiographic examination or the diagnosis of cirrhotic cardiomyopathy may be missed and a label of a hyperdynamic well functioning heart erroneously applied. The ventricular systolic dysfunction may only be demonstrated after induced stress. This cardiomyopathy worsens with increasing liver failure.

On electrophysiological examination a prolongation of the QT interval (> 0.44s) is frequently seen and this may be associated with the degree of liver dysfunction. It is associated with an increased risk for ventricular tachyarrhythmias and may be an important diagnostic indicator of cirrhotic cardiomyopathy. The sudden onset of atrial fibrillation may also be an indicator of underlying cardiomyopathy.

The beta-adrenergic receptor impairment seen with cirrhosis may be an early sign of cardiomyopathy. (Lee et al. 1990). There is a decrease in chronotropic and inotropic responses to beta-adrenergic receptor stimulation. This maybe due to a reduction in both receptor density and function and is found in all patients with cirrhotic cardiomyopathy. Cardiac contractility in cirrhosis is impaired especially when exposed to stress. Other contributing factors include ventricular overload from the hyperdynamic circulation and volume overload, circulating humoral factors and cardiac cellular membrane changes.

The cirrhotic cardiomyopathy does improve after liver transplantation with disappearance of diastolic dysfunction, and normalization of the cardiac response to stress.(Liu & Lee,

2005). The key to diagnosis of cirrhotic cardiomyopathy when baseline ventricular function may appear normal or hyperdynamic is to stress the heart and reveal the cardiac contractile impairment.

3. Hepatopulmonary syndrome

Hepatopulmonary syndrome (HPS) is characterized by pulmonary arteriolar endothelial dysfunction associated with liver disease, resulting in intrapulmonary vascular dilatations. These vascular dilatations result in a shorter transit time for red blood cells to traverse alveolar capillaries and therefore create a shunt causing an increase in alveolar to arterial (A-a) oxygen gradient. The alveolar oxygen being unable to completely traverse the dilated alveolar capillary, resulting in some deoxygenated blood reaching the systemic circulation, further increases the ventilation perfusion mismatch. If the size of the A-a gradient is > 15 mmHg the criteria for HPS are met. Clinically the hypoxemia may range from mild to being very severe requiring supplemental oxygen. The shunts most commonly are found diffusely throughout the lung (Type 1 HPS) but occasionally a discrete arteriovenous malformation may develop (Type 2 HPS), bypassing the alveolar capillaries completely. This type of discrete shunt will not pick up extra oxygen if supplemental oxygen is provided as it completely bypasses the alveoli. The more diffuse pathology will respond to supplemental oxygen.

The diagnostic criteria for HPS are: (Rodriguez-Roisin & Krowka, 2008).

1. The presence of liver disease usually with portal hypertension and cirrhosis.
2. An A-a oxygen gradient > 15 mmHg.
3. Pulmonary vascular dilatation demonstrated by:
   a. A delayed, contrast enhanced (agitated saline) echocardiogram showing contrast in the left heart chambers 4 to 6 cycles after their appearance in the right heart chambers.
   b. Brain uptake >6% following ^{99m}Tc macroaggregated albumin lung perfusion scan.

The screening test for all liver transplant candidates should be pulse oximetry in the sitting position followed by contrast enhanced transthoracic Doppler echocardiography if hypoxemia (hemoglobin saturation < 92%) is detected. If there is delayed appearance (over 4 to 6 cardiac cycles) of contrast in the left heart then HPS should be considered. If contrast appears immediately in the left heart then there is probably a direct communication and transesophageal echocardiography should be performed to determine the diagnosis.

If a discrete arteriovenous shunt exists it may be ameliorated by coiling in interventional radiology. Hepatopulmonary syndrome is a progressive disease and is an indication for liver transplantation. It resolves in approximately 6 months after liver transplantation. The clinical signs and symptoms that develop with HPS include digital clubbing, cyanosis, spider angiomata, exertional dyspnea and platypnea (a worsening of dyspnea on moving from lying to standing). This is the complete opposite to most other causes of dyspnea where the patient is more comfortable breathing sitting up. Frequently the patient will also develop a more severe hypoxemia on sitting up (orthodeoxia).

Hepatopulmonary syndrome is found in approximately 30% 0f liver transplant candidates. In a recent study where patients were screened with contrast enhanced echocardiography 46% of patients had pulmonary vascular dilatations but had not developed hypoxemia. (Fallon et al. 2008). There may be other reasons for hypoxemia in the liver transplant candidate, and these reasons may also increase the severity of hypoxemia in HPS patients.

These may include hydrothorax, intrinsic lung disease, atelectasis and other ventilation diffusion perfusion abnormalities. The early use of Doppler echocardiography can facilitate the diagnosis of HPS. Following liver transplantation intensive respiratory therapy may be necessary to prevent further hypoxia developing because of atelectasis, fluid overload, aspiration and other pulmonary complications. (Gupta et al, 2010). However liver transplantation is the only therapy that will cure HPS and therefore it is indicated for this condition. (Swanson et al. 2005).

4. Portopulmonary hypertension and pulmonary hypertension

The pulmonary vasculature is highly distensible and can accommodate the hyperdynamic circulatory state usually seen in patients with advanced liver disease with only a minimal increase in pulmonary artery pressures. The endothelial dysfunction that occurs with liver disease may present in the pulmonary circulation as predominantly vasodilatory causing HPS, but alternatively hyperplasia of the media may be found together with vascular smooth muscle proliferation, vasoconstriction, intimal proliferation and eventual fibrosis, all presenting as an obstructive pathology causing an increased resistance to flow. This may result in pulmonary hypertension and if associated with portal hypertension it is termed portopulmonary hypertension (POPH).

The diagnostic criteria for POPH include a mean pulmonary artery pressure (mPAP) > 25 mmHg at rest, and a pulmonary vascular resistance (PVR) > 240 dyn.s.cm^{-5}. The transpulmonary gradient (TPG) > 12 mm Hg, (mPAP – PAOP [pulmonary arteriolar occlusion pressure]) reflects the obstruction to flow and distinguishes the contribution of volume and resistance to the increase in mPAP.

The right ventricle (RV) is a thin wall chamber with little muscle power to overcome an increased resistance to forward flow. In the presence of a cirrhotic cardiomyopathy, volume overload and an increased *afterload* the RV will become dysfunctional, dilate and may fail. If the RV begins to fail the central venous pressure will rise and the liver will become congested. In better circumstances if the increase in PVR develops slowly the RV may hypertrophy and be able to cope with the increased workload. Survival of the patient and also the liver graft in the transplant recipient depends on the ability of the RV to cope with the increased workload. Therefore in the patient presenting for liver transplantation with POPH a careful assessment of RV function by Doppler echocardiography is essential.

Portopulmonary hypertension has been classified into mild (mPAP 25-35 mmHg), moderate (mPAP >35 and < 45 mmHg), and severe (mPAP > 45 mmHg). Mild POPH is not associated with an increased mortality at liver transplantation although the immediate recovery period may be challenging if there is a significant increase in cardiac output after reperfusion of the new graft. Moderate and severe POPH are associated with significant mortality at transplantation. The key factor is not the mPAP but the RV function.

All patients being assessed for liver transplantation should be screened for pulmonary hypertension. Approximately 20% of candidates will have pulmonary hypertension but this is usually the result of volume overload, cirrhotic cardiomyopathy, cardiac failure and the high output circulation. These patients will have a normal PVR and TPG. True POPH is found in approximately 5% of transplant candidates, and it is essential for it to be diagnosed prior to the start of the transplant procedure.

The assessment screen is as follows:

1. All potential transplant candidates screened with transthoracic Doppler echocardiography.
   a. Right ventricular systolic pressure (RVSP) > 50 mmHg a right heart catheterization required to characterize the pulmonary hemodynamics.
   b. If diagnosed in the operating room just prior to the start of transplant surgery the RV function must be assessed by TEE. Only proceed if RV function good and withstands a stress test.
2. mPAP < 35 mmHg
   a. PVR < 240 dyn.s.cm^{-5}
   b. Good RV function
   c. Place on transplant waiting list and start pulmonary vasodilator therapy
   d. Reassess every 6 months
3. mPAP 35-40 mmHg
   a. PVR > 240 dyn.s.cm^{-5}
   b. Good RV function that withstands stress test consider placing on transplant list
   c. Start pulmonary vasodilator therapy
   d. If RV dilated and function poor do not list until effective therapy has allowed RV to improve.
4. mPAP > 40 mmHg
   a. Assess RV function but even if good do not list until patient has undergone a period of vasodilator therapy.
   b. If RV function poor do not transplant. Allow time to improve with therapy.
   c. Consider a liver bilateral lung transplant.
5. All patients with POPH should be reassessed by TEE every 6 months.

Transthoracic Doppler echocardiography is a good assessment screening tool but it does require the presence of a tricuspid regurgitant jet to make the estimate of RVSP. This jet may not be present in 10 - 20% of patients. The RVSP is calculated from the peak tricuspid regurgitant velocity (TRV) using the modified Bernoulli equation and estimating right atrial pressure (RAP):

$$RVSP = 4(TRV)^2 + RAP$$

This algorithm has a 97% sensitivity and a 77% specificity for diagnosing moderate and severe POPH. (Kim et al. 2000).

A more accurate screening algorithm has been reported by measuring the increased PVR utilizing the ratio of peak TRV to the RV outflow tract velocity time integral (VTI_{RVOT}). The sensitivity and negative predictive values are reported at 100%. (Farzaneh-Far et al. 2008)

An accurate assessment of RV function as determined by TEE is essential to the management of the liver transplant recipient. The success of the transplant will depend on the RV maintaining good function during and after the procedure despite all the increases in cardiac output, volume and PVR. If RV dysfunction or failure occur then graft congestion with possible failure and serious morbidity including mortality may occur. The intraoperative course can be more optimally managed under TEE guidance.

The role of liver transplantation in the management of POPH is not well defined. Some patients will reverse quickly after transplant, others may require months or years of ongoing vasodilator therapy. Still other patients may continue to progress and eventually develop RV failure. There are even patients who will develop pulmonary hypertension after liver transplantation. Liver transplantation offers the best outcome to patients with POPH that is responsive to vasodilator therapy.

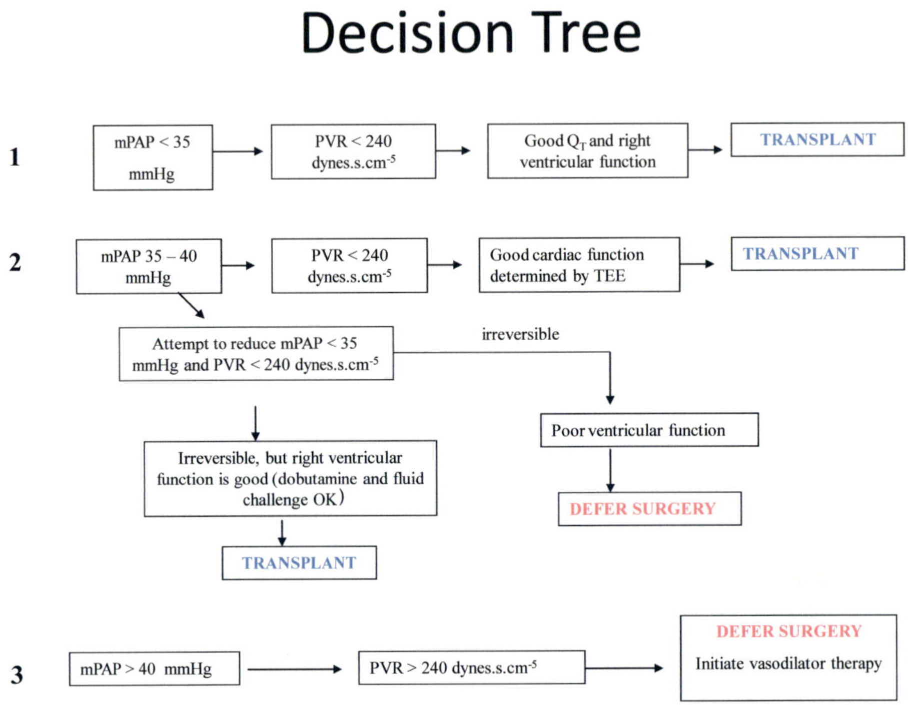

Fig. 1.

5. The role of Doppler echocardiography during liver transplantation

Many patients undergoing liver transplantation have varying degrees of cirrhotic cardiomyopathy, volume overload and significant stresses on the cardiovascular system. The addition of TEE to routine monitoring provides much essential information that can assist in patient management. The transgastric view may not be always available because of the placement of surgical retractors but the 4-chamber view can give a good assessment of preload, cardiac function and detection of air emboli and clot emboli. The filling pressures are not an accurate measure of preload especially if there is diastolic dysfunction present.

The postreperfusion syndrome following the opening of the blood supply to the new liver may be severe and better managed with the information provided by the TEE. The effects of acute acidosis, hyperkalemia and hypothermia compounded by an ischemia/reperfusion injury may result in severe arrhythmias, hypotension and cardiovascular collapse. (Ramsay, 2008).

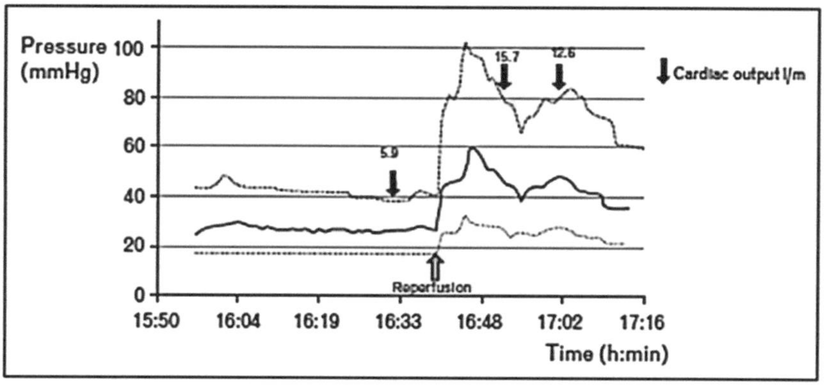

PA2-S, pulmonary artery pressure–systolic; PA2-D, pulmonary artery pressure–diastolic; PA2-M, pulmonary artery pressure–mean. Reproduced with permission from [2]. ...., PA2-S; ———, PA2-D; ...., PA2-M.

Fig. 2. Increase in cardiac output with concomitant increase in pulmonary artery pressures at reperfusion of the liver graft

End-stage liver disease is associated with increased risk of coronary artery disease. (Ehtisham, 2010). The incidence of coronary artery disease in liver transplant candidates over the age of 50 years has been reported as high as 28%. (Carey et al, 1995). Patients with risk factors for coronary artery disease should be screened pretransplant and if indicated they should be revascularized. The safety of percutaneous bare metal stent placement in this patient population has been demonstrated. (Azarbal et al, 2011).The dobutamine stress echocardiography has been advocated as the assessment tool of choice in this patient group. (Plotkin et al. 2000). The positive predictive value of this test has been questioned as many of these end-stage liver patients are receiving beta adrenergic blockers and cannot achieve the maximum predicted heart rate and rate pressure product. However there has been demonstrated a high negative predictive value of this test. (Umphrey et al. 2008).

6. Conclusion

The Doppler echocardiograph technology provides for a better assessment and management of the liver transplant patient. Its routine use in this patient population is to be recommended.

7. References

Azarbal B, Poommipanit P, Arbit B, Hage A, Patel J, Kittleson M, Kar S, Kaldas FM, Busuttil RW. Feasibility and safety of percutaneous coronary intervention in patients with end-stage liver disease referred for liver transplantation. *Liver Transpl* 2011, in press.

Carey WD, Dumot JA, Pimental RR, Barnes DS, Hobbs RE, Henderson JM et al. The prevalence of coronary artery disease in liver transplant candidates over age 50. *Transplantation* 1995, 59:859-864.

De Wolf AM, Aggarwal S. Monitoring preload during liver transplantation *Liver Transplantation* 2007; 14:268-269.

Ehtisham J, Altieri M, Salame E, Saloux E, Ollivier I, Hamon M. Coronary artery disease in orthotopic liver transplantation: pretransplant assessment and management. *Liver Transpl.*2010;16:550-557.

Fallon MB, Krowka MJ, Brown RS, Trotter JF, Zacks S, Roberts KE, et al. Impact of hepatopulmonary syndrome on quality of life and survival in liver transplant candidates. *Gastroenterology* 2008; 135:1168-1175.

Farzaneh-Far R, McKeown BH, Dang D, Roberts J, Schiller N, Foster E. Accuracy of Doppler-Estimated pulmonary vascular resistance in patients before liver transplantation. *Am J Cardiol.* 2008; 101:259-262.

Gupta S, Castel H, Rao RV, Picard M, Lilly L, Faughnan ME et al. Improved survival after liver transplantation in patients with hepatopulmonary syndrome. *Am J Transplantation* 2010; 10:254-263.

Kim W, Krowka M, Plevak D et al. Accuracy of Doppler echocardiography in the assessment of pulmonary hypertension in liver transplant candidates. *Liver Transpl* 2000; 6:453-458.

Lee SS. Cardiac abnormalities in liver cirrhosis. *West J Med* 1989; 151: 530-535.

Lee SS, Marty J, Mantz J, Samain E, Braillon A, Lebrac D. Desensitization of myocardial B-adrenergic receptors in cirrhotic rats. *Hepatology;* 1990; 12:481-485.

Liu H, Lee SS. What happens to cirrhotic cardiomyopathy after liver transplantation? *Hepatology,* 2005;43:1203-1205.

Plotkin JS, Johnson LB, Rustgi V, Kuo P. Coronary artery disease and liver transplantation: the state of the art. *Liver Transpl* 2000;6(suppl 1): S53-S56.

Ramsay M. Portopulmonary hypertension and right heart failure in patients with cirrhosis. *Curr Opin Anesthesiol* 2010; 23:145-150.

Ramsay M. The reperfusion syndrome: have we made any progress? *Liver Transplantation* 2008;14:412-414.

Rodriguez-Roisin R, Krowka MJ. Hepatopulmonary syndrome: a liver-induced lung vascular disorder. *N Eng J Med* 2008;358:2378-2387.

Swanson KL, Wiesner RH, Krowka MJ. Natural history of hepatopulmonary syndrome: impact of liver transplantation. *Hepatology* 2005; 41:1122-1129.

Umphrey LG, Hurst RT, Eleid MF, Lee KS, Reuss CS, Hentz JG, Vargas HE, Appleton CP. Preoperative dobutamine stress echocardiographic findings and subsequent short-term adverse cardiac events after orthotopic liver transplantation. *Liver Transpl* 2008;14:886-892.

Van der Linden P, Le Moine O, Ghyseis M, Ortinex M, Deviere J. Portopulmonary hypertension after transjugular intrahepatic portosystemic shunt: effects on right ventriculat function. *Hepatology* 1996;23:982-987.

Woitas RP, Heller J, Stoffel-Wagner B, Spengler U, Sauerbruch T. Renal functional reserve and nitric oxide in patients with compensated liver cirrhosis. *Hepatology:* 1997; 26: 858-864

Zardi EM, Abbate A, Zardi DM, Dobrina A, Margiotta D, Van Tassel BW, et al. Cirrhotic cardiomyopathy. *J Am Coll Cardiol* 2010; 56:539-549.

12

Echocardiography in Rheumatoid Arthritis (RA)

Małgorzata Wisłowska
Head of Clinic of Rheumatology & Internal Medicine of Central Clinical Hospital of Ministry of Internal Affairs and Administration in Warsaw, Warszawa
Poland

1. Introduction

The results of numerous clinical studies confirm the presence of cardiac abnormalities in patients with rheumatoid arthritis. Their authors emphasize the utility of echocardiography in detecting heart muscle damage, pericardial involvement and valvular heart disease in RA. Bacon and Gibson, using one-dimentional imaging mode, found mitral valve changes in 6.9% of their patients and ascribed it to the systemic spread of the disease. Prakash, Nomeir and MacDonald noted mitral valve defects in 25, 30 and 10% of RA individuals, respectively. Using two-dimensional technique Mody discovered the same disorder in 13% of his RA cases and additionally aortic valve insufficiency in a small percentage of this subset. Toumanidis et al. revealed mitral valve and aortic cusps derangements in about 24% of their RA patients. In Wisłowska's study mitral valve insufficiency was present in 8.6% of RA patients and occurred more frequently in them than in the controls. One must take into consideration, however, that mitral valve prolaps is observed in up 18% of healthy individuals, and therefore can not be regarded an RA characteristic.

Echocardiography also revealed discrepancies in heart muscle structure and function between RA patients and the control groups. Wisłowska found left ventricular mass in RA individuals significantly greater then in the controls. The same concerned intraventricular septum end diastolic thickness, LV posterior wall end diastolic thickness and the aortic root diameter. The ejection fraction was significantly lower and isovolumetric relaxation time (IVRT) and deceleration time significantly longer in RA patients compared to the controls. These findings are in accordance with Alpaslan, Di Franco and Levendoglu's results, that revealed significant differences in LV diastolic function (peak E velocity, E velocity/A velocity ratio, IVRT, myocardial performance index [MPI] and transmural flow propagation velocity [TFPV]) between RA group and the control subjects. The results of these studies indicate to the presence of subclinical myocardial involvement in RA, which can be ascribed to nonspecific myocarditis observed in this disease. Nevertheless different other risk factors for cardiac muscle impairment are usually present in RA individuals and therefore it is uncertain, whether heart pathology in rheumatoid arthritis is due to inflammation itself or is secondary to other process or to drug use in this disease.

Although pericardial effusion is considered the most common heart complication in RA, Wisłowska et al. observed it only on 4% of cases in echocardiography image. Pathologists find it in about 30% of RA cases post mortem, but clinical manifestation of pericarditis is rare in this disease. It's life-threatening complications such as constrictive pericarditis or tamponade were reported in very few RA cases, to date.

Rheumatoid arthritis (RA) is a connective tissue disease predominantly affecting joints and periarticular structures. Inflammatory process within the skeletal system - a source of patients' main complaints and eventual disability – draws the attention of medical service to the extent that sometimes results in negligence of other aspects of the systemic disorder. These in turn can be of importance, since inflammation in RA, as in other connective tissue diseases is widespread and affects such vital tissues and organs as those of the cardiovascular system, for instance. Extraarticular manifestations in RA however develop slowly and are poorly manifested. Their symptoms tend to be are assigned rather to patient's general malaise and the lack of fitness. Heart involvement is often asymptomatic or causes mild ailments, frequently disregarded by affected persons, because RA individuals are generally not energetic and avoid to move too much. Chest pain or fatigue in them happens to be contributed to skeletal system involvement rather then to other pathological process. These are perhaps the reasons why at least twice as many changes in RA hearts are recognized post-mortem then during the patient's' lifetime. One of the current issues in rheumatology therefore is to recognize the presence, type and the extend of heart involvement in RA and to search for correlations of their appearance and intensity with the disease clinical picture. Echocardiography appears to be of much help in this aspect. The development of this domain improved cardiological diagnostics, providing a valuable tool to assess the condition of heart structures and their functional properties. It enabled detecting even minor cardiac muscle, valvular and pericardial aberrations, also in asymptomatic individuals. Based on these observations numerous clinical studies to date focused on echocardiography application in RA and it's utility in diagnosing cardiovascular complications of the disease.

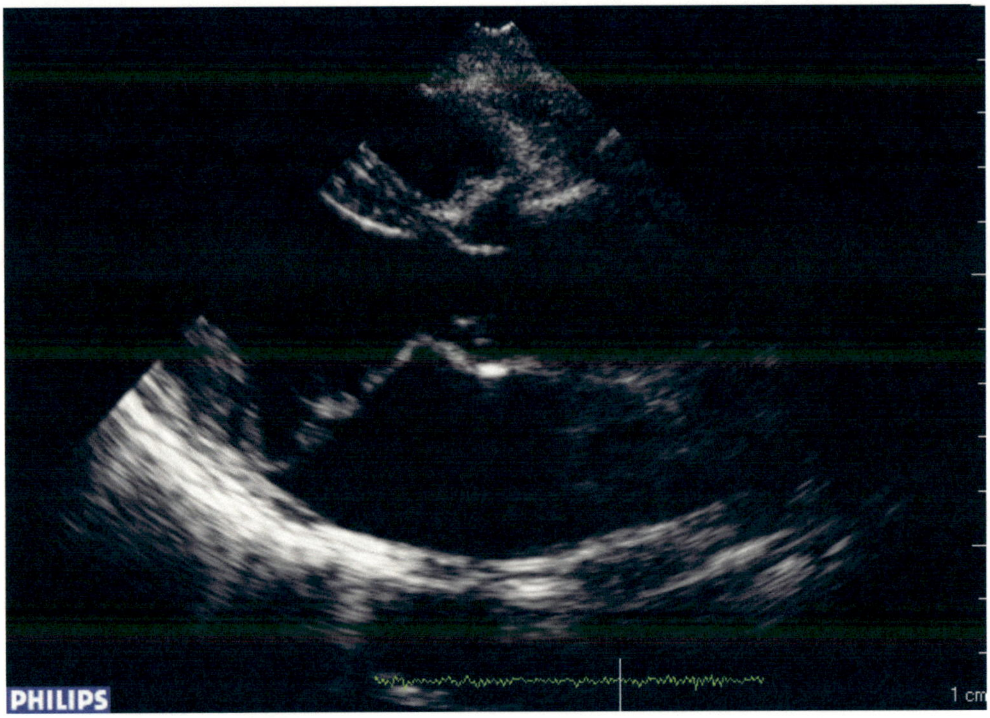

Fig. 1. Echocardiogram of RA patient LP female, age 46 - mitral valve prolaps

One of the firsts to examine echocardiography images RA patients were Bacon and Gibson [1]. In their one-dimentional examination of 44 individuals with classical or definite RA - 22 with palpable rheumatoid nodules and 22 without them - they demonstrated the presence of pericardial effusion in 34% of patients. It was detected in 50% of those with nodular and in 18% of those with non-nodular disease course. In most cases the fluid did not cause symptoms of pericarditis, although in several patients it was 1-2 cm in depth. No correlation could be seen between the appearance of effusion and the disease duration and pericardial pathology was not detected in age-matched controls with noninflammatory osteoarticular pathology. Bacon and Gibson also found mitral valve changes in 6.9% of their RA patients. In their study the average mitral diastolic closure rate in the control group was 116 mm/s (range 75 to 180; normal range over 80 mm/s). It was significantly lower in nodular RA group (63 mm/s), then in the non–nodular one ($p<0.05$) and in the controls ($p<0.001$), and only in 5 nodular patients the values were normal. In 3 nodular patients they were markedly decreased (less then 30 mm/s), symptomatic for severe rheumatic stenosis. In non-nodular group mean mitral diastolic closure rate was 94 mm/s (range 40-200) and only in 4 cases the values were below normal range. The frequency of diminished rate of mitral valve movement in this study increased with age in RA individuals, but not in the controls and increased with RA duration. The recording of a diminished rate of spontaneous mitral valve movement during the mid-diastolic partial closure period was a new observation. The correlation of decreased mitral diastolic closure rate with the duration of the disease, it's coincidence with severe nodular process and pericardial effusion was, according to authors, a strong argument for considering this parameter representative for a systemic RA manifestation.

Other investigators in 70-ties (Prakash et al. [2], Nomeir et al. [3] and MacDonald et al. [4]) reported mitral valve derangements in 25, 30 and 10% of RA patients, respectively. Prakash et al. [2] performed a prospective echocardiography study to search for cardiac abnormalities in 1 female and 15 male American patients (11 white and 5 black persons), free of cardiac symptoms. 44% of them had evidence of posterior pericardial effusion, not detected by electrocardiogram nor by the chest X-ray study. The E to F slope of the anterior leaflet of mitral valve was reduced in 25% of patients, which according to authors, could be due either to rheumatoid involvement of the mitral valve cusps or to changes in left ventricular compliance, both common in people with long-standing rheumatoid arthritis. The study revealed high prevalence of mitral valve and pericardial involvement in RA patients, previously only found in post-mortem studies and confirmed the utility of echocardiography in RA diagnosis.

In 1973 Nomeir et al. [3] studied the nature and extent of cardiac involvement in RA patients. Physical examination of 30 Americans with classic RA did not show any significant cardiac abnormalities, while echocardiography revealed pericardial effusion in 46.6% and mitral valve defects in 30% of patients, therefore demonstrating the presence of one of these pathologies in quite a large number of RA individuals. Although there was no correlation between different modalities of the study, echocardiography was claimed by the authors the most sensitive method of detecting cardiac complications of RA at early disease stage.

In 1975 in turn, Davia et al. [5] examined 35 consecutive American RA patients, submitting them to echocardiography to evaluate the motion of the anterior mitral valve leaflet. In contrast to previous results, through analysis they revealed normal valve motion and a normal E/F slope in as many as 31 of them. The authors discovered, that falsely low E/F slope values were noted only when the technique applied was not sufficiency meticulous, while the improvement of method resulted in normalization of these values. Their conclusion therefore was that anterior mitral valve leaflet abnormalities rarely if ever are seen in RA patients, provided that careful attention to recording technique is observed.

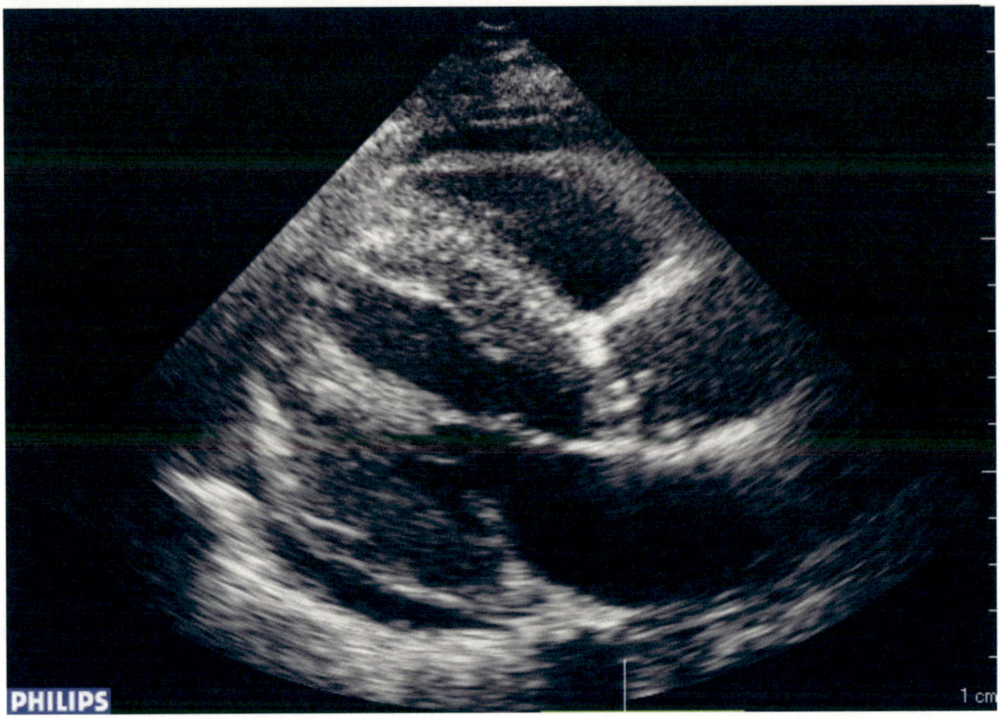

Fig. 2. Echocardiogram of RA patient AM female, age 58 - pericardial effusion

The results obtained by Nomeir et al. [6] in their subsequent study initially showed that 18 out of 30 their RA patients had cardiac involvement arising from the disease at baseline of the examination [3]. Abnormalities detected by echocardiography comprised mitral valve disease or pericardial alterations, or both. All patients were then followed up for 4 years from the initial workup. At the end of the study mitral valve abnormalities were still seen in 63% of those in whom they were previously present and pericardial effusion remained in 20%. Pericardial thickening persisted in 6 out of 7 patients. There was no definitive correlation between the protraction of these abnormalities and other clinical data, but it was noticed that patients who retained pericardial effusion and mitral valve abnormalities showed a higher number of joints involved and a higher erythrocyte sedimentation rate. It is worth mention that none of the patients developed constrictive pericarditis nor the heart failure and that all abnormalities detected remained clinically insignificant. The results of the study suggest that an impressive number of RA patients suffer from cardiac abnormalities related to their disease which may be clinically undetectable and are rarely life- threatening or requiring surgery support.

MacDonald et al. [4] performed clinical, electrocardiographic (ECG) and echocardiography examinations in 51 American outpatients with RA. 31% of patients had echocardiographic evidence of pericardial effusion and in 2 patients pericardial thickening was demonstrated. Mitral valve E/F slope was normal in as many as 46 out of 51 persons and left ventricular performance was depressed only in a few cases. The authors concluded that in unselected outpatients with RA pericardial abnormalities detected by echocardiograph are common although usually clinically unapparent.

Toumanidis et al. [8] visualized mitral and aortic cusps changes in about 24% of their patients.

In the Hungarian study of Nagyhegyi et al. [9] 100 of patients suffering from ankylosing spondylitis (AS) and 100 patients with RA were examined by clinical, non-invasive cardiological, radiological and laboratory methods to determine the prevalence of cardiac and cardiopulmonary disorders. 14 patients with AS and 24 with RA had several valvular abnormalities. Among those without valvular defects, myocardial systolic dysfunction was detectable in 15 AS and 11 RA cases and cor pulmonale was diagnosed in 16 and 7 patients, respectively. Conduction disturbances were demonstrated in 17 AS and 14 RA individuals.

Mody et al. [7] from South Africa examined their Negro-Caucasoids patients with RA seen in the rheumatic diseases unit during a 16-months period preceding the study. The authors aimed at determining the prevalence of cardiac abnormalities in RA. They used random tablets to select a group out of 330 persons and finally 101 of RA individuals underwent clinical and echocardiography examination. Adequate two-dimentional assessments were obtained in 84 patients and adequate M-mode recordings in 77. 31patients (37%) had 45 echocardiographic abnormalities, in 5 patients (6%) pericardial effusion was detected. 11 abnormalities of mitral valve noted in 10 (13%) patients: 3 had mitral valve prolaps, 1 - aortic incompetence and flutter on the mitral valve, in 5 patients mitral annular calcium was detected and 1 patient had hypertrophic obstructive cardiomyopathy and mitral calcium deposits. The reduction in E/F slope was noted in 12 patients, 7 of whom had associated cardiac disease, 1 patient had sinus tachycardia and 4 (5%) - a mild reduction of E/F slope without any other cardiac abnormality. The authors concluded that apart from the presence of pericardial effusion in 6% and minor abnormalities of the E/F slope in 5% of patients, all other significant echocardiographic abnormalities could be related to the presence of associated cardiac disease.

In 1983 Villecco et al. [10] from Italy confirmed the utility of echocardiography in detection of cardiac lesions in RA patients. In order to verify the frequency and the extend of heart pathology, the authors performed mechanophonocardiographic studies and simultaneous mono- and bi-dimentional echocardiography in 28 RA individuals. They showed an increase in the PEP/LVET ratio on the polycardiogram in 1 case and echocardiographic alterations in 18 (64.3%) of patients. Pericardial effusion was noted in 21.4%, the thickening of pericardium in 14.3%, alterations of mitral valve (the reduction in protodiastolic closing velocity of the anterior edge of the large mitral valve) in 35.7% and thickening of the interventricular septum in 17.9% of cases. The authors reckoned all measurements results to be good indicators of cardiac complications in RA. According to them such examinations allow to identify a group of patients suffering from abnormalities otherwise undetectable.

Wisłowska et al. [11,12] in Poland observed higher frequency of valvular heart disease, especially mitral insufficiency in RA patients than in the control group. Echocardiographic examinations were carried out in 100 patients (age<65 years) with rheumatoid arthritis (stages II–IV according to Steinbrocker's criteria). The control group consisted of 100 patients with osteoarthrosis, spondyloarthrosis and painful shoulder matched for age, sex and body surface area (BSA). All patients with myocardial infarction, hypertension, rheumatic fever or a history of diabetes were excluded from the study. Echocardiographic examination revealed more cases of valvular heart disease, especially mitral insufficiency, in

RA patients then in the control group. Mitral valve prolaps was noted in 6% of RA individuals and pericardial effusion in 4%, whereas it was absent in the control group and in all patients during of clinical assessment prior to echocardiography imaging. In all 4% the volume of fluid was less then 300 ml, which was considered neglectable. Patients with RA had greater diastolic left ventricular diameter and aortic root diameter, as well as a smaller ejection fraction, mean velocity of cimcumferential fibre shortening and fractional shortening than the control individuals. The comparison of results of the echocardiographic measurements on different RA stages or in relation to the functional index, seropositivity and seronegativity and in person of different disease duration did not reveal any statistically significant discrepancies. In 39% of RA patients and 19% of the controls valvular heart disease was discovered by echocardiographic examination (p<0.05). Mitral valve insufficiency (I and II degree) was noted in 29% of RA patients and in 10% of the controls (p<0.005), aortic insufficiency (I and II degree) in 8 RA patients and 4 of the control group (NS), tricuspid insufficiency in 3 RA individuals and in 2 control subjects (NS) and mitral stenosis in 1 RA patient. In total, valvular heart disease was seen in 47 RA cases and in 19 control subjects. Only in 4% of cases pericardial effusion was detected, though this abnormality is considered the most common heart complication in RA.

There is much controversy in literature, regarding the frequency of mitral valve prolaps in general population, where it fluctuated from 3–8% up to 18% in different clinical studies [13,14], as well as in RA patients [6]. In Wisłowska's nodular group the prevalence of this abnormality was 8.6% [12]. Such discrepancies make impossible to classify it as an RA characteristics.

In another study Wisłowska et al. [12] compared the results echocardiographic examinations in 35 patients with nodular and 35 with non–nodular RA. The groups were matched for age, sex and the BSA. 35 patients with osteoarthrosis and spondyloarthrosis matched with both RA groups formed a control group. Patients with history of myocardial infarction, hypertension, rheumatic fever and diabetes were excluded from the study. Echo-Doppler cardiography and echocardiographic Holter monitoring revealed cardiac involvement in 71.9% of patients with nodular RA and 42.9% of non–nodular cases compared to 22.9% of the control group (p<0.0002). Echocardiographic examination revealed more cases of valvular heart abnormalities, especially mitral insufficiency, in nodular RA patients than in non-nodular and the controls. Both mitral valve prolaps and pericardial effusion were noted in 8.6% of nodular subjects. Patients with nodular RA also had greater aortic root diameter, a smaller ejection fraction, and smaller mean velocity of circumferential fiber shortening and fractional shortening compared to ones non-nodular and to the control group subjects.

In another study concerning systolic and diastolic heart function in RA patients Wisłowska et al. [15] found left ventricular (LV) mass index in RA significantly greater than in the control group. The same concerned intraventricular septum end-diastolic thickness, LV posterior wall end-diastolic thickness and the aortic root diameter. The ejection fraction in RA patients was significantly lower than in the control group. The assessment of diastolic function parameters revealed significantly longer isovolumetric relaxation time and deceleration time in RA patients.

Similar results were presented by Alpaslan et al. [16], Di Franco et al. [17], and Levendoglu et al. [18]. In their studies echocardiographic indices of LV diastolic function (peak E velocity, E velocity/A velocity ratio, isovolumetric relaxation time [IVRT], myocardial performance index [MPI] and transmural flow propagation velocity [TFPV]) in RA group were significantly different from those of the controls. The reported finding indicate to the presence of subclinical myocardial involvement in RA, which is most probably due to the nonspecific myocarditis observed in these patients. Such myocardial involvement was elsewhere described as asymptomatic, rarely influencing cardiac size or function, predominantly affecting LV diastole, usually of diffuse pattern and scarcely clinically significant. It is not know to date, however, to what extent cardiac pathology in RA emerge from inflammatory myocarditis itself or is secondary to other pathology or drug use in this disease.

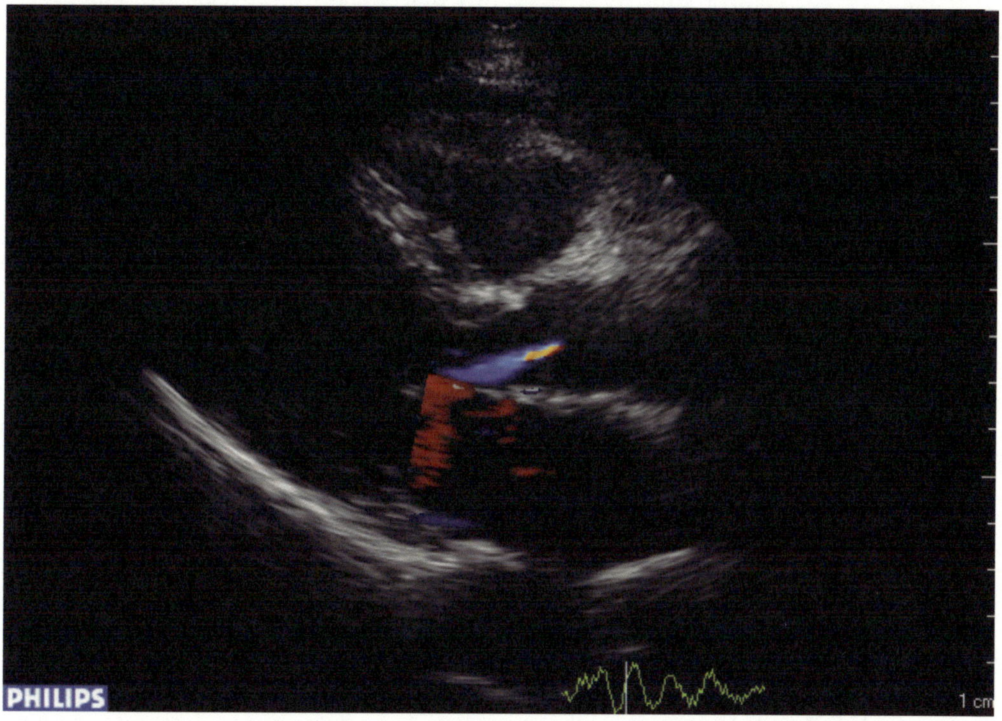

Fig. 3. Echocardiogram of RA patient BS female, age 50 - aortic valve insufficiency

Toumanidis et al. [8] examined a Greek population to evaluate early morphological and functional heart abnormalities. The examined group was free of risk factors for coronary artery disease and without any clinically evident cardiac manifestations. Echocardiography examination was performed in 62 patients with collagen disease, 15 with rheumatoid arthritis and in 40 healthy individuals. The imager was taken from apical four-chamber view at rest and during the end of a 3- minute isometric exercise with handgrip. Global and regional ejection fraction (EF) of left ventricle were calculated. In the RA group the EF was 62.38±6.88% vs 61.47±8.52% in the controls. Regional EF analysis revealed a major dysfunction of the proximal segment of interventricular septum in all groups and reduced separation of mitral and aortic valve leaflets in RA.

In Maione et al. [19] echocardiography examination of consecutive 39 Italian RA and 40 control subjects the occurrence of anatomic lesions was lower then that observed in other studies. No differences in mean values of left and right ventricular diastolic function indices obtained by Doppler echocardiography were found between patients and the controls.

However, in 26% of patients with RA, left ventricular abnormalities, probably secondary to myocardial fibrosis were detected. Pericardial effusions (less than 300 ml) were found in 3 RA patients (7%) and in none of the controls. Pericardial adhesion was seen in 1 RA patient only. Valvular involvement (1 case of mitral stenosis and 1 case of aortic stenosis) was detected in 2 RA cases, both having had suffered from rheumatic heart disease in the past. Moreover, the prevalence both: minor changes of mitral valve and trivial regurgitation was similar in the investigated groups. Left atrial or left ventricular dilation was found in 5 RA patients out of whom 3 were affected by coronary artery disease and 2 by valvular disease and in none of the control subjects. Left ventricular hypertrophy was present in 2 RA patients, both suffering from essential hypertension and in none of the controls. EF was normal in all except 3 RA patients, all of whom with ECG evidence of previous myocardial infarction. To investigate diastolic heart function the observers excluded persons with arterial hypertension, diabetes and valvular heart disease (4 RA cases and 1 from the control group). To further exclude the presence of occult heart disease patients and the controls underwent an echo-dobutamine provocative test. Afterwards echocardiographic indices of LV and RV diastolic function were calculated in 35 RA and 39 control subjects. The authors found no statistically significant differences in mean values of the parameters examined. Nevertheless diastolic function abnormalities consisting of IVRT prolongation and inverted E/A ratio were pointed out in 9 out of 35 (26%) RA cases and in 2 out of 39 (5%) controls. The difference was statistically significant (Fisher exact test, p=0.019) and considered due to the decrease in peak early diastolic velocity of the mitral valve. An inverted E/A ratio of the tricuspid flow velocity profile was detected in 3 RA patients, all with LV filling abnormalities, and was not detected in the controls.

Di Franco et al. [17] studied an Italian population to evaluate the LV filling parameters by the analysis of transmitral flow and pulmonary venous flow with special regard to patients' age and the disease duration. 32 RA cases without evidence of concomitant cardiac disease were selected and compared to matched control subjects. All patients and the control group were submitted to M-mode, two-dimensional Doppler and color Doppler (continuous and pulsed wave) echocardiography. Diastolic parameters evaluated comprised transmitral flow (E/A ratio), pulmonary venous flow (S/D ratio), a-Pw, IVRT and deceleration time (DT). In RA LV filling disturbances were apparent and characterized by a reduced E/A ratio (mean SD 1.16 [0.31] vs 1.37 [0.32] in the controls) (p= 0.02) and increased S/D ratio (1.43 [0.40] vs 1.22 [0.29] in the controls) (p=0.017). In this group of patients the correlation between E/A ratio and the disease duration (r=0.40, p=0.01 Spearman rank correlation) was also noted. The authors concluded that RA patients, in absence of overt heart disease, show diastolic function characterized by impaired E/A and S/D ratio. According to them it's relation to the disease duration suggests the presence of subclinical myocardial involvement.

In another Italian study Corrao et al. [20] investigated and verified diastolic abnormalities in rheumatoid patients, without clinically evident cardiovascular disease and other confounding complaints, by using pulsed Doppler examination of transmitral blood flow. They selected 40 patients fulfilling revised American Rheumatism Association (ARA) criteria for the diagnosis of rheumatoid arthritis with no symptoms of cardiac disease, nor clinical findings of other extracardiac pathology, matched with 40 healthy volunteers as a control. An echocardiographic examination was carried out in each subject. LV structural and functional measurements were obtained. Intraventricular septum thickness and LV mass index were significantly higher in rheumatoid patients than in the control. RA patients had higher mean values of peak A velocity and A/E ratio. When multiple linear regression data analysis was performed, an independent relationship only between A/E ratio and LV mass was found. The results confirmed the presence of diastolic abnormalities in rheumatoid patients and pointed out that these abnormalities also affect echo-Doppler parameters of LV filling. The study results further suggest that structural LV changes can be responsible for LV filling impairment.

One more Italian study was carried out by Montecucco et al. [21] who used digitized M-mode and Doppler echocardiography to assess LV function in 54 patients (mean age 50 years) suffering from active RA, without obvious cardiovascular disease. The group was compared with 54 age and sex matched normal subjects. No differences were found in LV end-diastolic diameter, systolic function and parietal thickness between patients and the controls. However, a significant reduction of various indices of LV diastolic function was recorded, including E/A ratio and the peak lengthening rate of the LV diameter (an index of relaxation evaluated by M-mode echocardiography). The former was correlated with patients' age and was independent of disease duration while the latter was more markedly correlated with the disease duration then with the patients' age. The authors suggested that the observation of relationship between diastolic impairment and the disease duration in active RA may open new perspectives for the study of RA-associated cardiovascular disease.

Voipio-Pulkki and Saraste [22] examined a Finish RA population. LV function was studied in 182 outpatients with rheumatoid arthritis compared with 182 controls matched for age and sex. Patients with RA showed mild but definite tachycardia and lower systolic and diastolic blood pressures at rest. PEP/LVET was equal in both groups and LV mass assessed by echocardiography tended to be increased in males with seropositive disease, while no differences were found in ejection fractions. Mean velocity of cimcumferential fibre shortening (VCF) was significantly higher in female patients then in the controls. As VCF corrected for heart rate showed no difference between patients and controls, this apparently reflected an adequate response to the higher pulse rate. Taken together, the results do not support the concept of LV dysfunction in chronic RA, but rather an altered haemodynamic state caused by the disease itself or by it's treatment.

The next Finish study performed by Mustonen et al. [23] concerned cardiac performance in 12 asymptomatic male patients with RA and 14 control subjects. It was planed to elucidate early disturbances in cardiac function in these subsets. In echocardiography, an IVRT and peak filling rate lower in RA patients then in the controls, which apparently reflected an impairment in LV diastolic function. LV diastolic function assessed by radionuclide angiocardiography at rest and during exercise was similar in both groups. There were no differences between the patients and the control subjects, as regards the heart rate, systolic blood pressure and oxygen uptake during peak exercise. LV diastolic function was impaired in spite of normal LV systolic function in RA patients without clinically evident cardiovascular disease and the authors suggested that the excess of cardiovascular mortality in RA patients can be ascribed to this phenomenon. They emphasized the importance of further epidemiological studies to elucidate this matter.

Kozakova et al. [24] performed echocardiographic, electrocardiographic and roentgenologic examinations in 50 Czech patients with RA and no clinical signs of pericardial effusion. Using one-dimentional echocardiography, pericardial effusion was detected in 27 (54%) subjects. Neither valvular involvement nor specific changes in myocardium were found. In sera of patients with pericardial effusion the presence of rheumatoid factor was significantly more frequent then in patients without effusion. Patients on steroid therapy for the primary disease had statistically lower incidence of pericardial involvement than patients who were subjected to other forms of treatment. Again, echocardiography proved to be the only sensitive non-invasive method capable of detecting small and medium-sized effusions in pericardial cavity.

In the next Czech echocardiography study of Alusik and Skalicka [25] pericardial effusion was detected in 35 out of 104 RA patients. The amount of fluid was small in 29, medium in 3 and large in 3 of them. The thickening of pericardium was seen in 4 patients, mitral valve prolaps in 22 and thickened mitral valve in 10. In 24 patients the authors found a small regurgitation at the mitral valve in 10 patients it was more significant. Thickened aortic valve was seen in 14, a small regurgitation though the valve in 8 and a significant one in 4 patients. The LV dilatation was detected in 13 subjects, it's hypertrophy in 12 and an impaired kinetics in another 12 individuals. Dilatation of the RV was seen in 15 and it's hypertrophy in 3 patients. Ventricular hypertrophy and dilatation as well as an impaired LV were interpreted as consequences of valvular involvement and of associated diseases.

Alpaslan et al. [16] examined a Turkish population of RA patients to assess ventricular function by measurement of myocardial performance index (MPI) and transmitral flow propagation velocity (TFPV), which they reckoned better indices of ventricular function than hithero utilized pulsed-Doppler echocardiography of LV inflow, the results of which were affected by changes in pre- and afterload, tachycardia or first degree A-V block as well as pseudonormalisation phenomenon. 32 patients with long-standing RA and 32 control subjects participated in the study. Systolic function was assessed by subjective evaluation of wall motion for both ventricles and by the assessment of fractional shortening of the LV. LV diastolic function was evaluated by standard pulsed-wave Doppler echocardiography, the MPI and the TFPV. RV function was evaluated by MPI. No subject has signs nor symptoms of clinically overt heart failure. Systolic function was normal in all of them. Echocardiographic functional indices of LV diastolic performance: the peak E velocity, E/A velocity ratio, IVRT, MPI and TFPV in the RA group were significantly different from those of the controls ($p<0.05$). However, the authors did not observe any significant difference in RV echocardiographic indices between the two groups. Their results show, the presence of LV diastolic dysfunction in patients with long-standing RA. The lack of history of cardiotoxic antirheumatic drug use suggested that this abnormality was due to RA itself. The study showed that LV MPI and TFPV, both easily obtained and not affected by ventricular geometry, well identify the presence of LV diastolic dysfunction in patients with long-standing disease. The findings were in accordance with the results of classic measurements methods of LV function: decreased E/A ratio and prolonged IVRT.

Levendoglu et al. [18] in the study on Turkey population tried to evaluate cardiac involvement in patients with active rheumatoid arthritis. 40 of them participated in the study. All were submitted to standard Doppler echocardiography and MPI grading, which revealed LV and RV diastolic function abnormalities with LV MPI significantly higher than in controls ($p<0.05$). A relationship was also found between LV E/A ratio, IVRT and the disease duration ($r=-0.47$ and $p=0.002$, $r=0.618$ and $p=0.000$, respectively). Diastolic function was impaired in both ventricles and a direct relationship between some of the parameters of LV diastolic function and the disease duration was observed, too. The findings suggest the presence of subclinical myocardial involvement in RA patients. The earliest deterioration in cardiac disease is an impaired diastolic function. Such abnormalities have been reported in a number of conditions such as arterial hypertension, coronary artery disease and in elderly subjects, yet the authors selected patients without no evidence of heart problems and impaired ventricular function was observed at all ages in RA, contrary to the control group. Another Turkish study performed by Arslan et al. [26] was planned to evaluate LV diastolic function in patients with active RA by the analysis of conventional Doppler and tissue Doppler echocardiographic imaging (TDI). 52 patients with active RA and 47 healthy persons were included in this study. All were evaluated by M-mode, two-dimentional conventional Doppler echocardiography and the TDI. Late diastolic flow velocity (A) and deceleration time (DT) values were higher in patients with RA than that in the control group ($p<0.001$) and E/A ratio was lower in RA than in the controls ($p<0.001$). Among TDI parameters mitral annular early diastolic velocity (Em) and Em/Am (mitral annular late diastolic velocity) ratio were lower in RA patients then in the control group ($p<0.001$). The correlation was found between A ($r=0.43$, $p=0.001$), DT ($r=0.30$, $p=0.03$), E/A ratio ($r=0.409$, $p=0.004$), Em ($r=0.32$, $p=0.02$), Em/Am ratio ($r=0.30$, $p=0.03$) and E/Em ($r=0.32$, $p=0.02$) and the RA duration. The authors concluded, that patients with active RA in absence of clinically evident heart disease show diastolic dysfunction characterized by impaired E/A ratio, Em/Am ratio and the DT. The relation between diastolic dysfunction and the disease duration suggests a subclinical myocardial involvement.

The Turkish study of Rexhepaj et al. [27] was aimed the assessment of prevalence of diastolic LV and RV dysfunction in patients with rheumatoid arthritis. The authors tried to estimate whether there is a correlation between the duration of RA and the degree of LV diastolic failure. 81 patients (61 females and 20 males) with RA and without clinically evident heart disease (group 1) and 40 healthy subjects (29 females and 11 males) (group 2) were matched for age and sex. Echocardiographic and Doppler studies revealed significant differences in E, A and E/A ratio (0.68 ± 0.19 m/s vs. 0.84 ± 0.14 m/s, $p<0.001$; 0.73 ± 0.15 m/s vs. 0.66 ± 0.13 m/s, $p=0.01$; and 0.97 ± 0.3 vs. 1.32 ± 0.37, $p<0.001$, respectively) between RA patients and the controls. Significant difference between groups was also noted in RV early diastolic (Er)/atrial (Ar) flow velocities (Er/Ar ratio) (1.07 ± 0.3 vs. 1.26 ± 0.3, $p=0.002$) and weak correlation was observed between transmitral E/A ratio and the duration of RA ($r=-0.22$, $p=0.001$). The MPI appeared to differ little in patients with RA as compared to the control group (0.51 ± 0.1 vs. 0.52 ± 0.2, p=NS). In RA individuals without clinically evident cardiovascular disease the LV and RV diastolic function were reduced. LV wall thickness, it's dimensions, systolic function and the MPI remained normal.

Another Turkish investigators Yazici et al. [28] suggested that RA is associated with increased risk of cardiovascular mortality. Considering that cardiovascular findings are mostly subtle and diastolic function abnormalities are one of the earliest manifestations, they aimed at determining diastolic abnormalities in RA at baseline and after a 5-year follow-up. 72 RA patients without any known cardiac disease and 67 controls were recruited for the study. Disease activity score (DAS), blood lipids and C-reactive protein (CRP) levels were determined. LV mass, IVRT, E and A were determined by M-mode two-dimensional color Doppler echocardiography. Mitral annular early (E') and late (A') diastolic velocities were also checked by TDI. 24 RA patients were reevaluated after 5 years for DAS, biochemical variables and echocardiography. In 57 out of 72 (76%) of them and in 12 of the 67 (18%) controls diastolic dysfunction (DD) was diagnosed. In 7 out of 10 patients with DD at baseline it remained in the follow-up, while in 8 patients normal diastolic function sustained. DAS and lipid values did not altered during the follow-up and CRP levels decreased significantly ($p<0.05$). In conclusion, RA patients are prone to develop diastolic function abnormalities in comparison to healthy controls. A 5-year follow-up of this group showed that although clinical response was unsatisfactory, cardiac function was conserved without a major deterioration. Moreover, disease-modifying antirheumatic drugs (DMARDs), such as anti-TNF alpha agent, did not seem to have a major adverse effect on cardiac findings in patients.

The Turkish study of Birdane et al. [29] was aimed at the comparison of standard Doppler and TDI results in RA patients. In 60 such individuals with longstanding disease LV and RV parameters were assessed by standard pulsed-wave Doppler echocardiography, the color M-mode flow propagation velocity and the TDI. LV TDI was achieved at 4 different sites (lateral, septal, anterior and inferior walls) and RV TDI - through the tricuspid lateral annulus. The analysis of the results showed that the basal clinical and echocardiographic parameters: E, A, diastolic velocities of atrioventricular valves, E/A ratio and pulmonary venous Doppler parameters were similar in both groups. The values of LV and RV E/wave deceleration times and IVRT of RA patients were greater then in healthy controls ($p<0.05$). RA patients also had significantly lower color M-mode flow propagation velocity ($p<0.05$), while S' peak and E' peak, two of the LV and RV parameters were similar in both groups. Furthermore A' peak, E'/A', and E/E' values showed statistically significant differences among RA patients. The results confirmed the presence of LV and RV impairment in RA.

In another Turkish study Seyfeli et al. [30] investigated RV diastolic function in RA and it's relationship with LV function and pulmonary involvement. 35 RA patients and 30 healthy controls were submitted to conventional Doppler (CE) and tissue Doppler echocardiography (TDE) to assess LV and RV systolic and diastolic function and to estimate maximal arterial systolic pulmonary pressure (PAP). To detect pulmonary involvement, pulmonary function tests and high-resolution computed tomography (HRCT) scans were performed in all RA individuals. An abnormal RV filling, as expressed by an inverted tricuspid (Tr.) E/A ratio, was detected in 12 (34%) of RA patients and in 2 (7%) of controls ($p<0.004$). The prevalence of RV diastolic abnormalities was higher in RA patients examined by TDE, than by CE (RV annulus Em/Am ratio <1 in 31 (89%) of patients) ($p=0.002$). 22 (63%) RA subjects had abnormal HRCT findings. Pulmonary involvement with pulmonary hypertension (PHT) (36±5 mmHg) was detected in 10 (29%). In this group an increased RV annulus and basal Am wave, decreased Tr. E/A ratio and the decreased RV annulus Em/Am ratio were statistically significant compared to RA patients with pulmonary involvement, who had normal PAP (19±5 mmHg: 12 [34%] of 35), $p=0.014$, $p=0.006$, $p=0.015$, $p=0.049$, respectively). The study revealed an impaired RV filling in a significant part of RA patients without overt heart failure. Impairment of RV diastolic function can be a predictor of subclinical myocardial and pulmonary involvement in RA.

The aim of the next Turkish study of Guyler et al. [31] was the assessment of P wave dispersion (PWD) as a sign for the prediction of atrial fibrillation (AF) and it's relation to clinical and echocardiographic parameters in RA patients. 30 patients (mean age 49±10 years) and 27 healthy controls (mean age 47±8 years) were included in the study and electrocardiography and Doppler echocardiography was performed. Maximum and minimum P wave duration were obtained from electrocardiographic measurements. PWD defined as the difference between maximum and minimum P wave duration was calculated. Maximum P wave duration and PWD were higher in RA patients than in the controls ($p=0.031$ and $p=0.001$, respectively), however there were no significant correlation between PWD and disease duration ($r=0.375$, $p=0.009$) and IVRT ($r=0.390$, $p=0.006$). P wave duration and PWD was higher in RA patients than in the controls and was closely associated with the disease duration and LV diastolic dysfunction.

In the last Turkish study Canturk et al. [32] evaluated diastolic functions in patients with RA by assessment of propagation velocity and intraventricular dispersion of E wave velocity. 34 RA cases without evidence of cardiac disease and LV systolic impairment were enrolled in the study. Echocardiographic examinations were performed for the evaluation of diastolic dysfunction (DD) in all of them. Propagation velocity in RA patients was significantly lower than in the control group (42±16 cm/s, 54±15 cm/s, p=0.002). There was significant intraventricular dispersion of E wave velocity towards the cardiac apex in RA patients (p<0.001) compared to the controls (p=0.79). There was also a significant correlation between intraventricular dispersion of E wave velocity and diastolic dysfunction in the patients in which the duration of illness was longer than 10 years (p<0.001). The authors concluded that an impaired LV relaxation in RA, correlated with the duration of the disease might be due to structural myocardial abnormalities. Furthermore, the combined use of propagation velocity and intraventricular E wave dispersion measurements can help in early determination of diastolic functions in RA patients.

The Russian publication of Krasnosel'skĭ et al. [33] concerned the use of tissue dopplerography (TDG) in detection of myocardial involvement in RA by assessment of the velocity of myocardial movement. TDG was carried out in 22 patients with verified RA (age 33-66, mean age 45.2±7.4 years) and in 20 healthy volunteers (age 29-58, mean age 44.6±8.4 years). Modules of velocities of systolic and early diastolic peaks in LV wall at basal level and at levels of upper, middle and lower thirds were calculated in all patients. In some LV segments the results correlated with CRP and ESR in RA (r from 0.29 to 0.46) and were diffusely lowered in this disease, which on author's opinion reflected the participation of inflammatory process in development of asymptomatic diffuse myocardial damage in RA.

Gonzales-Juanatey et al. [34] examined Spanish population towards the frequency of echocardiographic and Doppler abnormalities in long-term treated RA patients without clinically overt heart disease. 47 such individuals, treated for at least 5 years with 1 or more DMARDs were recruited. Those with cardiovascular risk factors, cardiovascular or cerebrovascular events were excluded from the study. 47 healthy persons formed the control grouping patients with RA. The presence of aortic regurgitation (17%) and tricuspid regurgitation (17%) was higher than in the controls (15% and 6%, respectively). Pulmonary artery systolic pressure was higher in RA patients (30.3±8.0 mmHg) compared to the in control subjects (26.2±4.8) (p=0.004). The incidence of pulmonary artery systolic pressure above 35 mm Hg was significantly higher in RA patients (21% versus 4% in controls; p= 0.03), diastolic dysfunction caused by impaired relaxation was more common in patients with RA (66%) than in controls (43%) (p=0.02) and more frequent in older patients. Extraarticular manifestations were more common in patients with RA in whom diastolic dysfunction was recognized (p=0.05). This study confirmed a high frequency of LV diastolic dysfunction and pulmonary hypertension in patients with RA without evident cardiovascular disease.

In French patients Meune et al. [35] were determined the sensitivity and accuracy of tissue-Doppler echocardiography (TDE) to assess myocardial contractility. The stimulus of this study was an observation that heart failure was one of the determinants of the excess mortality in RA patients. Consecutive 27 RA individuals with normal results of cardiac clinical examination were prospectively included and compared to 27 controls. All underwent conventional echocardiography, furthermore their systolic and diastolic strain rate (SR) were determined by TDE. When compared to the controls RA patients had increased LV mass (99±24 vs 80±25g/m^2, p=0.009), and a trend towards left atrial enlargement (31±3 vs 29±6 mm, p=0.006). Fractional shortening and systolic SR did not differ between groups. Diastolic function, as estimated by the E/A Doppler velocity ratio was similar in both populations (p=0.18). However, diastolic SR was strikingly reduced in patients with RA versus controls (3.7±1.3 vs 5.5±1.1 s-1, p <0.001). In 18 out of 27 RA patients markedly reduced diastolic SR (SR<4s-1) was noted, too. None of the RA characteristics was associated with significant differences in TDE measurements. This study confirmed that TDE enable to identify impaired diastolic function in RA even in cases where it can not be detected by conventional measurements.

An Indian project of Uddayakumar et al. [36] was one of the in numerous studies on the prevalence of diastolic dysfunction in RA from Indian subcontinent. The aim of it was to evaluate LV filling abnormalities in RA patients without clinically evident cardiovascular manifestations and to search for their correlation with the disease duration. 45 such patients affected by RA diagnosed according to ARA criteria were selected and compared with age and sex matched control subjects. All were submitted to M-mode, two-dimensional and Doppler echocardiography. E, A, E/A ratio, IVRT, EF and fractional shortening were evaluated. In RA patients LV filling abnormalities were characterized by a reduced E/A ratio (mean [SD] 0.98 [0.22]) compared to the controls (1.09 [0.11]; p-value equals 0.004), prolonged IVRT (75.77 [8.12] ms versus 70.43 [2.94] ms; p-value equals 0.001) and increased late diastole flow velocity (76.91 [11.61] cm/s versus 70.11 [5.32] cm/s; p-value equals 0.001). A negative correlation was found between E/A ratio and the disease duration (Pearson correlation, r equals -0.56, p-value equals 0.001), indicating that diastolic dysfunction rate increased with disease duration. A strong correlation was also found between IVRT and the disease duration (r equals 0.66, p-value equals 0.01) and between late diastolic flow velocity and the disease duration (r equals 0.61, p-value equals 0.001). The study confirms a high frequency of LV diastolic dysfunction characterized by impaired E/A ratio, prolonged IVRT and increased late diastole flow velocity in patients with RA without evident cardiovascular disease. The correlation between transmitral flow alteration and the disease duration suggests a progressive subclinical myocardial involvement with the disease progression. This may be relevant to high incidence of cardiovascular deaths observed in patients with RA.

Honda et al. [37] from Japan performed in 1981 studied cardiac function and vascular hemodynamics by non–invasive means in order to assess LV performance in 50 RA patients and 30 healthy controls. They did not find significant difference in LV end-diastolic dimension, LV posterior wall thickness, LV posterior wall excursion and mean posterior wall velocity between groups, yet the ejection fraction and ejection time/preejection period were significantly decreased. Hemodynamic status in patients with advanced RA in this study was characterized by mild tachycardia and a mild decrease of LV function, pericardial effusion was also noted in these individuals.

Echocardiography, a rapidly developing diagnostic procedure enable to examine heart structure and function in different clinical setting. It can be particularly useful in connective tissue diseases, such as rheumatoid arthritis. Generalized inflammatory process in these conditions affects heart muscle directly and through changes in tissue vasculature induced by cytokins and other inflammatory mediators of prothrombotic and atherogenic properties. Inflammatory vasculitis, another well-known complication of RA, especially of long duration, also contribute to heart damage in this disease. Cardiac muscle fibrosis and amyloidosis, that develop as further sequels of rheumatoid arthritis, add to cardiovascular system, especially diastolic function, impairment. Thrombus formation at heart valves with consecutive stenosis and/or regurgitations is an independent factor that disturb heart function in RA individuals.

Furthermore, one must not neglect the deleterious effects of drugs used to combat RA on cardiopulmonary system. Non-steroid anti-inflammatory agents with their water-retention and renal-toxic effects can induce or exacerbate hypertension and heart failure. So can cause corticosteroids, yet these are also known to strongly enhance atherogenesis and thrombosis. Methotrexate, the most popular and most effective of conventionally used DMARDs is able to induce lung fibrosis and therefore cause pulmonary hypertension, moreover it is renal-toxic. Chloroquine exerts proarrhytmic effect and cyklosporin induce hypertension. Gold salts, as well as D-penicillamine are also known to be capable of causing vasculitis and adversely affect patients' cardiovascular risk factor profile.

All these data clearly indicate to high risk of cardiovascular diseases in RA patients. Echocardiography in turn enables to detect early pathological changes of this kind and therefore can be helpful in prevention of the development of life-threatening complications. The results of studies presented in this topic confirm the utility of different echocardiography techniques in detecting heart damage in RA patients. Echocardiography visualizes for example decreased LV diastolic performance, as the earliest predictor of development of left ventricular heart failure, different kinds of valvular defects, pulmonary hypertension and the presence of pericardial effusion. The last one, although rarely clinically significant and only scarcely causing life-threatening complications is tamponade or constrictive pericarditis. Pericarditis is nevertheless present in about 30% of RA cases post-mortem [38]. It's appearance during patient's diagnostics could therefore be useful in recording cardiovascular involvement by RA, difficult or impossible to visualize by conventional methods. Another echocardiography application in RA is to investigate correlations between heart changes and the disease duration and activity, as well as with the patient's age. The discovery of such dependences can be helpful in prediction and therefore prevention of heart damage and perhaps other complications of RA.

Taken together - echocardiography is a chance for improving diagnostic methods in RA, yet further investigations are needed to work out techniques and medical standards in such patients. Hagendorff and Pfeiffer [39] focused on echocardiography application in modern diagnostics of connective tissue diseases, with special regard for rheumatoid arthritis. The authors concluded, that the prerequisites for successful diagnostic echocardiography in RA are the knowledge of modern echocardiographic techniques like tissue Doppler and contrast echocardiography and clinical experience with patients with rheumatoid arthritis. The standardization of procedures is important for reproducibility and comparability of results.

2. References

[1] Bacon PA, Gibson DG. Cardiac involvement in rheumatoid arthritis. An echocardiographic study. *Ann Rheum Dis* 1974; 33: 20-24.

[2] Prakash R, Atassi A, Poske R, Rosen KM. Prevalence of pericardial effusion and mitral valve involvement in patients with rheumatoid arthritis without cardiac symptoms. *N Engl J Med* 1973; 289: 597-600.

[3] Nomeir AM, Turner R, Watts E, Smith D, West G, Edmonds J. Cardiac involvement in rheumatoid arthritis. *Ann Int Med* 1973; 79: 800-806.

[4] Mac Donald WJ Jr, Crawford MH, Klippel JH, Zvaifler N, O'Rourke R. Echocardiographic assessment of cardiac structure and function in patients with rheumatoid arthritis. *Ann J Med* 1977; 63: 890-896.

[5] Davia JE, Cheitlin MD, de Castro CM, Lawless O, Niemi L. Absence of echocardiographic abnormalities of the anterior mitral valve leaflet in rheumatoid arthritis. *Ann Int Med* 1975; 83: 500-502.

[6] Nomeir AM, Turner RA, Watts E. Cardiac involvement in rheumatoid arthritis. Followup study. *Arthritis Rheum* 1979; 25:561- 564.

[7] Mody GM, Stevens JE, Meyers OL. The heart in rheumatoid arthritis - a clinical and laboratory study. *Q J Med* 1987; 65: 921-928.

[8] Toumanidis ST, Papamichael CM, Antoniades LG, Pantelia MI, Saridakis NS, Mavrikakis ME, Sideris DA, Moulopoulos SD. *Cardiac involvement in collagen diseases Eur Heart J* 1995; 16: 257-262.

[9] Nagyhegyi G, Nadas I, Banyai F, Luzsa G, Geher P, Molnar J, Velics V, Gomor B, Weisz M, Antaloczy Z. Cardiac and cardiopulmonary disorders in patients with ankylosing spondylitis and rheumatoid arthritis. *Clin Exp Rheumatol.* 1988;6:17-26.

[10] Villecco AS, Ferri S, de Liberali E, Ferrari G, Marsigli R. Apport de l'echocardiographie au depistage des lesions cardiaques dans la polyarthrite rhumatoide. *Revue du Rhumatisme* 1983; 50: 187-193.

[11] Wislowska M, Sypuła S, Kowalik I. Echocardiographic findings, 24-hour electrocardiographic Holter monitoring in patients with rheumatoid arthritis according to Steinbrocker's criteria, functional index, value of Waaler-Rose titre and duration of disease. *Clin Rheumatol* 1998;17:369-377.

[12] Wislowska M, Sypuła S, Kowalik I. Echocardiographic findings and 24-h electrocardiographic Holter monitoring in patients with nodular and non-nodular rheumatoid arthritis. *Rheumatol Int* 1999; 18: 163-169.

[13] Barlow JB, Pocock WA. Mitral valve prolapsed, the specific billowing mitral leaflet syndrome, or an insignificant non-ejection systolic click. *Am Heart J* 1979; 97:277-285.

[14] Leatham A, Brigden W. Mild mitral regurgitation and the mitral prolapsed fiasco. *Am Heart J* 1980; 99: 659-664.

[15] Wislowska M, Jaszczyk B, Kochmański M, Sypuła S, Sztechman M. Diastolic heart function in rheumatoid arthritis patients. *Rheumatol Int* 2008; 28: 513-519.

[16] Alpaslan M, Onrat E, Evcik D. Doppler echocardiographic evaluation of ventricular function in patients with rheumatoid arthritis. *Clin Rheumatol* 2003; 22: 84-88.

[17] Di Franco M, Paradiso M, Mammarella A, Paoletti V, Labbadia G, Coppotelli L, Taccari E, Musca A. Diastolic function abnormalities in rheumatoid arthritis. Evaluation by echo Doppler transmitral flow and pulmonary venous flow: relation with duration of disease. *Ann Rheum Dis.* 2000;59:227-229

[18] Levendoglu F, Temizhan A, Ugurlu H, Ozdemir A, Yazici M. Ventricular function abnormalities in active rheumatoid arthritis: a Doppler echocardiographic study. *Rheumatol Int.* 2004;24:141-146.

[19] Maione S, Valentini G, Giunta A, Tirri R, Giacummo A, Lippolis C, Arnese M, de Paulis A, Marone G, Tirri G. Cardiac involvement in rheumatoid arthritis: an echocardiographic study. *Cardiology* 1993; 83: 234-239.

[20] Corrao S, Sallì L, Arnone S, Scaglione R, Pinto A, Licata G. Echo-Doppler left ventricular filling abnormalities in patients with rheumatoid arthritis without clinically evident cardiovascular disease. *Eur J Clin Invest.* 1996;26:293-297.

[21] Montecucco C, Gobbi G, Perlini S, Rossi S, Grandi AM, Caporali R, Finardi G. Impaired diastolic function in active rheumatoid arthritis. Relationship with disease duration. *Clin Exp Rheumatol.* 1999;17:407-412.

[22] Voipio-Pulkki LM, Sarate M. Left ventricular function in rheumatoid arthritis. *Eur Heart J* 1987; 8 (Supplement J), 105-107.

[23] Mustonen J, Laakso M, Hirvonen T, Mutru O, Pirnes M, Vainio P, Kuikka JT, Rautio P, Länsimies E. Abnormalities in left ventricular diastolic function in male patients with rheumatoid arthritis without clinically evident cardiovascular disease. *Eur J Clin Invest.* 1993;23:246-53.

[24] Kozakova M, Hradec J, Petrasek J, Kolbel F, Urbanova M, Dostal C. Cardiac involvement in progressive polyarthritis - an echocardiographic study. *Cor Vasa* 1985; 27: 54-59.

[25] Alusik S, Skalicka H. Cardiac involvement in rheumatoid arthritis - an echocardiographic study. "R", 1991, 21: 17-21.

[26] Arslan S, Bozkurt E, Sari RA, Erol MK. Diastolic function abnormalities in active rheumatoid arthritis evaluation by conventional Doppler and tissue Doppler: relation with duration of disease. *Clin Rheumatol.* 2006 ;25:294-299.

[27] Rexhepaj N, Bajraktari G, Berisha I, Beqiri A, Shatri F, Hima F, Elezi S, Ndrepepa G. Left and right ventricular diastolic functions in patients with rheumatoid arthritis without clinically evident cardiovascular disease. *Int J Clin Pract.* 2006;60:683-688.

[28] Yazici D, Tokay S, Aydin S, Toprak A, Inanc N, Khan SR, Fak AS, Direskeneli H. Echocardiographic evaluation of cardiac diastolic function in patients with rheumatoid arthritis: 5 years of follow-up. *Clin Rheumatol.* 2008;27:647-650.

[29] Birdane A, Korkmaz C, Ata N, Cavusoglu Y, Kasifoglu T, Dogan SM, Gorenek B, Goktekin O, Unalir A, Timuralp B. Tissue Doppler imaging in the evaluation of the left and right ventricular diastolic functions in rheumatoid arthritis. *Echocardiography.* 2007;24:485-493.

[30] Seyfeli E, Guler H, Akoglu S, Karazincir S, Akgul F, Saglam H, Seydaliyeva T, Yalcin F. Right ventricular diastolic abnormalities in rheumatoid arthritis and its relationship with left ventricular and pulmonary involvement. A tissue Doppler echocardiographic study. *Int J Cardiovasc Imaging* 2006; 22: 745-754.

[31] Guyler H, Seyfeli E, Sahin G, Duru M, Akgul F, Saglam H, Yalcin F. P wave dispersion in patients with rheumatoid arthritis: its relation with clinical and echocardiographic parameters. *Rheumatol Int* 2007;27:813-818.

[32] Canturk F, Yazici M, Alayli G, Menekse EB, Demircan S, Ibrahimli F, Menekse S. Combined use of propagation velocity and intraventricular dispersion of E wave velocity for the evaluation of diastolic functions in patients with rheumatoid arthritis. *Int J Cardiovasc Imaging.* 2006;22:369-376.

[33] Krasnosel'skĭ MI, Bratanova MZ, Polupan AA, Tsurko VV. Tissue dopplerography of the myocardium in diagnosis of myocardial involvement in patients with rheumatoid arthritis. *Kardiologiia.* 2007;47:59-62.

[34] Gonzalez-Juanatey C, Testa A, Garcia-Castelo A, Garcia-Porrua C, Llorca J, Ollier WE, Gonzalez-Gay MA. Echocardiographic and Doppler findings in long-term treated

rheumatoid arthritis patients without clinically evident cardiovascular disease. *Semin Arthritis Rheum*. 2004;33:231- 238.

[35] Meune C, Wahbi K, Assous N, Weber S, Kahan A, Allanore Y. Myocardial dysfunction in rheumatoid arthritis: a controlled tissue-Doppler echocardiography study. *J Rheumatol*. 2007;34:2005-2009.

[36] Udayakumar N, Venkatesan S., Rajendiran C. Diastolic function abnormalities in rheumatoid arthritis: relation with duration of disease. *Singapore Med J*. 2007;48:537-542.

[37] Honda M, Muraki N, Takahari O, Nohira K, Matsui N, Hirai A. Cardiac function and vascular hemodynamics in rheumatoid arthritis. *Revue du Rhumatisme* 1981; (numero special Juin) 0320.

[38] Leibowitz WB. The heart in rheumatoid arthritis (rheumatoid disease). A clinical and pathological study of 62 cases. *Ann Int Med* 1963; 58: 102-123.

[39] Hagendorff A, Pfeiffer D. Echocardiographic functional analysis of patients with rheumatoid arthritis and collagen diseases. *Z Rheumatol*. 2005; 64: 239-248.

Part 5

Nuclear Cardiology

13

Fleming-Harrington Redistribution Wash-in Washout (FHRWW): The Platinum Standard for Nuclear Cardiology

Richard M. Fleming and Gordon M. Harrington
FHHI, UNI
USA

1. Introduction

Since its advent in 1925, Nuclear Cardiology has undergone multiple changes in technology including detectors, computers, changes in protocols, various approaches to stress including physiologic and pharmacologic methods, changes in the type of isotope utilized and finally concerns over the distribution of radioactive isotopes and efforts to improve the detection of heart disease while reducing radiation dosage to both patients and health care workers alike. We will divide this chapter into five Sections. First, we will review the work that led to the discovery that the technetium-99m isotopes, like thallium-201, redistribute. Secondly, we will look at currently employed Cardiac imaging using Single Photon Emission Computed Tomography (SPECT) cameras for detecting technetium-99m isotopes (principally Sestamibi). Thirdly, we will consider how these isotopes are injected, distributed and redistributed within Cardiac tissue. Fourth, we will look at how single injection stress-stress imaging can not only increase the accuracy of SPECT imaging of the heart, detecting the most critically diseased coronary vessels while reducing the amount of radioactive isotope injected into the patient, who will subsequently expose others to this radiation and finally, we will look at how rest-rest comparisons of isotope redistribution can be used to differentiate between viable and non-viable damaged myocardial tissue using SPECT cameras.

At the completion of this chapter, clinician and scientist alike, will (1) better understand the physics of SPECT imaging of the heart, (2) will better understand the kinetics of technetium-99m isotopes (which are applicable to thallium-201 and other isotopes, given differences in redistribution times), (3) be able to better detect heart disease with special emphasis placed on ischemic heart disease, while addressing issues of patient radiation safety (4) be able to differentiate viable from non-viable cardiac tissue and (5) be able to utilize SPECT cameras to extract both anatomic and physiologic information, not currently possible with single isotope injection, single camera imaging systems, including Positron Emission Tomography (PET), Magnetic Resonance Imaging (MRI) and/or Computed Tomography (CT). Currently, imaging with PET cameras, cannot be completed rapidly enough to allow for measurements of redistribution properties of PET isotopes, nor is it clear if any of these isotopes (ammonia, FDG, Rb-82, etc) actually have redistribution properties, while MRI and Coronary CT currently are only able to yield anatomic information and are unable to measure physiologic redistribution of isotopes. This chapter will describe the recent advances in single isotope injection, single camera imaging (FHRWW) while explaining why the practice of rest-stress imaging has failed to deliver on the promises made.

2. Discovering the redistribution properties of technetium-99m isotopes

The development of Nuclear Cardiology (discussed in detail later in this chapter) evolved through the utilization of Thallium-201 (Tl-201) by the 1970's. The protocol at that time consisted of stressing the patient and injecting 1-3 mCi (74-111 MBq) intravenously into the patients venous system and continuing to exercise the patient for an additional minute prior to ceasing exercise (Fleming, 1991a, 1999a). The patient was then "recovered" and underwent "stress" imaging one hour after initiation of the patients exercise session. While imaging one hour after exercise is clearly not a period of time when the individual is "stressed", the terminology persisted since this image was the first image obtained following the stress. Subsequently, these images became known as "stress" images. Over time, thallium distribution changed and consequently the appearance of the images themselves changed. This became known as "redistribution" since the distribution of Th-201 changed with time. For lack of a better term, this second image was coined a "resting" image and their comparison was used to define changes, which were thought to represent ischemia and possibly infarction. As we shall see in subsequent sections, neither Blumgart (1926) nor Gorlin (1959) considered this to be so and a better understanding of their work might have saved Nuclear Cardiology decades of misdirection. However, the actual ability to detect infarction was not through the rest image obtained in this manner; but rather, a resting (Parkey 1976, Ahmad 1979, Walsh 1977) image obtained by using Tc-99m pyrophosphate (Tc-99 PYP), which required imaging of the heart within 48-72 hours of the time of infarction to accurately detect. Efforts to replace Tc-99m PYP with newer imaging agents (Khaw 1999) not only emphasize the limitations of timing and possible overlap of bone activity; but, the importance of utilization of resting images and not stress images to determine the presence or absence of damaged (infarction, stunned, hibernating) myocardium, as emphasized by Blumgart (1926) and Gorlin (1959).

Over time, the lessons of Blumgart and Gorlin were all but forgotten and the terms "stress" and "rest" anthropomorphically took on a life and meaning of their own. Instead of viewing comparative Nuclear images obtained under same state conditions at two different points in time, which could then be compared to look for changes in distribution of isotope scintillation consistent with changes in supply (blood flow) and function (cellular, including mitochondria), the introduction of technetium-99m isotopes were introduced with directions by the manufacturers that clinicians and scientists needed to give two injections (rest stress), instead of one (stress-redistribution) used for Tl-201. In the first instance, teboroxime (Fleming 1991a) was reported as having too rapid a "washout" (another term for redistribution), which would prevent multiple imaging given the camera acquisition speed of the time, while Sestamibi would be promoted as having no washout allowing one to chose when they wanted to image the patient; a property which would be warmly welcomed by nuclear medicine departments concerned with the number of studies being ordered and nuclear departments scheduling issues. Truly, this alleged property of Sestamibi was a welcomed relief for such scheduling issues. This misinformation continued to drive the market reducing study accuracy despite multiple studies reporting that Sestamibi did in fact redistribute. By using this redistribution property, investigators have been better able to define heart failure (Hurwitz 1993, 1998, Saha 1994, Giubbini 1995,

Sugiura 2006, Kumita 2002), cardiomyopathy (Matsuo 2007, Ikawa 2007, Meissner 2002) and coronary artery vasospasm (Ono 2002, 2003). Perhaps the most compelling work was published by Maublant (1988), prior to the introduction of Sestamibi into the United States. This work revealed that Sestamibi has a 28 minute washout under non-ischemic conditions while the work of Crane (1993), which was funded by the pharmaceutical company itself, demonstrated that under ischemic conditions, the washout of Sestamibi occurred more rapidly due to mitochondrial calcium overload. This information, to date, continues to appear within package inserts as shown in Figure 1 and is now described as having "minimal cardiac redistribution," encouraging physicians to use multiple doses for studies.

	REST				**STRESS**			
	Heart		**Liver**		**Heart**		**Liver**	
Time	**Biological**	**Effective**	**Biological**	**Effective**	**Biological**	**Effective**	**Biological**	**Effective**
5 min.	1.2	1.2	19.6	19.4	1.5	1.5	5.0	5.8
30 min.	1.1	1.0	12.2	11.5	1.4	1.3	4.5	4.2
1 hour	1.0	0.9	5.6	5.0	1.4	1.2	2.4	2.1
2 hours	1.0	0.8	2.2	1.7	1.2	1.0	0.9	0.7
4 hours	0.8	0.5	0.7	0.4	1.0	0.6	0.3	0.2

A study in a dog myocardial ischemia model reported that Technetium TC99m Sestamibi undergoes myocardial distribuion (redistribution), although more slowly and less completely than thalous chloride Tl-201. A study in a dog myocardial infarction model reported that the drug showed no redistribution of any consequence. Definitive human studies to demonstrate possible redistribution have not been reported. In patients with documented myocardial infarction, imaging revealed the infarct up to four hours post dose.

Fig. 1. Cardiolite US PI 513121-0309 (3-16-2009 package insert)

After our initial work (Fleming 1991a) with these Tc-99m isotopes in 1989, we published several papers (Fleming 1995, 1998, 1999a-b, 1992a-b, 2000a-b, 2002a-b) under the misinformation that two injections of these compounds were required and like many others we failed to fully understand the work of Blumgart and Gorlin. By 1999-2000, Sestamibi was being used for the detection of breast cancer. The company involved with this work (under the trade name Miraluma) was concerned that clinicians were not ordering the study due to what was perceived as incorrect results. Studies performed show "abnormal" results without the detection of biopsy proven breast cancer. However, the tissue while not cancerous was not "normal" either and considerable confusion existed at the time. We were asked to conduct breast imaging studies and developed a method for simultaneous detection of both heart disease and breast disease. The results were published (Fleming 2002c-e, 2003a-c) and presented at several meetings as shown in Figure 2. While beyond the scope of this text, it resulted in our looking more closely at the information, which the nuclear computer was seeing (Fleming 2003d) and which we were not; viz. the actual scintigraphic counts from regions of interest (ROIs) as shown in Figure 3 for the breast and Figure 4 for the heart. This approach not only gave us a greater insight as to the cause of angina, viz. regional blood flow differences (Fleming 2003d); but, it allowed us to additionally see for the first time detectable evidence of an activated thymus gland (Fleming 2003e) with enlargement and increased isotope uptake associated with coronary artery disease/inflammation (Fleming 1999c, 2003e, 2008a) and providing further evidence of underlying coronary artery disease. This same state physiologic approach allowed us to compare images of the heart taken at 5 minutes and 60 minutes following pharmacologic stressing of the heart utilizing a single injection of the isotope Sestamibi. These rather crude early findings (Figure 5) clearly demonstrated that individuals with ischemic heart disease revealed different distribution patterns of Sestamibi within cardiac tissue at 5 and 60 minutes post stress, proving that Sestamibi in fact "redistributes" within the heart and confirmed the information reported by others as noted above and as we will see in the remainder of this chapter, it has been confirmed by others world wide as well as recent work out of both UCLA and Harvard (Sheikine 2010). We have also demonstrated (Fleming 2009) that technetium-99m tetrofosmin (trade name Myoview) similarly redistributes. Since it is imperative that comparison images be performed on the same SPECT camera to allow meaningful comparisons of the two images, we will now turn our attention to the details of when nuclear SPECT cameras provide us the information we are seeking and when they do not.

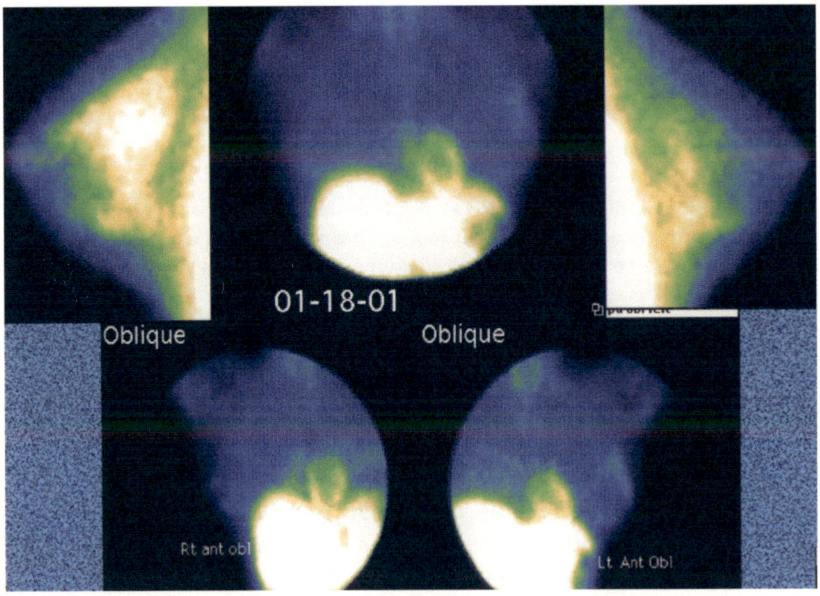

Fig. 2. Acquisition of Heart and Breast Image 5 Minutes After Stress Injection

Information obtained from the package insert of this product reports that "Definitive human studies to demonstrate possible redistribution have not been reported." The information provided as discussed in the text and literature clearly shows this not to be the case.

Following pharmacologic stress and injection of sestamibi, images of cardiac and breast tissue were acquired using a SPECT camera 5-minutes after cessation of stress. Detection of thymic tissue, while not noted in this individual, has been published by us elsewhere (Fleming 2003e).

Here breast enhanced scintigraphy test (BEST) images from three different women are quantified using regions of interest (ROIs) and compared with results (immediately below each image) obtained by Dr. William Dooley using ductoscopy. The results of tissue specimens were confirmed pathologically as representing inflammatory tissue and cancer respectively as shown in the images. This study provided further information as to the ability to reliable "quantify" differences on Nuclear imaging using ROI and the role of scintigraphy measurement in diagnosing both heart disease and breast cancer.

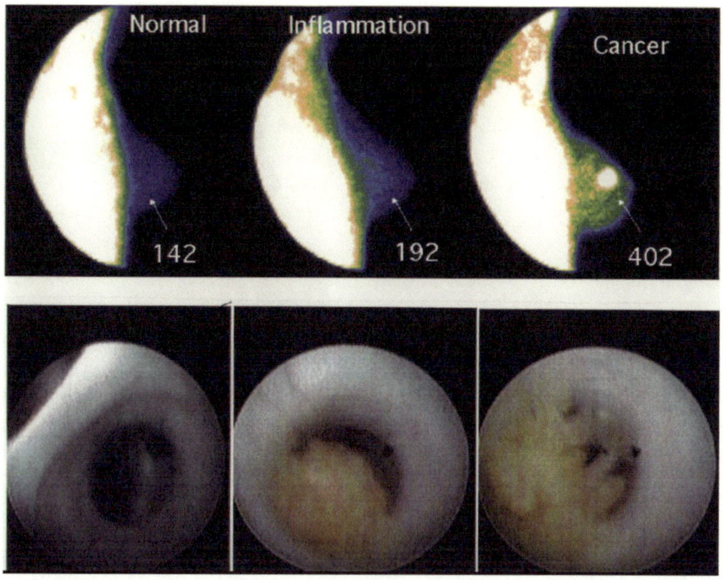

Fig. 3. Analysis of regions of interest (ROIs) of breast tissue

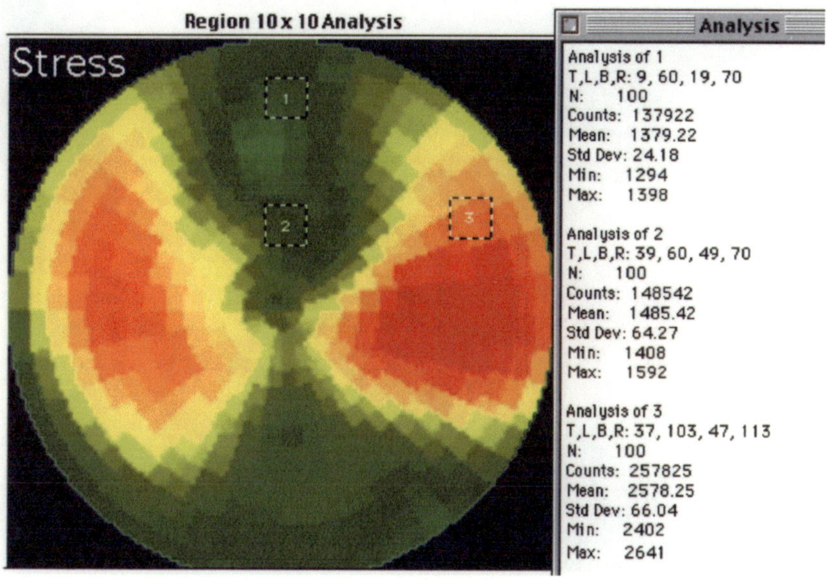

Fig. 4. Analysis of regions of interest (ROIs) from Cardiac bullseye images

While qualitative Gestalt of images are frequently utilized for both clinical and scientific work, regions 1 (mean count of 1379.22) and 2 (mean count of 1485.42) represents an almost 8% difference in count activity which cannot be appreciated visually. The quantification of the differences in regions (ROIs) of interest (Fleming 2003d) was utilized to demonstrate that angina is not the result of narrowed arteries; but rather, the reduced ability of diseased arteries to vasodilate to the extent that non-diseased coronary arteries can dilate (viz. regional blood flow differences) under the influence of pharmacologic stress.

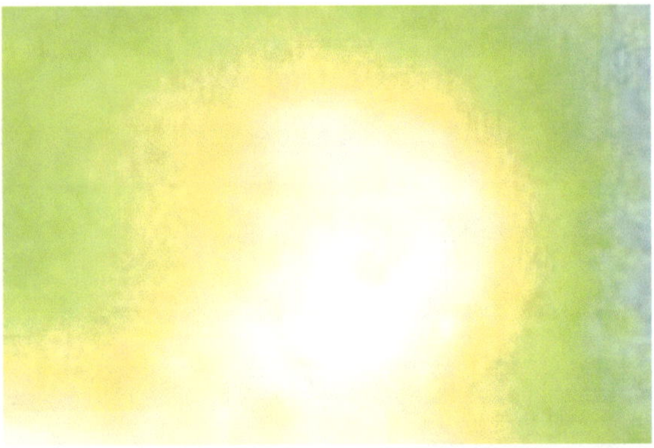

a) 5 Minute post-stress image taken on NucLear MAC SPECT Camera

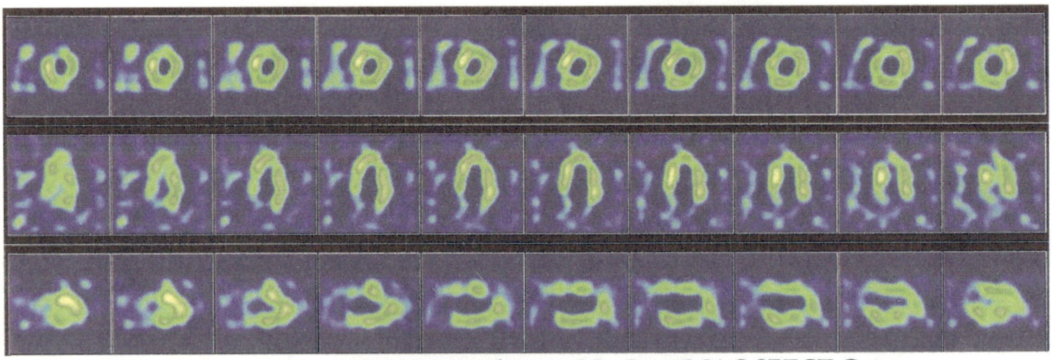

b) 60 Minute post-stress image taken on NucLear MAC SPECT Camera

c) Washout of Sestamibi as determined by NucLear MAC Spect Camera system

Fig. 5a-c. Early comparisons of coronary artery disease showing differences in Sestamibi distribution at 5 and 60 minutes post stressing of the heart

This early study SPECT camera image reveals an anterior image of the heart acquired 5 minutes after peak cardiac stress and Sestamibi injection, demonstrating no regional defects in isotope activity.

This qualitative study, performed in 2001 of the same patient in figure 5A, shows washout of Sestamibi compared with the 5-minute image. Here there are both distal anterior and apical reductions in isotope in addition to a dilated right ventricle. Clearly, these early 2001 studies demonstrated that Sestamibi redistributes throughout cardiac tissue with different results seen at 5 and 60 minutes post-stress. This is confirmed in the "washout" study seen in Figure 5C. Bullseye definition of "washout" made by the same SPECT camera system using it's computer software to compare the two sets of images shown above (5A and 5B). The results show a qualitative (blue) redistribution/washout in the distal anterior and apical regions. Clearly, these 2001 images show differences in isotope distribution between the 5 and 60-minute images. Similar findings have now been reported by others, including researchers at UCLA and Harvard Universities (Sheikine 2010).

3. The Fleming-Harrington nuclear imaging uncertainty principle. Understanding the physics of how nuclear SPECT cameras really work?

Abstract: The introduction of the Heisenberg Uncertainty principle and Nuclear Cardiology occurred simultaneously in 1925-1927. Thirty years later the Anger gamma camera would allow for a more sophisticated radioactive isotope counting to determine the presence or absence of disease. When employed with technetium-99m isotopes, ischemic heart disease can be inferred by differences in visual appearance of cardiac images. These gestalts of imaging results have been separated from the quantitative information recorded by the cameras computer. We investigated whether current camera and computer systems are sophisticated enough to quantify differences between images to be clinically relevant. Our study demonstrated that efforts to "sharpen" image appearance does so at a reduction in "accuracy". Like Heisenberg, this work shows that one cannot know the exact location and the amount of activity simultaneously and that a decision must be made for accuracy over image sharpness if one is to truly quantify differences in isotope concentration between images.

In 1927, Werner Heisenberg (Heisenberg 1927), published his "Uncertainty principle" which in brief states that it is impossible to simultaneously know both the position and momentum of an electron or any other particle with any degree of accuracy or "certainty." To define the location of an electron required interaction with it. This interaction would result in movement of the electron and as a result, would move the electron. The best one could achieve is knowledge of where the electron was at the time of interaction.

The first utilization of nuclear isotopes for medical imaging and evaluation of heart disease was conducted by Blumgart (1926) in February of 1925 when he injected himself with Radium C, which emits alpha and beta particles and gamma rays. As such, the Geiger counter chamber developed by Blumgart and Yens, could detect the passage of blood carrying the radium. The studies would first be published in 1926 (Blumgart 1926) and become known as "circulation time" and would dynamically define myocardial contractility by comparing changes in count activity over time.

In 1957, Hal Anger (1957) demonstrated the first gamma camera designed to detect the emission of radioactive decay emanating from the patient. In essence, a modern Geiger counter which could be held some distance from the chest to measure isotope decay while present in cardiac tissue. The decay (scintillation) is detected by the camera after being absorbed by the camera crystal (usually sodium iodide) with the subsequent release of an electron from the sodium iodide, which is subsequently detected by a photomultiplier (PMT) tube as shown in Figure 6. These scintillations are tallied by the computer. These anger cameras have been used to image various regions of the body using radioactive isotopes which are known to localize to the tissues in question. For cardiac disease this has primarily included thallium-201 and technetium-99m.

The utilization of these cameras have been assumed to be able to detect changes in isotope availability by "counting" the amount of radioactivity as described and translating this information into a black and white or color format image for human viewing and interpretation of disease. However, to the best our knowledge, no such experimentation has been carried out to determine if today's gamma cameras can in fact accurately count radioactive decay required for image comparison. This quantification is necessary to compare redistribution of isotopes and to avoid errors in interpretation. This requires more than simply the ability to produce pictures of different brightness; it requires actual ability to measure differences in isotope decay (scintillation), as did Blumgarts Geiger counter. This is the basis of devices used to determine human radiation exposure and is a requirement in diagnostic imaging. To investigate this we conducted a series of experiments with known quantities of Tc-99m and utilized two different matrixes commonly employed in clinical cardiology to determine if the cameras are able to accurately measure radioactive decay.

The acquisition of technetium-99m isotopes for diagnostic purposes results from the radioactive decay of the parent compound (Molybdenum) to the daughter compound (technetium-99m) is shown in Figure 7. The half-life for technetium-99m is 6.01 hours as shown in Figure 8. Each sample of technetium-99m contained 10.1 mCi (37.37 MBq) of radioactive compound. Each sample was sealed in a syringe preventing any leakage of material. If the cameras are able to accurately measure isotope decay, the camera should reveal a 10% reduction in count activity from the first image and the second image taken 55 minutes later. Utilizing a Philips Forte Dual head single photon emission computed tomography (SPECT) camera with general all purpose collimators, the camera was set to (1) a 64 x 64 matrix and (2) 128 x 128 matrix settings. As shown in Figure 9A-C, the greater the matrix (pixel) settings per image, the greater the localization of isotope emission within the field of view and the sharper the image. However, for each pixel, there are surrounding septa of lost information forming the border of the pixel. The question is whether the increase in image "sharpness" comes at the expense of "accuracy" of radioactive isotope count activity, which is the basis for image comparisons.

As shown in Figure 10A, the initial radioactive count obtained over 5 minutes from a syringe of 37.37 MBq of radioactive tc-99m using a 64 by 64 pixel matrix was 1,405,721. Using the same matrix and imaging 55 minutes later, Figure 10B shows the counts collected over 5 minutes were 1,251,359. The decay curve for tc-99m means that there should have been a 10% reduction in count activity. In this instance, there was a 10.98% reduction in measured isotope activity. When efforts to improve image "sharpness" were made by changing the matrix to 128 x 128, Figure 10C shows the initial count activity measured over 5 minutes was 3,473,001. When the syringe was reimaged 55 minutes later using the 128 x 128 matrix, the counts collected over a 5 minute period, as shown in Figure 10D, were 2,966,394 . While there was an increase in actual radioactive count activity compared with the 64 x 64 matrix, this came at a cost of accuracy with a 14.59% reduction in radioactive count activity. This is 4.68 times the data lost as was seen with the 64 x 64 matrix.

While the visual appearance desired by most clinicians to make diagnostic decisions is important, images can be manipulated to confirm what the diagnostician is looking for. These adjustments may lead to incorrect conclusions and visual interpretations alone may lead to incorrect conclusions. When done at social gatherings, these visual illusions as shown in Figure 11 can be entertaining. When done to determine if someone has ischemic heart disease, such illusions can be more distressing. For that reason, multiple researchers have been trying to develop algorithms, which will reduce this human error. It is impossible to reduce this human error, if Section of the error is the result of instrumentation.

These findings have demonstrated that independent of the visual image seen by the clinician, this information is dependent upon the accuracy of the computers ability to detect the radioactive decay of isotope needed to make image comparisons. Like, Heisenberg's uncertainty principle, this uncertainty principle comes at a cost. The ability to detect the location of the emission of the gamma ray is influenced by the matrix surrounding the acquired image of the heart. This precision of location comes at the cost of lost accuracy as to the number of gamma rays being emitted. Given this spatial limitation (sharpness) versus accuracy, like Heisenberg we are left with a dilemma. Do we sacrifice accuracy for "sharpness" or should we be more concerned with the necessary accuracy required to compare images (Fleming 2009b, 2010a-b, Sheikine 2010), thereby reducing errors made in evaluation of the extent of ischemic heart disease?
Now that we have defined the limitations and accuracy of our SPECT cameras to define the presence or absence of disease, we can now turn our attention to understanding the kinetics of nuclear isotopes, with particular attention to technetium-99m compounds (viz. Sestamibi) to better understand how to best study the heart using our SPECT cameras.

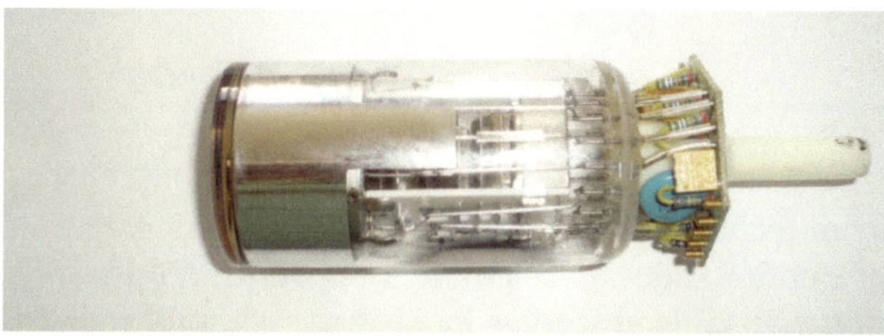

Fig. 6. Photomultiplier (PMTs) Tube

As shown, PMTs are composed of glass tube with a vacuum inside. Photons leaving the patient would approach the PMT from left to right, striking the photocathode material first. This results in electrons being produced as a consequence of the photoelectric effect. The focusing electrode subsequently directs these toward the electron multiplier composed of a series of electrodes (dynodes), each with a more positive voltage than the next. The electrons are accelerated toward the first dynode, arriving with a greater energy. This results in low energy electrons being generated by the first dynode, which are in turn accelerated toward the second dynode and so on. The process is known as secondary emission and results in an amplification of the original scintillation. The electrons finally reach the anode (far right Section of PMT) where the accumulated charge results in a sharp current pulse indicating the arrival of the photon at the photocathode.

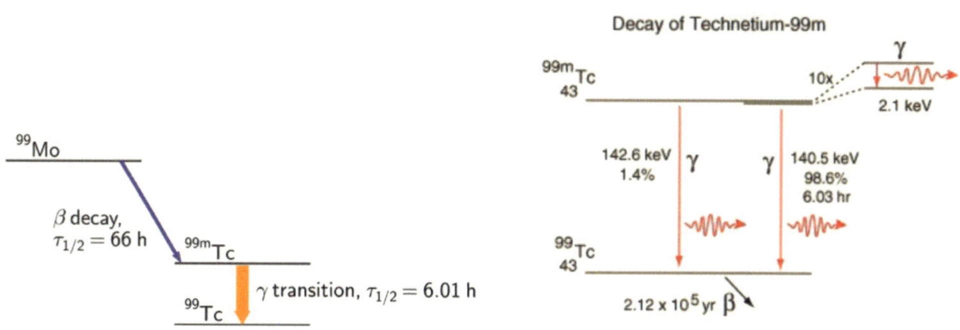

Fig. 7. Decay of Technetium-99m

The production of technetium by bombardment of a molybdenum atom with deuterons was first documented by Carol Perrier and Emilio Segre in 1937. Technetium-99m (meta stable) decays to Technetium 99 through the release of a gamma (photons) rays of 140.5 keV (98.6%) and 142.6 keV (1.4%) as shown. The final result is Technetium-99 (Tc-99) with a half-life of 210,000 years.

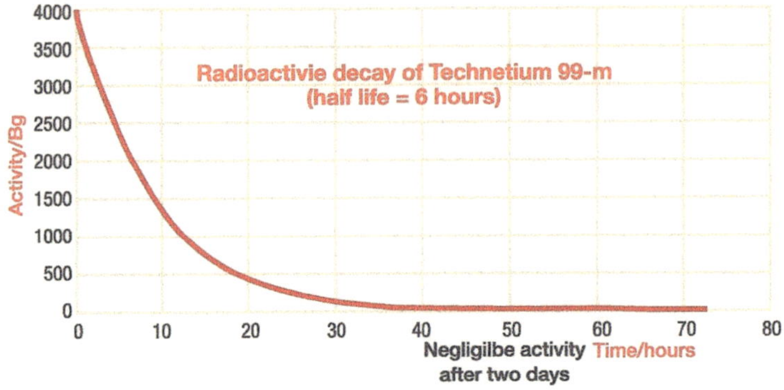

Fig. 8. Radioactive decay curve of Technetium-99m

The radioactive decay of technetium-99m is shown. The physical half-life for Tc-99m is 6.01 hours. Given this information, one can calculate that over the course of 55 minutes there is a 10% decay of the isotope. In clinical studies looking at sestamibi redistribution to determine ischemia (Fleming 2009b, 2010a) the initial stress imaging is made at 5 minutes with the second imaging at 60 minutes.

An effort to improve image "sharpness" (Figure 9A) is the result of increasing the number of pixels in a given field. Cameras set up with a 64 x 64 matrix (pixel) resolution, will result in a more blurred image, while a matrix of 128 x 128 (pixels) will increase image "sharpness." As seen in Figures 9B and 9C, the cost of increasing "sharpness" occurs at the cost of more septa separating each pixel, which reduces the area available for information acquisition. Each septa itself is excluded from acquiring information on radioactive decay, exchanging information for sharpness.

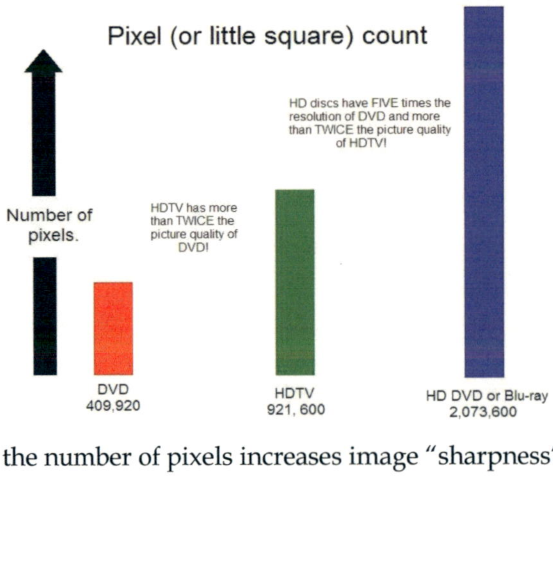

Fig. 9a. Increasing the number of pixels increases image "sharpness"

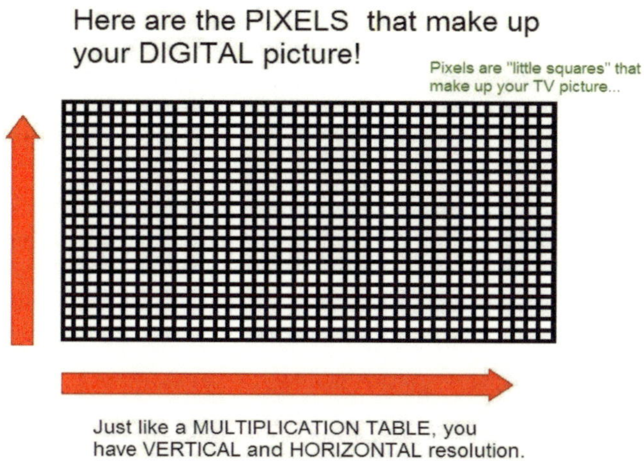

Fig. 9b. Fewer pixels reduce "sharpness" while increasing scintillation detection

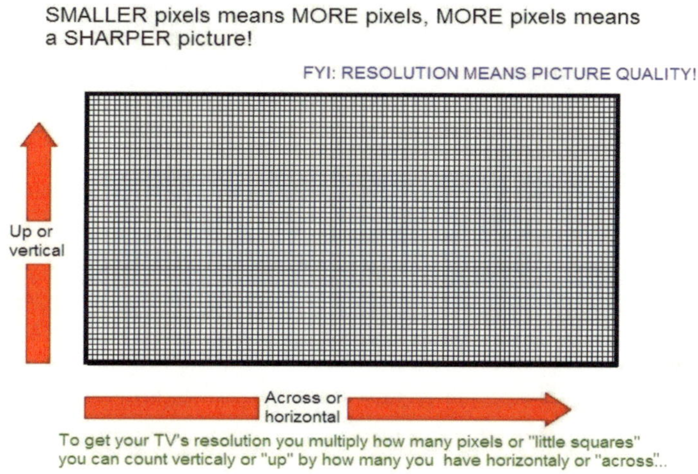

Fig. 9c. More pixels increase image "sharpness" but at the expense of scintillation detection

Fig. 9a-c. The greater the number of pixels, the "sharper" the image "appears"

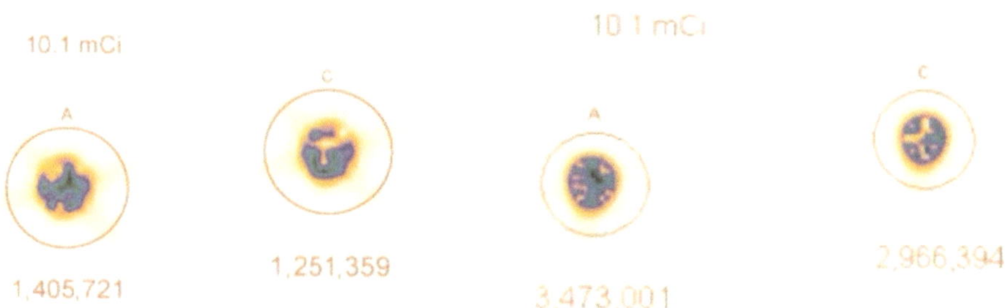

a) b) c) d)

Fig. 10. Verification of Technetium-99m-Sestamibi Count Imaging

A 37.37 MBq syringe of technetium-99m-sestamibi is placed under the camera and counts acquired over 5 minutes. The same syringe is reimaged 55 minutes later for an equal amount of time. When the 64 x 64 matrix was used, the original count was 1,405,721, the second image count was 1,251,359, representing 89% of the original count activity. When the resolution was increased to 128 x 128 matrix, there was an additional 50% loss in data, with a 5-minute image (different syringe sample) count of 3,473,001. The second image count 55 minutes later was 2,966,394, representing a count decrease of 14.6%, 4.6 % more than should have been shown. This reduction is due to data lost as a result of increased grid lines forming the increased number of pixels per image. Subsequently, total information is lost at the gain of localization information (FH Uncertainty principle). Since we are looking for total cell uptake of the tracer, one must use the 64 x 64 matrix as a better index of isotope activity in exchange for resolution.

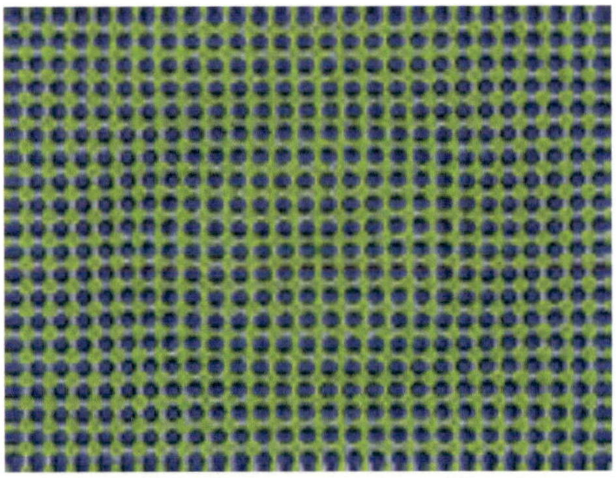

Fig. 11. The importance of recognizing visual illusions

Visual illusions such as this shown here can result in incorrect diagnostic decisions when depended upon by the clinician. This particular illusion demonstrates visual problems resulting from pixel information. When these illusions are the result of instrumentality, diagnosticians cannot reliably use them to make clinical decisions and the utilization of attenuation algorithms cannot reliably reduce these errors, making it even more important that we know what our nuclear cameras are truly capable of measuring and how to most accurately use them.

4. The kinetics of radioactive isotope distribution from vein to heart to cells to redistribution

Imaging protocols are frequently employed by clinicians with an incomplete understanding of the kinetics of a given isotope. Consequently, patients receive more isotope than may be necessary and under the wrong conditions for detection of the question at hand. E.g. the utilization of stress-rest OR rest-stress imaging, frequently results in two injections of radioactive isotope, when only one is needed, resulting in comparing apples and oranges. Resting images as discussed elsewhere in this chapter are useful only for determining tissue viability and do not augment coronary artery blood flow (viz. coronary or stenosis flow reserve) as discussed in Figure 14 below and elsewhere in this chapter and as such cannot be used to determine the presence or absence of ischemia. Similarly, resting images are not helpful for comparison with stress images as discussed in Section IV of this chapter and results in failure to accurately detect ischemia along with assignment of ischemia to the wrong regions of myocardium, leading to continued frustration for those using stress-rest protocols. In this Section of the chapter, we will review the process by which nuclear isotopes are injected, delivered and redistributed throughout the myocardium allowing us to better understand how we can take advantage of these properties to increase our detection of ischemia and as we shall see in Section V, the ability to detect myocardial viability.

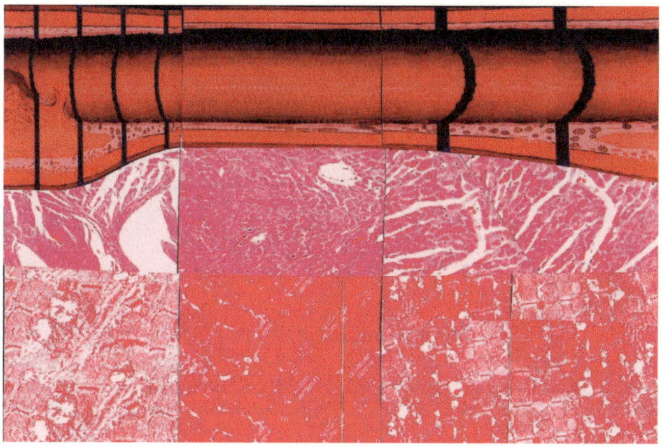

Fig. 12. Diagram of coronary artery prior to injection of radioactive isotope

Figure 12 represents an artery with the lumen of the artery at the top of the image. On the left side is a critically narrowed artery with a vulnerable plaque, the region immediately below that represents myocytes when ischemic as seen under the microscope. Immediately below this is the appearance of mitochondria under severe ischemic conditions. Note the reduction in myofibrils and mitochondria under severe ischemic conditions. In the middle third of the image, at the top, lies a normal appearing coronary lumen with normal appearing myocyte with normal concentration of mitochondria immediately below the myocytes image. The right Section of the image represents diseased artery initially represented by extension outward as first demonstrated by Glagov (1987) from pathology specimens with encroachment into the lumen as we proceed from left to right. Immediately below the artery is the microscopic appearance of mildly damaged myocytes with the lower Section of the image revealing a reduction in the numbers of mitochondria present in regions with mild to moderate ischemia, but, more than the region of vulnerable plaque (left side of image) where severe ischemia is present.

Figure 13 shows the longitudinal and cross-sectional effects of an artery without disease on the left and a region of artery with inflammatory coronary artery disease resulting in ischemia. Arteries free of disease can vasodilate upon command to increase coronary blood flow while arteries with inflammation are unable to dilate to the same degree. These differences can be detected and measured in the nuclear laboratory as we have shown (Fleming2008a).

Figure 14 shows the relationship between coronary (stenosis) flow reserve and percent diameter narrowing. As established by Gould (1990) in dogs and in humans by Fleming (1991b, 1994) the greater the amount of inflammatory coronary artery disease (ischemia), the less the flow reserve and the greater the reduction in an arteries ability to carry blood flow along with radioactive isotopes to a region of myocardium where the isotope can cross the capillary membrane and migrate into myocytes for uptake and detection. These differences in flow were first established by Poiseuille (1840) in the laboratory.

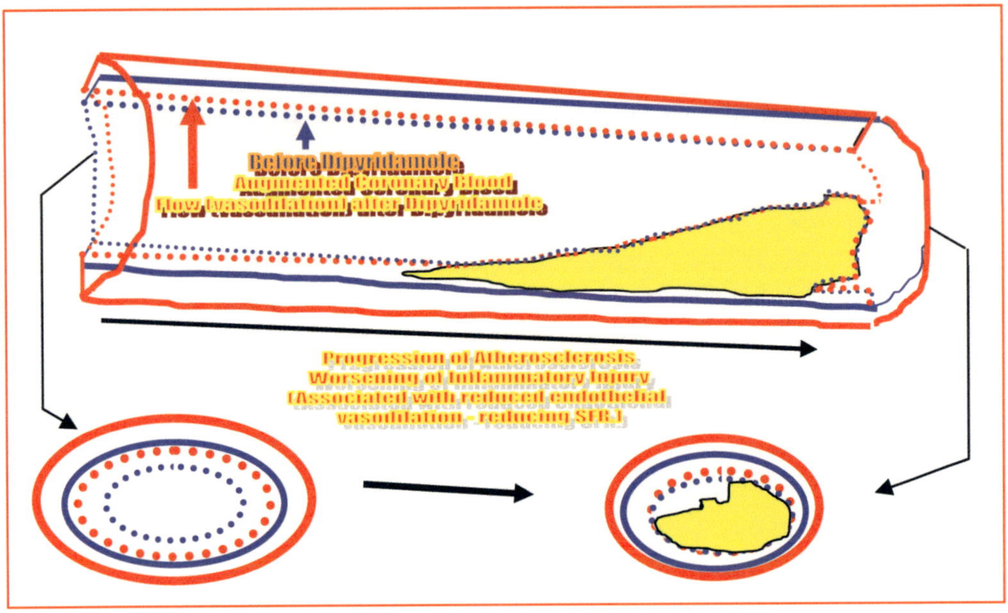

Fig. 13. Demonstrates the capability of coronary arteries to dilate to increase coronary blood flow, viz. stenosis (or coronary) flow reserve, to meet increased myocardial oxygen and nutrient demands with "stress"

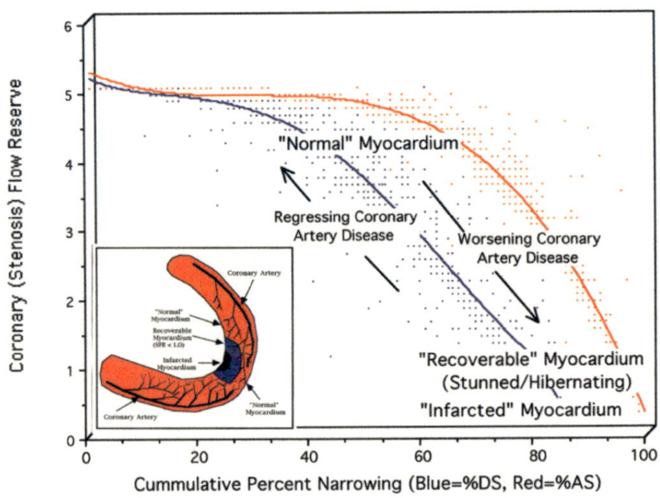

Fig. 14. Actual coronary flow reserve in humans as influenced by anatomic narrowing of coronary arteries

Figure 15 shows the injection of sestamibi into the right antecubital region immediately following stress. The radioactive material can be measured as documented by Blumgart (1926) to determine circulation time and myocardial status.
Figure 16 shows the same artery from Figure 12, with the initial pass of radioactive isotope material through the lumen.

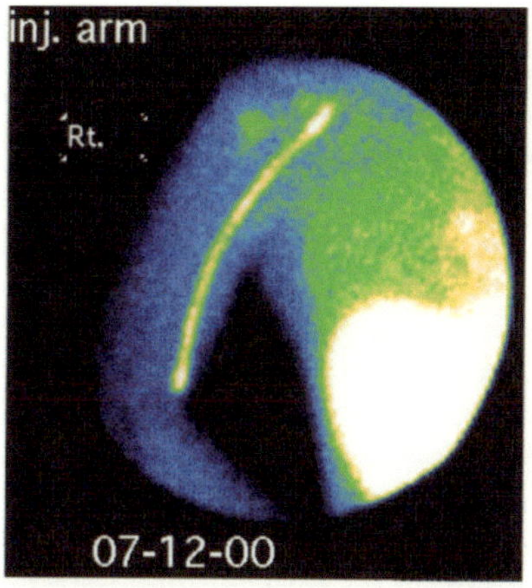

Fig. 15. Initial injection of technetium-99m into the right antecubital vein

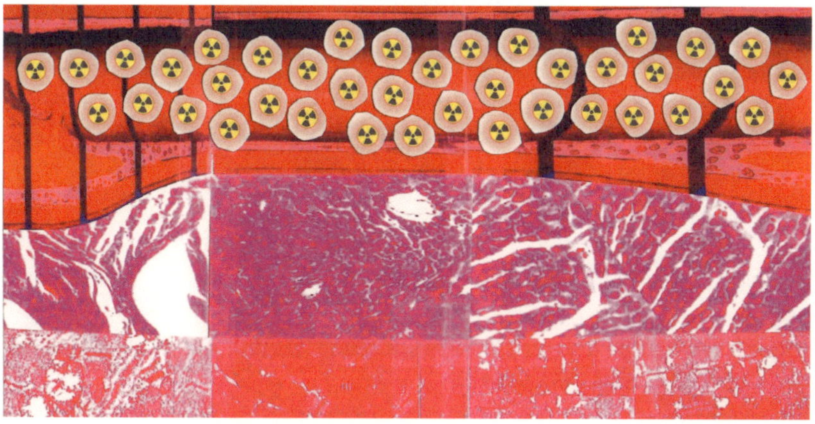

Fig. 16. Cartoon depiction of radioactive isotope initially entering a coronary artery.

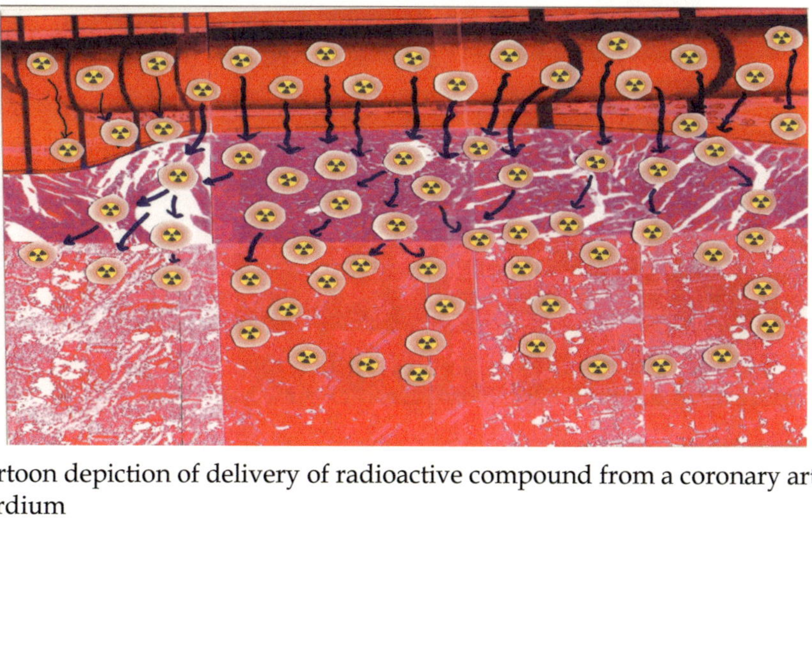

Fig. 17. Cartoon depiction of delivery of radioactive compound from a coronary artery into the myocardium

This figure shows the passage of radioactive isotope (sestamibi) from the lumen into the myocardial tissues 5 minutes after injection into the venous system following "stress". Passage from lumen to tissue is dependent upon four variables. First, when there is a region of artery is inflamed, there is (a) reduced passage of material through the region from the narrowing as well as a reduction in the dilatation of the artery to carry radioactive material as described in Figure 14. Secondly, as the wall of the artery is inflamed and thickened, there is an increased impediment to the movement of sestamibi through such a region in contrast to a non-inflamed region. Thirdly, as a region becomes ischemic, the mitochondria are less able to retain the sestamibi due to calcium overload (Crane 1993, Lenzi 2003, Kodavanti 2008) and there are fewer mitochondria to retain the sestamibi. Finally, sestamibi is a lipophilic compound (Maublant 1988) which when passing through (a) a lipid laden plaque and (b) an inflamed region or region with increased mitochondrial activity (Fleming 2000c) due to the white blood cells (greater mitochondrial concentration is required of these cells if they are to be able to respond to inflammatory stimuli including diseased arteries or bacteria which may or may not play a role in a disease artery) will have a greater uptake (Fleming 2002c-e, 2003a-c) of sestamibi, reducing the amount of radioactive tracer passing through the lumen into myocardial tissue with its mitochondria.

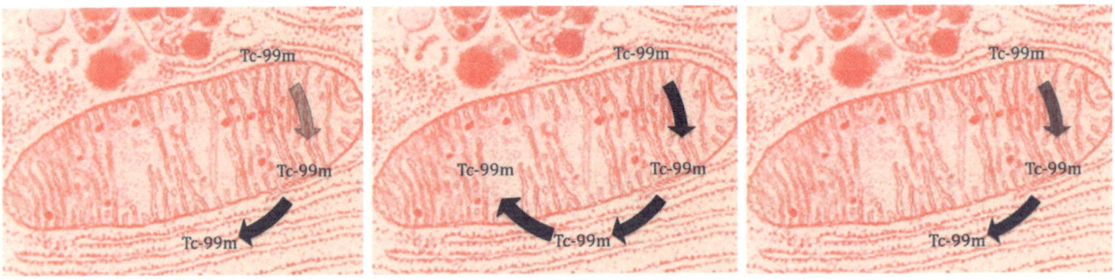

Fig. 18. Electron microscopic images of mitochondria showing the outer and inner membranes along with cristae and matrix

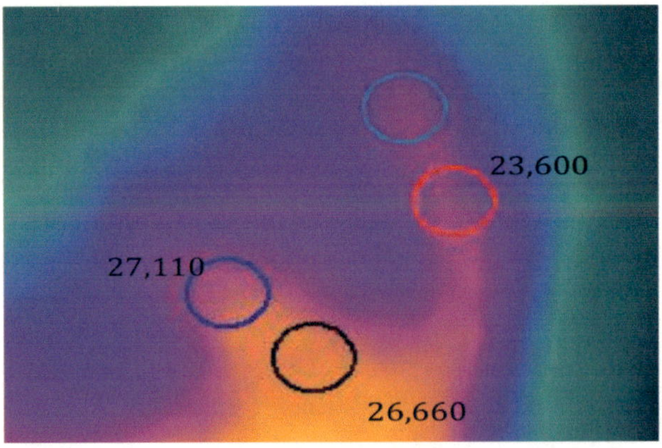

Fig. 19. SPECT image of distribution of Sestamibi within myocardial tissue which can be qualitatively Gestalted or quantitatively measured as done here

Figure 18 shows three mitochondria under different sets of conditions, as shown in Figure 17. The far left mitochondria shows the reduced delivery of sestamibi in a region of vulnerable plaque where the reduced lumen size, reduced flow reserve ability, the increased

lipid laden material will result in a reduction in delivery of sestamibi to the mitochondria in the region. The middle panel shows a mitochondria receiving maximum delivery of sestamibi from an artery, which is able to vasodilate and carry maximum amount of isotope with no impedance to delivery of the isotope to the mitochondria and non-ischemic mitochondria. The far right panel shows more sestamibi delivery than the region with vulnerable plaque, with reductions due to limitations in lumen size and reduced flow reserve, but, not as limited as that occurring with the region of vulnerable plaque.
Figure 19 shows an actual myocardial perfusion image obtained 5 minutes after injection of sestamibi with three regions of interest (ROIs) measured in regions of (a) a vulnerable plaque (23,600), (b) a normal region (27,110) and finally (c) a region with ischemia without critical narrowing or vulnerable plaque (26,660).

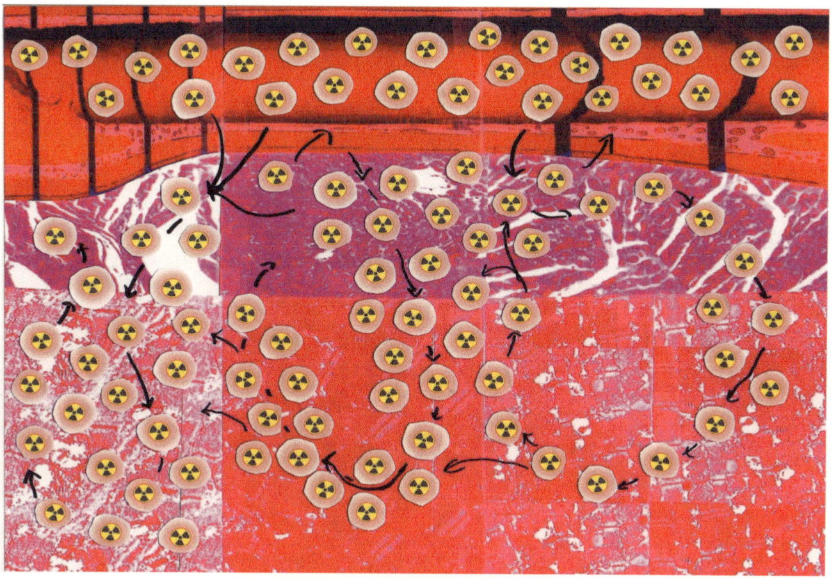

Fig. 20. Coronary artery cartoon showing redistribution of radioactive isotope (in this instance sestamibi) with time

Figure 20 shows the effect of 55 additional minutes (60 minutes post-stress) of perfusion of tissue with sestamibi. During this time, there has been additional delivery of sestamibi to each of the regions of the heart. As established by Maublant (1988), the washout for sestamibi is 28 minutes. Crane(1993) established that ischemia affects the calcium concentration within mitochondria resulting in calcium overload and decreased potentiation for sestamibi retention. Between these two factors in addition to the four reasons discussed with Figure 17, regions of critically narrowed arteries or arteries with vulnerable plaque, as shown in the left side of the figure will have an increase in radioactive (sestamibi) count (concentration) at 60 minutes compared with that seen at 5 minutes. In the middle of the figure, the region of myocardium supplied with a normally functioning artery without narrowing sees a constant uptake and washout of Sestamibi (Maublant 1988) with the expected decay in isotope of 10% as shown in Figure 21. During this time, the greater amount of radioactive material present in the normal region provides a concentration gradient for increased delivery of isotope (sestamibi) to the region with critical narrowing and/or vulnerable plaque, adding to the increased delivery in isotope in this region over time. This increased delivery of isotope is defined as washin as will be discussed below. The far right hand Section of the diagram shows the effect of decreased retention of sestamibi by ischemic mitochondria (Crane 1993) with a greater than expected (10% by technetium-99m isotope decay) reduction in isotope concentration returning from the mitochondria into regions of normal tissue with a greater capacity to retain sestamibi for a greater period of time, or return of the isotope into the vascular space where isotope is delivered for excretion (Sattari 2001) from the body.

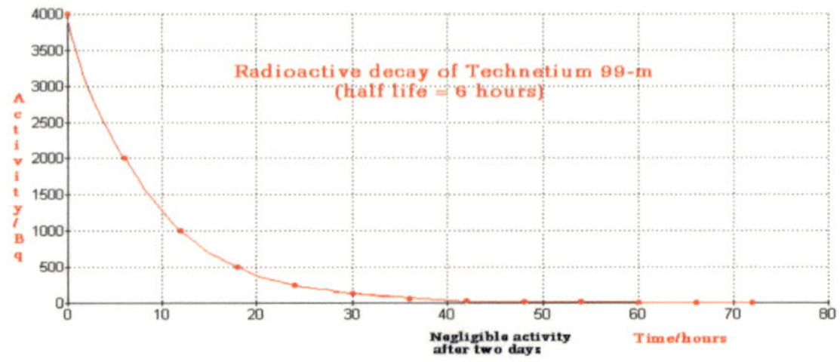

Fig. 21. Decay curve of technetium-99m

Figure 21 shows the decay curve seen for technetium-99m compounds. Over the course of 55 minutes (the time difference between imaging at 5 minutes and 60 minutes), there is a 10% isotope decay, which will result in the "normal" reduction in isotope seen over a 55-minute period of time.

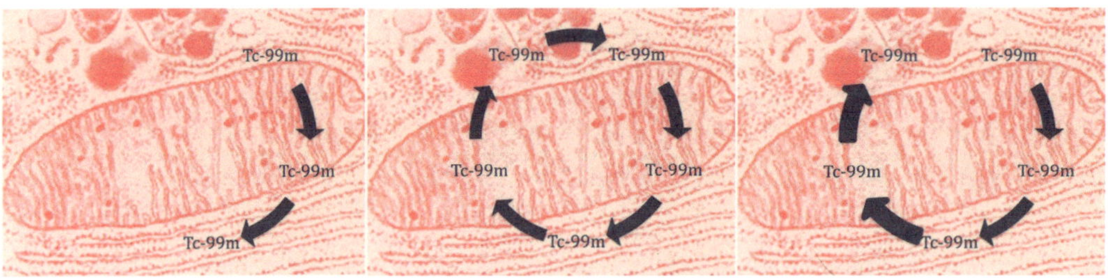

Fig. 22. Changes in mitochondrial movement (redistribution) of sestamibi over time

Figure 22 shows the uptake/release of sestamibi by mitochondria at 60 minutes post-stress. When compared with Figure 18, it is clear that mitochondria (far left) in the critically narrowed/vulnerable plaque regions are now receiving greater concentrations of sestamibi as described in Figure 20. The mitochondria in the middle image shows continual uptake and release of sestamibi given the unimpaired delivery of the isotope and normal mitochondrial calcium levels leaving an unimpeded mitochondrial uptake and release of sestamibi. The far right panel reflects the findings noted in Figure 18, where there is relatively unimpeded delivery of sestamibi to the mitochondria, with increased release due to the effect of ischemia upon mitochondrial calcium concentration and mitochondrial function.
Figure 23 shows the results of sestamibi concentration and measurement of radioactive levels of sestamibi at 60 minutes post-stress. These results show what is described above, viz. and increase in concentration in the region of the vulnerable plaque/critically narrowed coronary artery with a count of 30,470. The region with normal blood flow and normal functioning mitochondria shows a count of 25,472 while the ischemic region without a critical narrowing or vulnerable plaque shows impairment in mitochondrial function as described above with a count of 15,407 despite reasonable delivery of the radioactive isotope sestamibi. This single

60-minute image minus the actual ROI counts, appears completely normal qualitatively leading one to detect no ischemia when it is used for rest to stress comparisons, which Gorlin (1959) demonstrated could not be used as a method for detecting ischemia.

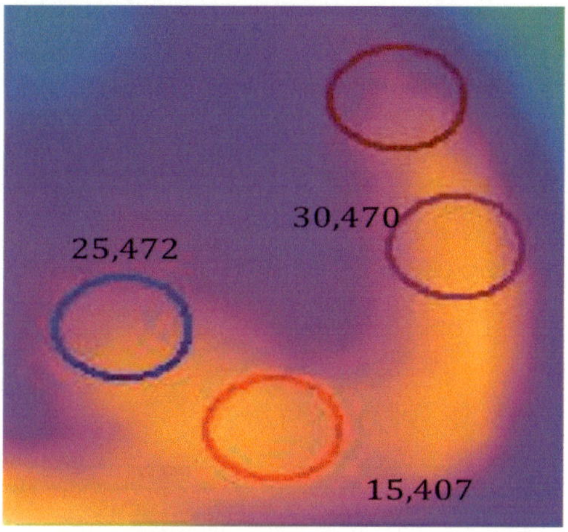

Fig. 23. Measurement of sestamibi redistribution as quantitatively measured, allowing for assessment of both physiologic and anatomic information, which cannot be determined by comparing images using a visual Gestalt

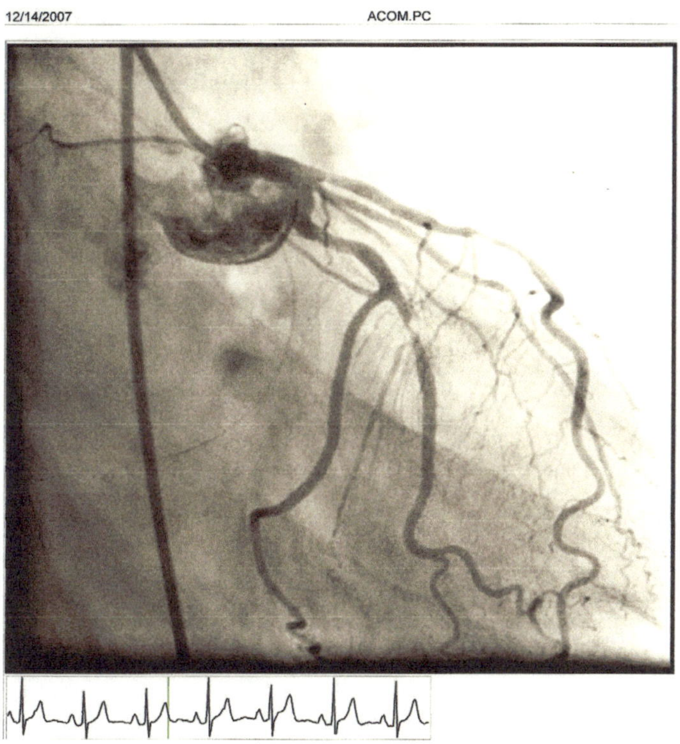

Fig. 24. Anatomic information obtained from coronary angiography which was compared with physiologic information obtained from Sestamibi redistribution

Figure 24 shows the results of coronary angiography with detection of vulnerable plaques, normal arterial regions and regions of ischemia matching the findings of wash in and washout; but, not matching the results of the single 60-minute image displayed in Figure 23 when using only a qualitative method in stark contrast to a comparison of change seen between the 5-minute and 60-minute images above.

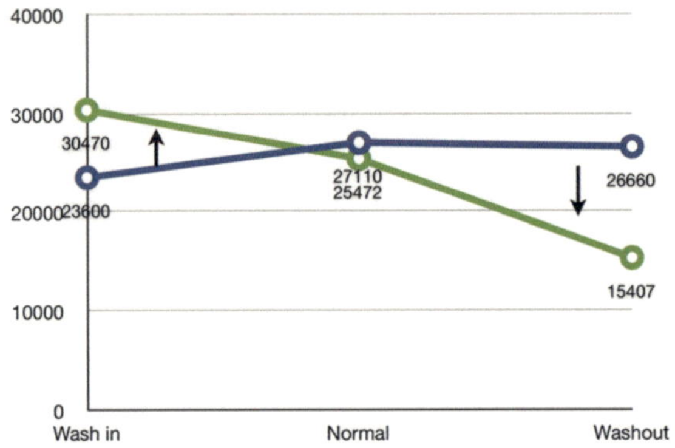

Fig. 25. Comparing quantitative sestamibi information between stress-stress imaging

Figure 25 represents the results of what is seen when the quantitative measurement of ROIs are compared for (a) regions of critically narrowed/vulnerable plaque regions (wash in) where radioactive concentration is seen to increase between the 5 and 60-minute images, (b) when disease is not present (both flow and mitochondrial function are unimpaired) and the change is count activity can be accounted for on the basis of isotope decay (Figure 21). As we have seen, the isotope (sestamibi) is not merely taken up and retained but as demonstrated by both Maublant (1988) and then Crane (1993), the isotope undergoes uptake and release, the rate of which is determined by ischemia and mitochondrial function. Finally, (c) washout is seen as an initial near normal delivery of isotope with impaired retention independent of the delivery of the isotope owing to mitochondrial calcium overload resulting from ischemia.

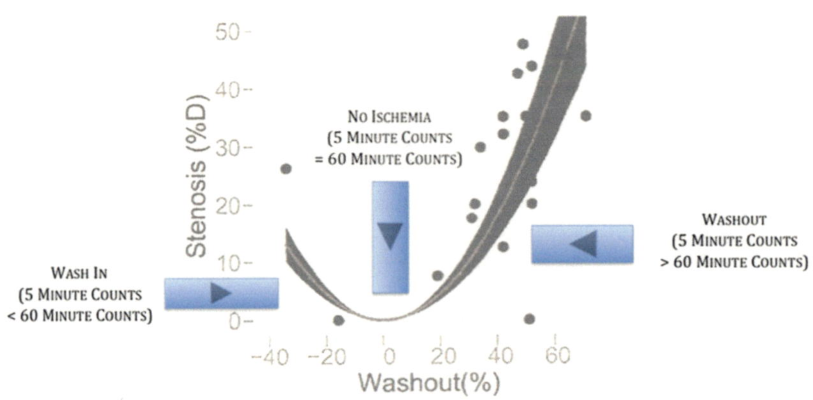

Fig. 26. Single injection, single camera imaging assessment of anatomic AND physiologic information obtainable by quantitative measurement of Sestamibi redistribution

Figure 26 summarizes all of the information seen both with changes in isotope concentration (washin, normal, washout); but, more importantly compares this with findings seen on coronary angiography, enhancing decision making capabilities from this physiologic change (Fleming 2008b, 2009a) in isotope over time.

Armed with the understanding of how our Nuclear SPECT cameras work and how these isotopes redistribute over time, we can now better understand the process by which we can best use our nuclear cameras to detect ischemic heart disease. It is estimated that in the United States alone, some 10 million nuclear heart scans are performed each yearly. Of these some 80,000 to 140,000 individuals will be told following their (Heart 2011) "rest-stress" SPECT myocardial perfusion imaging (MPI) studies, that they have no ischemic heart disease whatsoever. Of these 40,000 to 70,000 will go home and die from a heart attack. Evidence indicates that these individuals have "normal" appearing 60-minute post-stress studies and are only detected by finding a decreased uptake at 5-minutes post stress, viz. "wash-in." The "rest-stress" approach simply cannot detect these individuals. In the next Section of this chapter, we will look at the evidence proving this and scientifically establish why so many people are being misdiagnosed and what we can do about it.

5. Fleming Harrington Stress SPECT protocol reduces radioactive dosage and increases ischemia detection. The detection of ischemic heart disease is accomplished by comparing multiple images of the heart following stress. (ischemia equals stress imaging)

Background: Radioisotope manufacturers, nuclear camera manufacturers, standard guidelines for myocardial perfusion imaging, all assume rapid isotope uptake followed by an essentially static retention mechanism. Contrariwise, the historic first nuclear cardiology study found measurement of nuclear isotope blood flow kinetics to be diagnostic of heart disease. No clinical investigations appear to have followed that classic finding. We assessed the clinical diagnostic utility of time course myocardial perfusion measurements following single injections.

Methods: One hundred twenty patients suspected of having heart disease underwent Sestamibi stress images taken at 5 and at 60 minutes following completion of cardiac stress. Quantitative (FRHWW) redistribution differences between the images were assessed. FHRWW results were compared with angiographic findings.

Results: Parabolic regression of stenosis on redistribution yielded an effect size of R(CI95%) = 0.72 to 0.95, ($P=3.8\times10^{-8}$). Fifteen percent of individuals with "normal" appearing 60 minute SPECT images were noted to having coronary artery disease using both redistribution data and coronary angiography requiring stent placement. These individuals had "wash in" of Sestamibi (isotope uptake greater at 60 minutes than 5 minutes) and signaled patients at risk of undergoing an acute cardiac event due to vulnerable plaques or tight lesions placing significant amounts of myocardium at risk of infarction. One of the individuals who did not require cardiac catheterization based upon the FHRWW data, underwent coronary angiography based upon rest-stress results AND had a major adverse event as a result of the subsequent cardiac catheterization. There was no detectable CAD, confirming the FHRWW findings and the need for caution in individuals undergoing invasive procedures.

Conclusions: Dynamic "uptake / release" models appear to be a superior alternative to the common "uptake/retention" models of technetium-99m isotopes used in nuclear myocardial perfusion imaging. This sequential quantitative diagnostic model, reinforces the work by Blumgart, enabling more accurate diagnosis of coronary artery disease and providing for intervention in individuals requiring stents or bypass, whom would otherwise be missed on rest-stress imaging protocols while avoiding unnecessary coronary angiography among individuals with "normal" Sestamibi redistribution.

While diagnostic testing and decision making in the treatment of atherosclerotic coronary artery disease (ASCAD/CAD) tends to revolve around evidence of anatomic [cardiac catheterization (Fleming1991b), coronary computed tomography, intravascular ultrasound (Taki 2001, St Goar 1991), et cetera] disease, it has been well established that this inflammatory (Fleming 1999c, 2000c-d) process may smolder for years and that up to 85% of all myocardial infarctions occur with < 30% diameter narrowing. It is; therefore, important for us to look for new ways to uncover this smoldering inflammatory disease process when intervention may be more beneficial to the patient and potentially less costly to the patient and society at a time when health care costs are a major issue.

When teenagers learn to buy their first automobile, they learn an important lesson. Not every car that looks good runs well. This same lesson applies to the diagnosis and treatment of ASCAD. The lesson is to determine how well the car runs, or in this case, how well the heart runs. Hence the importance of physiologic testing; i.e. testing to see how well the heart runs. Prior to nuclear imaging of the heart, now called myocardial perfusion (Maddahi 2001, Kern 2006) imaging (MPI), patients ran on a treadmill (exercise stress testing/EST) under the belief that this would precipitate chest pain (angina) and perhaps electrocardiographic and hemodynamic changes which would indicate problems with coronary blood flow. Until recently, it was believed that this was purely the result of narrowing within the lumen of the artery. It has since been demonstrated that angina is the result of regional blood flow (Fleming 2000e, 2003d) differences; hence, the importance of quantifying such areas of the heart by analyzing regions of interest (ROI). These differences in regional blood flow work through mechanisms as of yet not completely understood. The ability to precipitate these differences in regional blood flow can be accomplished via the utilization of MPI and pharmacologic or exercise stress testing. A major limitation with utilizing single 60 minute images for interpreting the presence of ischemia on MPI are attenuation artifacts. Such artifacts include anterior attenuation from breast tissue, diaphragmatic attenuation from abdominal obesity, hypertrophic differences in walls of the heart, bundle branch anomalies, et cetera. These attenuation issues have not been significantly corrected with the addition of attenuation correction protocols. While nuclear tracers (isotopes) have improved over the years, many misconceptions (Beller 1990, Fleming 1991a, Sinusas 1994, Dahlberg 1994, Glover 1995, Hurwitz 1996, Husain 2007) have plagued the field limiting the accuracy of MPI with sensitivities and specificities remaining at 65-90% in most published investigations (Parameswaran 2006).

In 1926 Blumgart first proposed nuclear imaging techniques for the detection of heart disease. His method clearly proposed serial assessment of isotope count activity to determine cardiac function. Decades passed before Love (1965) discussed the potential future of Nuclear Cardiology and pointed out that rest images (Gorlin 1959) were useless in the detection of coronary artery narrowing. With the advent of technetium-99m- sestamibi, clinicians believed that the isotope was taken up by myocardial tissue within minutes of injection and remained fixed within myocytes. Crane (1993) demonstrated this was not so and demonstrated that retention of sestamibi was dependent upon ischemia and cellular viability. This opened the door to the discovery of changes in isotope count over the course of time and reinforced Blumgart's 1926 paper. During our initial (Fleming 2003e, 2008) efforts to better understand the underlying inflammatory component of CAD via MPI, five and sixty minute imaging revealed differences in the qualitative appearances of images seen following pharmacologic stressing of individuals as predicted by Blumgart (1926), Love (1965) and Crane (1993). As noted below, others have noticed these differences as well. Furthermore, comparisons of the initial 5-minute imaging with the 60-minute imaging demonstrated different results from the simple "uptake/retention" rest-stress model. Other investigators have noted similar differences between 5 minute and 60 minute imaging of the heart (Hurwitz 1993, 1998, Saha 1994, Giubbini 1995, Pace 2005) allowing for enhanced detection of congestive heart failure (Hurwitz 1998, Kumita 2002, Sugiura 2006, Matsuo 2007), cardiomyopathies (Meissner 2002, Ikawa 2007), Prinzmetal 's angina (Ono 2002, 2003) and underlying coronary artery disease (Meerdink 1990, Richter 1995, Shin 1995, Takeishi 1996, Takahashi 1996, Fujiwara 1998, Hurwitz 1998, Ayalew 2000, 2002, Liu 2001, Kumita 2002, Tanaka 2006, Fukushima 2007, VanBrocklin 2007) including evidence of wash-in (Meerdink 1990, Richter 1995) indicative of critical lesions not detected by conventional MPI. In the same way that thrombolysis in myocardial infarction (TIMI) flow is used to look for changes (sometimes subtle, sometimes not) in coronary blood flow in the catch lab, multiple imaging following pharmacologic or EST allows us to take a more advanced look at the physiologic function of the heart, unmasking ischemic heart disease missed by rest-stress imaging.

Given these recent investigations into improving the detection of ischemia by quantifying isotope counts on multiple (sequential) images following pharmacologic and exercise stress, we set out to determine (1) are nuclear cameras used in the "clinical" setting today able to detect differences in radioactive isotope counts over a period of time, which would allow these cameras to detect changes in flow and retention of isotope over time (2) what are the optimal imaging times for the detection of ischemia and (3) how do these changes in isotope counts compare with percent diameter stenosis as seen on coronary angiography?

5.1 Methods

5.1.1 Single Photon Emission Computed Tomography (SPECT) cameras

The Philips Forte Dual Head SPECT camera used general all (GAP) purpose collimators with the heads positioned at 90 degrees per manufacturers specifications. A 15% window was used with a 64 by 64 matrix. In the first Section of this study, we additionally looked at differences between 64 x 64 matrix and 128 x 128 matrix. Imaging occurred 5 and 60 minutes post stress with processing of images as described in the literature (Fleming 1991a, 2003e, 2008). Jet stream software was used per manufacturer's instructions to quantitatively measure regions of interest (ROIs).

The Picker Axis Dual Head SPECT camera used a low energy general all (LEGAR-PAR) purpose collimator with parallel hole positioning. The heads were positioned at 102 degrees per manufacturer specifications. Picker camera software was used for ROI measurements.

1. Determining if Nuclear Cameras used in "Clinical" Practice are able to detect changes in isotope count over time.

   Establishing technetium-99m decay by radioactive count measurement: Based upon the half-life of technetium-99m, a stable source representing the "uptake/retention" model (viz. a syringe filled with the isotope) has a 10% decay over 55 minutes with a retention of ~90% of the radioactive counts over a 55 minute (the difference between 5 and 60 minute images) span of time. In an effort to establish whether "clinically" used cameras are able to measure this physical decay in technetium-99m, we studied a 37.37 MBq (10.1 mCi) sample of sestamibi at baseline and again 55 minutes later. As shown in

Figure 10, the resting isotope count was 1,405,721 while the second image obtained 55 minutes later was 1,251,359 representing 89% of the original count activity. Independent of the actual amount of activity which is taken up by a region of myocardium, if the "uptake/retention" model was correct, images taken 55 minutes after the original image would yield counts of 90% of that seen in the first image.

Fleming-Harrington Redistribution Wash-in (FHRWW) Washout (Fleming 2009a-b, 2010a): Using Multiple SPECT Camera Images of the Heart to Determine Changes Between 5 and 60-Minute Images.

2. Optimal Timing to Measure Changes in Radioactive (Sestamibi) Isotope Activity.

   Measuring regions of interest (ROIs) to quantify changes in technetium-99m isotopes between 5 and 60-minute images to look for changes in isotope "uptake/retention." We began with the knowledge acquired from the first Section of this study, that we needed to use the 64 x 64 matrix to accurately measure changes in radioactive decay. We then proceeded to analyze ROIs at 5-minutes (Figure 27) and at 60-minutes (Figure 28). FHRWW calculations (discussed below) demonstrated that the "uptake/retention" model was clearly wrong as seen by the increase in count activity in the anterior wall (23,600 at 5-minutes and 30,470 at 60 minutes) while the inferior region without ischemia demonstrated a 6% reduction in count activity.

   Establishing the optimal time sequence for image acquisition to measure radioactive counts: Using this particular individual (Figures 27 and 28), during this second phase of the investigation, we additionally compared the basal anterolateral, mid anterolateral, basal anterior, mid anterior, basal inferior, mid inferior basal, inferoseptal and mid inferoseptal ROIs and compared the results with that obtained from coronary angiography. We then measured radioactivity in each of the 8 ROIs over the course of an hour, with the salient findings reported in Figure 29. These results were compared with our previous studies (Fleming 2003e, 2008) which revealed the ideal timing for detection of inflammatory changes and based upon the expected 10% decay of technetium-99m over a span of 55 minutes, the remainder of our work (FRHWW) focused on ROIs obtained at 5 and 60 minutes post stress. These results confirm that Sestamibi does NOT follow an "uptake/retention" model; but rather an "uptake/release" model consistent with Sestamibi redistribution (FHRWW).

5.2 Calculating FHRWW

By comparing 5 and 60-minute imaging, the expected decay of Tc-99m is 10%. Actual counts from individual ROIs can then be taken and actual redistribution (FHRWW) can be calculated as follows.

$$\text{FHRWW (Total Heart)} = \\ = \frac{\text{ROI counts (total heart) at 5 minutes} - \text{ROI counts (total heart) at 60 minutes}}{\text{ROI counts (total heart) at 5 minutes}} \times 100 - 10 \quad \text{(eq 1)}$$

Where 100 places the answer in percent minus the 10 % expected decay.

$$\text{FHRWW for a particular myocardial ROI} = \\ = \frac{\text{ROI counts (region) at 5 minutes} - \text{ROI counts (region) at 60 minutes}}{\text{ROI counts (region) at 5 minutes}} \times 100 - 10 \quad \text{(eq 2)}$$

This can be re-written as:

Let the 5 minute counts = 'x', let the 60 minute counts = 'y', and let % washout = '100 * w' (eq 3)

Then w = (x - y)/x - 0.1 = x/x - y/x - 0.1 = 1.0 - y/x - 0.1 = 0.9 - y/x = .9 – 60 minute counts/5 minute counts.

3. Comparing washout/wash-in results with coronary angiographic assessment of percent diameter stenosis.
   One hundred twenty patients (ages 25 to 82 years) with suspected coronary artery disease underwent myocardial perfusion imaging after signing informed consent per Institutional protocol following adenosine (n=30), lexiscan (n=61), dobutamine (Fleming 1995, 1999a, Calnon 1997, 1999, Matsunari 2001), n=4 or treadmill (Fleming 1991a, 1999a), n=25 stress. Following standardized protocols already published (Fleming 2009a-b, 2010a) MPI using both the rest-stress and stress-stress (FHRWW) approach were compared with coronary angiography (Fleming 1992a-b).
   Statistical Analysis. Quantification of isotope counts was made using the specific nuclear computer software provided by the nuclear camera companies. These quantified counts were recorded with calculations of FHRWW as noted above. Correlation coefficients, confidence intervals and p-value (significance levels) were determined between %DS and FHRWW using product-moment correlation and least squares regression fitting the hypothesized model of $y=cx^2$. Using the null hypothesis for n = 120 patients, we estimated odds ratios (ORs) for predicting final diagnosis from nuclear procedures. ORs were determined against coronary angiography results for both the rest/stress images and FHRWW images. Statistical analysis and graphics were developed using R-2.6.0 and GGobi software.

5.3 Results

To the best of our knowledge verification of the ability of a nuclear camera used for "clinical" purposes to measure sequential radioactive counts confirming differences in technetium-99m-sestamibi resulting from the physical decay of the isotope has not previously been reported in the literature. The first phase of this study was to confirm that cameras used clinically are able to detect differences in radioactivity accurately, assuming they employ the correct matrix to do so. To prove this, we used 37.37 MBq of technetium-99m-sestamibi with both a 64 x 64 matrix and a 128 x 128 matrix. The results of the 64 x 64 and 128 x 128 matrices are shown in Figure 10. Over a 55 minute period of time, the expected decay of technetium-99m would be 10%, leaving a residual activity of 90% of the original counts. This represents a true "uptake/retention" model since the radioactive compound is retained within the syringe. Using the 64 x 64 matrix, the radioactive counts went from 1,405,721 to 1,251,359 representing an 11% decay with a residual 89% of the original isotope activity. The 128 x 128 matrix reported 3,473,001 at baseline and a count of 2,966,394 55-minutes later for a decay of 14.6% with a residual of 85.4% of the original isotope activity. For this reason, the 64 x 64 matrix more correctly demonstrated the expected decay of the isotope based upon the physical half-life of Tc-99m and was therefore chosen as the standard for performing these studies.

The second question related to the timing of data collection. Prior studies (Fleming 2003e, 2008) demonstrated the ability to detect inflammatory markers on SPECT images at 5 minutes; but, not at later periods of time. Figure 29 displays the results of radioactivity measured using the clinical camera with a 64 x 64 matrix. As shown, the peak detectable radioactivity was measured between 5 and 10 minutes post injection for individuals with "no" coronary artery disease or coronary artery disease without "critical" lesions or "vulnerable" plaques. In individuals with "critical" lesions and/or vulnerable plaques, radioactive counts increase from 5 to 60 minutes, viz. wash-in (Fleming 2009a-b, 2010a). Combined with the results of instrumentation (Figure 10), the ability to detect ischemia based upon blood flow and cellular uptake and release of sestamibi, is best made by comparing counts at 5 minutes and 60 minutes.

The final component of our study compared results of rest-stress imaging and FHRWW with angiographic (%DS) data. There were no differences observed between individuals who were stressed either physically or pharmacologically. Outcomes were not changed by the stressor used, as the comparison between rest/stress and FHRWW determination of redistribution was independent of the type of stress. The use of regional wall motion information was used with both the rest/stress protocol and the FHRWW approach, which made it possible to look for wall motion abnormalities and ejection fraction using either approach. Since these observations are identical, regardless of which method was used to report ischemia, we do not report them here.

We analyzed the results of rest/stress image comparisons and FHRWW redistribution images and compared them with findings obtained from coronary angiography. For the rest/stress images, the OR for detecting ischemia was 4.9 with a CI (95%) of 2.3 to 10.3. For FHRWW, the OR was 56.8 with a CI (95%) of 27.5 to 117.2. When the results of these ORs were compared, the t value was greater than 6.6 ($P < .0001$). We obtained results of %DS for each of the epicardial arteries and their branches, and plotted these results against the redistribution results for each of the eight ROIs. This could only be done with the redistribution data, which provided quantitative results, which could be compared with the quantitative results obtained angiographically.

Comparison of the rest/stress image results with the angiographic results showed a sestamibi rest/stress imaging sensitivity of 67%. Of the false negative results (n = 22), 18% (n = 4) had critically narrowed arteries or arteries with vulnerable plaques whose 60-minute images appeared completely normal (Pace 2005, Fleming 2008). However, evaluation of the 5-minute images for redistribution (using FHRWW), revealed both qualitative and quantitative decreased uptake, demonstrating a washin effect. The 60-minute post stress images miss this washin phenomena when looked at independent of the 5-minute images, yielding incorrect results. The standard rest/stress images also yielded a specificity of 88%; of which, only one participant (0.8%) who underwent a coronary angiogram had an adverse outcome requiring cardiopulmonary resuscitation (Hurwitz 1993).

FHRWW calculation was made first by comparing the total radioactive counts of the heart at 5 minutes with the total counts of the heart measured at 60 minutes. The eight regions of interest (ROIs) were then compared using both the 5 and 60-minute image information. Analysis of eight ROIs appears to provide the optimal analysis of specific coronary artery beds (left anterior descending, circumflex and right). These regions include the basal anterior, mid anterior, basal anterolateral, mid anterolateral, basal inferior/posterior, mid inferior, basal inferoseptal and mid inferoseptal. Examples of some of these regions are shown in Figures 27, 28, 30A-C and 31A-D. These multiple examples show how, independent of different color scales and cameras used to qualitatively estimate ischemia; quantitative measurements can be made independently and without interference from hepatic and other tissue uptake. Washout (counts greater at 5 minutes than 60 minutes, excluding the expected isotope decay) and washin (noted counts greater at 60 minutes than

5 minutes) were plotted against the percent diameter stenosis (%DS) determined on coronary angiography. Washin was seen in 15% of the individuals studied and was associated with "normal" appearing 60-minute images. When the results of washout/washin were compared with %DS, a parabolic relationship (figure 6) was demonstrated with $F = 70.4$, $df(1,21)$, ($P=3.8\times10^{-8}$), $R(CI95\%) = 0.72$ to 0.95.

5.4 Discussion

The advent of nuclear cardiology by Blumgart beginning in 1925 yielded a new era of medicine with the use of radioactive materials to perform physiologic testing which requires sequential measurements as described by Blumgart to be performed correctly. Unfortunately, decades elapsed (Love 1965) before such nuclear materials were made readily available for "clinical" use. The first agent being Thallium-201 (Tl-201) was plagued with limitations including a long half-life (72 hours) resulting in the need to use relatively low doses (6.8-11.1 MBq) of the isotope. Given the limitations (Fleming 1992a, 1995) of Compton scatter, tissue attenuation and the emission of mercury x-rays from the isotope, cameras could not acquire adequate counts for imaging until 60 minutes had elapsed. Given the passage of time, much of what Blumgart discussed had been lost to history (Love 1965). With the advent of Molybdenum-99, Technetium-99m generators, the ability to perform clinical studies using technetium tagged agents (e.g. teboroxime, sestamibi, myoview, et cetera) with shorter half-lifes (6 hours) allowing greater doses (up to 1110 MBq) and less Compton scatter and tissue attenuation issues yielded what "appeared to be cleaner images". These images were still plagued with attenuation issues and were reported to be "taken up and retained" within minutes of intravenous injections. Despite the report by DuPont (Crane 1993) and multiple other research and clinical (Everett 1977, Fleming 1992b, 2003e, Aodah 2007, Fallahi 2008) studies discussed above and below, which have clearly established that these isotopes redistribute and do not "stick", most clinicians have continued to ignore Blumgart's teaching of performing sequential evaluations under same state conditions and have subsequently limited their investigation of coronary artery disease to single post-stress imaging despite the teaching of nuclear imaging which notes that "a better indicator of organ function is the change in the activity in a particular organ with time." Newer clinical observations and publications (Sheikine 2010) have since been made confirming our earlier observations from 2000-2001.

Inconsistencies in analysis of cardiac imaging have led some researchers (Fleming 2002b, Toriyama 2005, Oregon 2008) to recommend that these clinical studies be standardized quantitatively; something this study has accomplished. In medical school we were taught that there were two ways to understand the results of a test. The first is to compare it against the population (e.g. one obtains an electrocardiogram to look for evidence of ischemia or infarction), the second is to compare it with the results of that test which the patient had previously (e.g. poor R-wave progression may actually represent loss of R-waves and evidence of a prior anteroseptal injury/infarction which can be made more confidently in the presence of a change in the electrocardiogram for that patient, opposed to the confidence one has in making such a diagnosis when this is the first electrocardiogram). The same problem applies with looking at a region of the heart on a single 60 minute image post stress. Issues of tissue attenuation including (1) breast artifacts in the anterior wall, (2) diaphragmatic attenuation inferiorly, (3) differences in wall thickness (asymmetric septal hypertrophy) and (4) conduction disturbances influencing timing of systole (left bundle branch morphology) are examples of errors made when one region of myocardium is compared with another region (e.g. a single 60 minute image) instead of comparing a region with itself (5 and 60 minute images) and looking for change. Unless there is a change in breast tissue or abdominal obesity between the 5 and 60 minute image, errors resulting from soft tissue attenuation of photon activity are eliminated. The same applies for changes in wall thickness and conduction issues; unless there is a change between the 5 and 60 minute image, the region is being compared with itself and such artifacts are eliminated.

Despite an absence of research to support the ability of "clinical" nuclear cameras to accurately detect changes in radioactive counts which match the expected decay of the nuclear isotope in question clinicians have used these cameras to assess the presence or absence of disease in patients. As Archie Cochrane and history has taught us it is truly dangerous to assume that the way we have been doing something is the correct way to do it in the absence of data to confirm we are right. The first Section of this study demonstrated that the cameras we used in this study were able to accurately detect the decay of technetium-99m-sestamibi over a 10% decay. This was best appreciated using the 64 x 64 matrix. Even though manufactures support the use of 128 x 128 matrix as giving greater detail, the use of the 128 x 128 matrix reported a greater decay in the isotope than is physically possible suggesting that information is lost; perhaps as a result of "modulation transfer function" (a concept well known to photographers and imaging engineers).

During the second and third Section of our study we looked at the timing sequence, which would yield the most valuable information, not only regarding detecting changes in radioactivity with cardiac tissue, but the ability to detect markers of inflammation (Fleming 1999c, 2000c, 2003e, 2008, Kern 2006). Our previous findings clearly demonstrated the importance of looking for markers of inflammation when detectable, i.e. at 5 minutes post stress. During this study and our most recent work (Fleming 2009a-b, 2010a) we clearly demonstrated that in individuals who had ischemia with non-critical narrowing of arteries, that maximum radioactivity was present during the first 5 to 10 minutes. The inability to maintain the Sestamibi in regions of ischemia has previously been termed "washout" and represents an inability to retain the isotope within the mitochondria in the region. This clearly confirms the work of Crane (1993), who demonstrated that sestamibi redistributes AND is not retained in regions of "ischemia." Our studies also proved this to be the case, independent of which technetium-99m isotope (Fleming 2009a) was used or which form of stressor (Fleming 2009a-b, 2010a) was used. Our current study clearly demonstrates this to be true in the "clinical" setting and disproves the "uptake/retention" theory in favor of an continual FHRWW "uptake/release" model which would explain not only the loss of isotope to an ischemic myocardial region over time; but, also accounts for "wash-in." "Wash-in" was noted in 15% of the cases where regions of myocardium were supplied by "critically" narrowed arteries and arteries whose "vulnerable plaques" were ready to rupture. In these individuals the combination of severely disturbed flow through critically narrowed and/or unstable coronary lumen passages and relatively large regions of ischemic myocardium with impaired ability to accumulate sestamibi, results in a delay in initial isotope counts. From this perspective, uptake is a function of isotope availability (myocardial blood flow) and cellular health; retention is transient with release of the isotope back into the blood stream or redistribution to other cells, a function of cellular health and re-uptake subject to a cellular refractory period. As a result the delay in isotope delivery is not noted if stress imaging is limited to 60 minute imaging. These individuals, despite "normal" appearing 60 minute images, were at risk of experiencing an acute coronary event with loss of substantial amounts of myocardial tissue.

5.5 Conclusion

The standard "uptake/retention" model was observed only in subjects who demonstrated no evidence of coronary ischemia or infarction. In reality, such an "uptake/retention" model is simply an illusion. It is the rapid "uptake/release", "uptake/release", "uptake/release" in non-ischemic, non-infarcted myocardial tissue that makes it appear that the isotope is taken up and retained. In other words, if the amount being released and the amount being taken up are equal, one will not detect a change in isotope count over time, minus the slight decrease occurring from isotope decay. Such individuals would appear to have no change in isotope concentration despite continual turnover of isotope. "Uptake/release" was demonstrated via washout in individuals with coronary ischemia and a delayed "uptake/release" in individuals with washin due to critically narrowed and unstable plaqued regions supplying significant amounts of myocardium. Wash-in and washout are terms used to convey different types of CHANGE in isotope concentrations which occur over time at different rates to indicate the type of lesions present in the individual being studied. The results of these changes can be compared with changes found on cardiac catheterization as shown in Figure 32. As we continue to expand the number of individuals being studied with this method, it is clear that specific regional information can be determined from the parabolic equations used here and graphically displayed in Figure 32. The utilization of this knowledge will allow us to better determine which patients will benefit most from coronary angiography and has now been confirmed "qualitatively" by investigators at UCLA and Harvard Universities (Sheikine 2010). With the advent of nuclear cameras capable of faster image acquisition, we will undoubtedly be able to compare washout of the more rapidly redistributing technetium-99m compounds such as Teboroxime (Fleming 1990a-c, 1991a, 1992b, Goldstein 1991). Given the failure of rest-stress imaging to deliver on the promise of detecting ischemia and tissue viability due to their failure to image the heart as explained by Blumgart (1926) and Gorlin (1959), it is clear that FHRWW represents a superior method as we have already seen above and will see below.

We expect that the FHRWW protocol will replace other outdated and incorrectly proposed protocols due to its accuracy, simplicity, and reduction in amount of radioactive material used for imaging allowing for (1) a further reduction in the amount of radioactive material required for ischemic imaging, (2) faster imaging times (3) with FHRWW the ability to calculate %DS directly from nuclear imaging and (4) when coupled with previously published flow reserve equations (Figure 14), the ability to calculate stenosis (Fleming 1994) flow reserve directly from FHRWW. The Fleming Harrington Redistribution Wash-in Washout quantification of technetium-99m isotopes will allow for the first time (Fleming 2010c), the acquisition of both Anatomic and Physiologic data from a single radioisotope injection, single camera imaging system, including Positron Emission (PET) Tomography (Fleming 1999a), Magnetic Resonance Imaging, or Computed Tomography (CT).

As mentioned in the first Section of this chapter, the desire to know if the patient has undergone myocardial damage or injury (infarction, stunning or hibernation) has long been a question of interest. While, today it may appear to be much less of a concern given the increased availability to measure cardiac enzymes and look for evidence of regional wall motion abnormalities, either by echocardiography, nuclear, magnetic resonance or other imaging modalities, the detection of wall motion abnormalities and elevated cardiac enzymes does not tell us if the tissue damage is full thickness (Figure 14) and permanent, or partial thickness and recoverable. This is the true value of "resting" nuclear imaging. However, just like ischemic imaging, the detection of tissue damage, requires multiple same state condition (viz. rest-rest) imaging, which we will discuss in the next and final Section of this chapter.

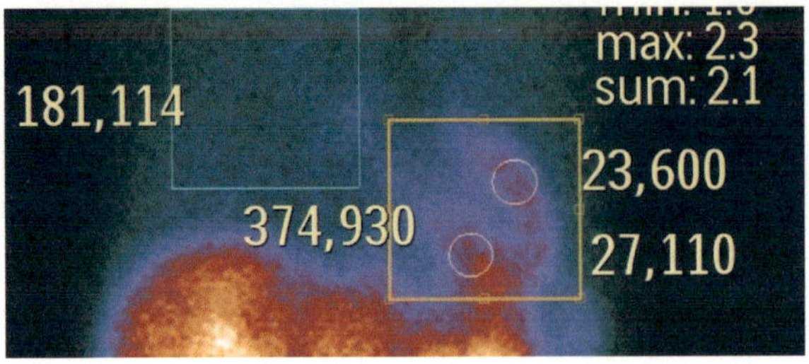

Fig. 27. SPECT image acquired 5 minutes post stress with regions of interest including the total heart, anterior and inferior myocardial regions

Static image acquired at 5 minutes with regions of interest (ROI) showing total heart count of 374,930. The anterior ROI representing the basal anterior region of the perfused by the left anterior descending artery shows 23,600 counts while the inferior ROI shows 27,110 counts.

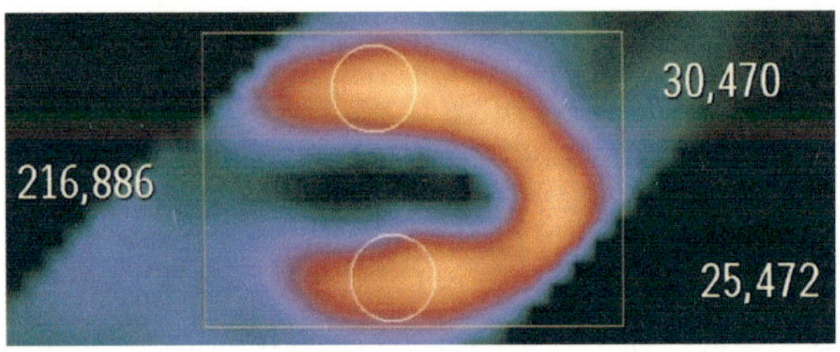

Fig. 28. SPECT image acquired 60 minutes post stress with regions of interest including the total heart, anterior and inferior myocardial regions

Reconstruction of the same myocardial regions noted in figure 2, this time taken from the dynamic image result obtained at 60 minutes post stress, showing a total heart count of 216,886. The anterior ROI shows an increase in count activity (wash-in) of 30,470 compared with the activity of 23,600 (Figure 2) obtained at 5 minutes. The inferior ROI shows a count of 25,472 compared with the count activity of 27,110 (Figure 2) obtained 5 minutes post stress.

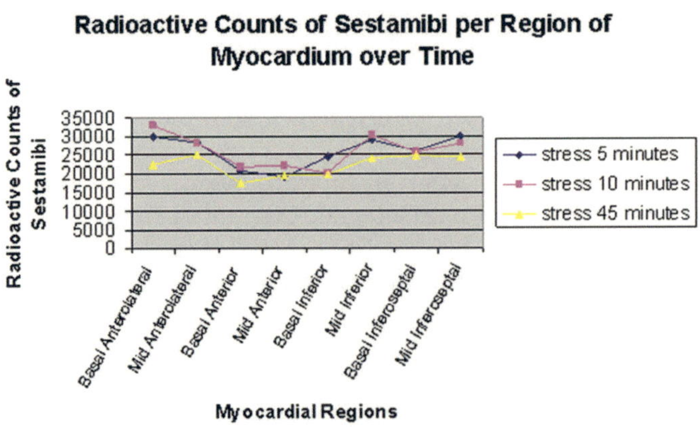

Fig. 29. Determination of Optimal Timing of Image Acquisition

The radioactive counts acquired in eight different myocardial regions vary with time and disease. This graphic demonstrates changes between 5, 10 and 45 minutes post stress. This graph demonstrates that the "uptake/retention" model of technetium-99m-sestamibi is incorrect and that "uptake/release" of technetium-99m-sestamibi occurs throughout the first 45 minutes following stress.

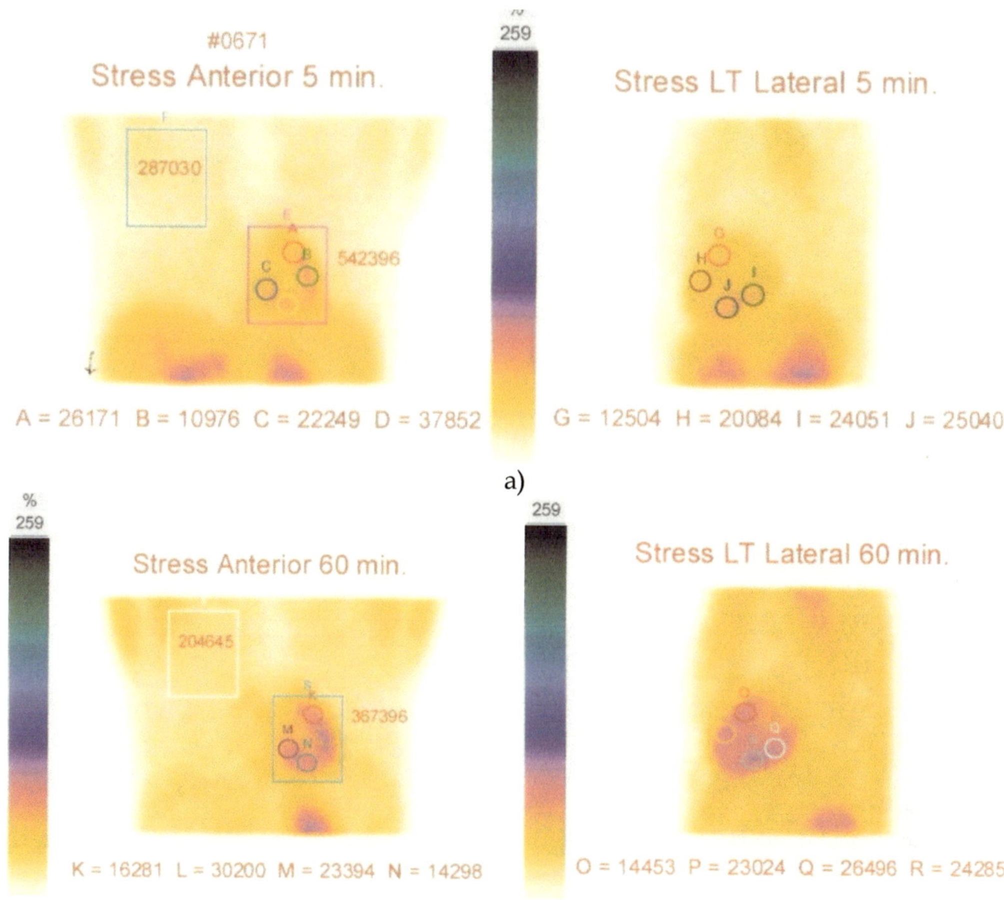

Fig. 30a-c. Radioactive Counts Acquired at 5 and 60 Minutes Post Stress

Anterior images reveal ROI counts at 5 and 60 minutes in the basal anterolateral (A, K), mid anterolateral (B, L), mid inferoseptal (D, N) and basal inferoseptal (C, M) respectively. The counts are shown below the images. The lateral images reveal ROI counts at 5 and 60 minutes in the basal anterior (G, O), mid anterior (H, P), mid inferior (J, R) and basal inferoposterior (I, Q) regions respectively. The total heart and lung counts are not shown or discussed in this paper; however, their ROIs are represented by square boxes of equal size in the anterior images.

Anterior images reveal ROI counts at 5 and 60 minutes in the basal anterolateral (1, 1), mid anterolateral (2, 2), mid inferoseptal (4, 4) and basal inferoseptal (3, 3) respectively. The counts are shown below the images. The lateral images reveal ROI counts at 5 and 60 minutes in the basal anterior (1, 1), mid anterior (2, 2), mid inferior (4, 4) and basal inferoposterior (3, 3) regions respectively. The total heart and lung counts are not shown or discussed in this paper; however, their ROIs are represented by square boxes of equal size in the anterior images.

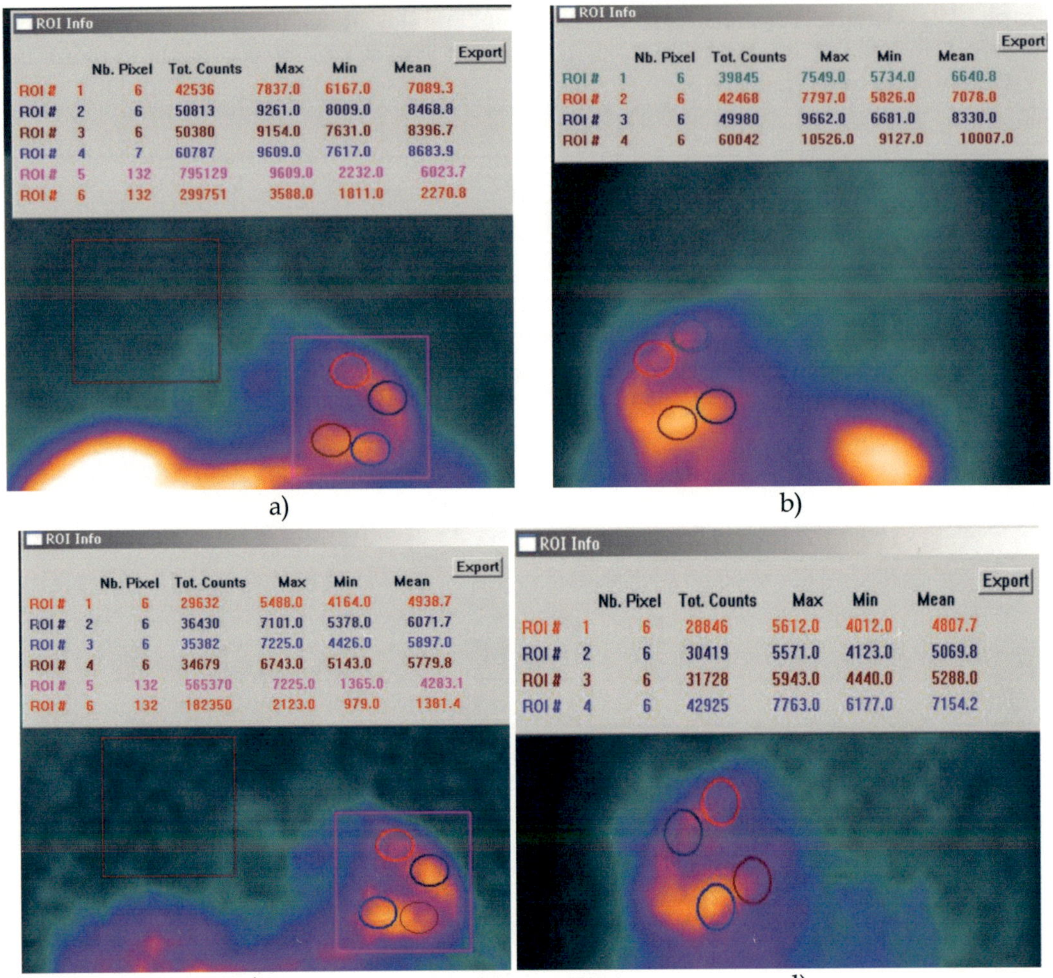

Fig. 31. Radioactive Counts acquired at 5 and 60 Minutes Post Stress

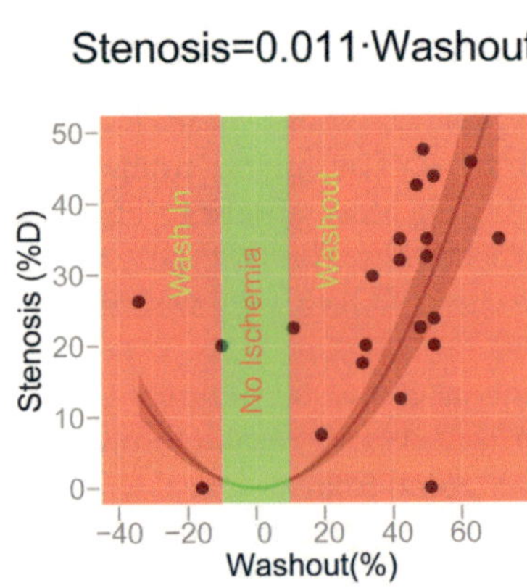

Fig. 32. Parabolic Regression of Washout on Percent Diameter Stenosis

Percent diameter stenosis noted on coronary angiography was plotted against the results of washout. Stenosis = $0.011 \times Washout^2$, F = 70.4, df(1,21), ($P=3.8\times10^{-8}$), R(CI95%) = 0.72 to 0.95, Graphic bands show the standard error of the fit. The region of "No Ischemia" is marked in green. "Wash in" is displayed in red to the left of the "No Ischemia" region, while "Washout" is to the right of the "No Ischemia" zone.

6. FHRWW rest-rest SPECT viability imaging - cardiac viability measured using resting FHRWW redistribution of sestamibi: the scientific evidence proves "sestamibi redistributes and is not mitochondrial superglue"

Abstract: Sequential imaging of the heart began in 1926 with the emphasis by Blumgart[1] on detecting changes in isotope over time. In recent years this change in isotope has been defined as "washout/wash in" and has been used to better define ischemia. Our investigations of sestamibi have demonstrated that not only can multiple post-stress images be used to more accurately define ischemia as defined below; but also, multiple resting images can be used to differentiate between viable and infracted myocardium.
The introduction of Nuclear Cardiology in 1926 by Blumgart (1926) established a protocol of sequential imaging/counts to differentiate people with heart disease from those without. In 1959 Gorlin demonstrated the importance of differentiating between resting studies, which provided information regarding tissue damage, from stress studies, which provided important information relevant to ischemia. With the introduction of technetium-99m compounds in the late 1980's, clinicians erroneously assumed that sestamibi was taken up by cardiac tissue within minutes and retained. Crane (1993) proved that the uptake of sestamibi by myocytes was dependent upon mitochondrial calcium, which in turn was dependent upon ischemia. This was confirmed clinically by Hurwitz (1998) and many (Ono 2002, 2003, Fleming 2008b, 2009) others. Our investigations have included initial observations regarding cellular viability. We present a case report of the promise of sestamibi in distinguishing between viable and infracted myocardium.
Case Report. Mr. JW is a 56 year-old Caucasian male who presented to the Emergency Department with chest pressure. His risk factors for heart disease included tobacco use, hyperlipidemia and borderline glucose intolerance. No electrocardiographic changes (Figure 33) were noted. Over the course of the next 24-36 hours both his Troponin and CK-MB levels were noted to be elevated and he was taken to the coronary angiography suite where a 100% occluded first obtuse marginal was stented. Also noted were a 20% mid-left anterior descending (LAD) and 50% distal LAD lesion, which were not treated.

6.1 Redistribution/washout information

The patient was brought to the nuclear laboratory 3 days after undergoing coronary angiography to evaluate the extent of myocardial damage. He was given an injection of 370 MBq (10 mCi) of sestamibi and had static images (FH Washout) taken 5-minutes and 60-minutes later (Fleming 2008b, 2009). Dynamic images were subsequently taken looking for wall motion abnormalities. The patient then underwent adenosine sestamibi (1110 MBq) imaging following the same protocol as that used for the resting images. The results of the counts obtained from the resting images are shown in Figure 34. The dynamic resting study demonstrated no regional wall motion abnormality and a near absence of isotope activity in the lateral wall. The dynamic stress study showed lateral wall hypokinesis.

In previous years, technetium pyrophospate was used and later abandoned to define the presence or absence of myocardial infarction (MI) when cardiac enzymes were obtained too late to determine non-q-wave MIs. Of great interest is the ability to determine if an area which appears infracted (Figure 35) on resting studies represents potentially viable tissue, which would benefit from revascularization. Clearly, sestamibi does not simply "stick" to myocardial cells; but, as emphasized by Crane[3] is dependent upon mitochondrial calcium, which is subsequently influenced by ischemia. Once cellular death has occurred, mitochondrial function ceases and mitochondrial calcium "overload" results.

In this patient the final 60 minute counts equaled that of the remaining "clearly viable" myocardium and as such is "viable" despite the appearance on the 60-minute resting dynamic study from which only infarction can be inferred. The 60-minute dynamic rest study revealed no regional wall motion abnormality while the dynamic stress study revealed "hypokinesis", not "akinesis". The initial 5-minute static resting counts demonstrated that either injury (viable) or infarction had occurred in the anterolateral region. It is the comparison of the two sets of resting image "counts" which allows the distinction between viable and infarcted tissue. Had the anterolateral region been infarcted, then the myocytes would not have been able to concentrate any sestamibi and both 5 and 60 minute counts would be lower than the remaining viable myocardium. These findings support the speculation by Crane in 1993, that "99m-sestamibi should not be retained in necrotic or irreversibly ischemic myocardium" and that by comparing results at 5 and 60-minutes, we can distinguish between viable and non-viable myocardium.

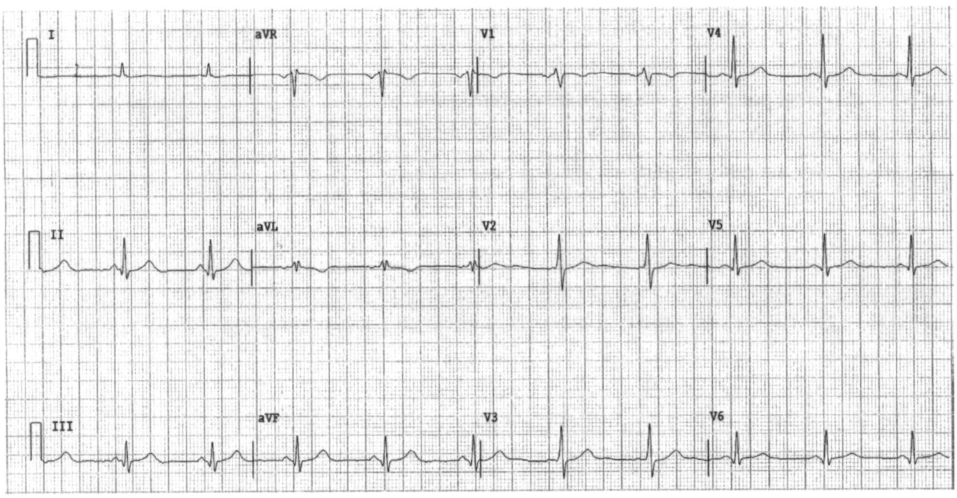

Fig. 33. Electrocardiogram

The patients resting electrocardiogram showed no evidence q-wave or ST changes.

The radioactive counts for each of 8 regions of myocardium are shown. The count activity present at 5 minutes is shown in blue and is greater than that seen for the count activity at 60 minutes. By 60 minutes, most of the myocardium had the same count activity despite the appearance present in figure 3. Note that the count activity in the anterolateral region is much lower initially than the count activity present in the remaining myocardium indicating that a non-q-wave myocardial "damage" has occurred in the anterolateral region. However, the presence of sestamibi activity at 5-minutes indicates viability anterolaterally.

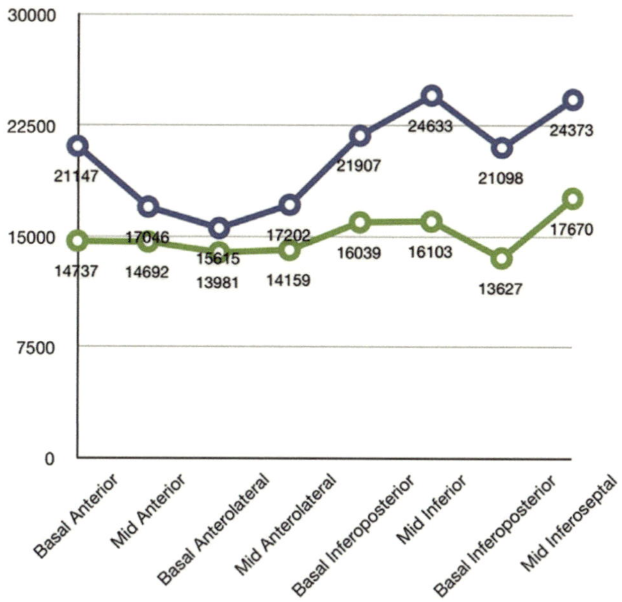

Fig. 34. 5 and 60-Minute Rest Image Counts

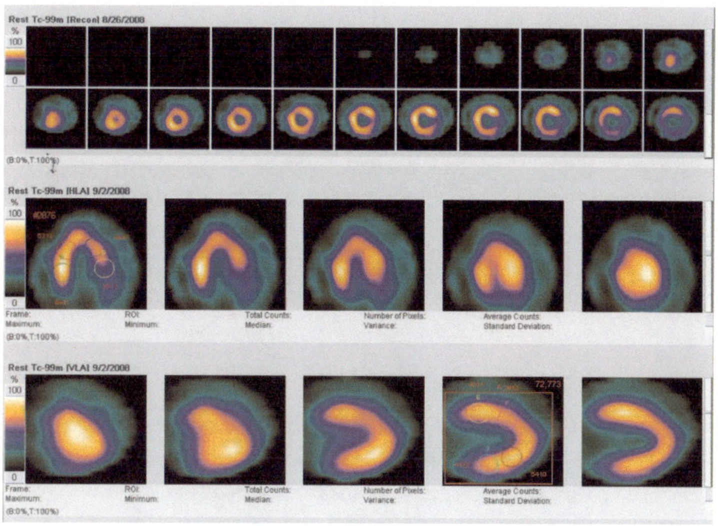

Fig. 35. Results of the dynamic 60-minute rest image

The resting image obtained 60 minutes post injection of isotope shows a significant reduction in isotope in the anterolateral wall despite similar count activity as shown in figure 2. The electrocardiogram in figure 1 shows no evidence of q-wave development or ST changes.

7. Conclusion

As this chapter has emphasized, the development of Nuclear Cardiology by Blumgart in 1926 saw a bright future allowing clinicians and scientists the opportunity to look within the body by detecting the emission of radioactive decay from tissue following its injection, distribution and redistribution. The radioactive compounds are not static and their movement (redistribution) allows us the unique opportunity to understand where there are and how they change position with time. This movement is a reflection of delivery (blood) and uptake (cellular and mitochondrial) and redistribution of the isotope over time. Just as the solutes within our cells and interstitial space are not static, so it is with the radioactive isotopes we inject. The movement of these radioactive isotopes over time allows us to understand both the Anatomy and the Physiology of the interior of our bodies. More importantly, understanding when to image and for what purpose is key to understanding what processes we are actually measuring (either qualitatively or quantitatively). In the case of ischemia, these comparisons must be made between "stress" images, while for tissue viability, these comparisons must be made under "resting" conditions. While Blumgart and Gorlin were clear as to these points, much of the energy expended in Nuclear Imaging of the Heart has failed to address these errors. As such, coronary arteriography has remained the "Gold" standard for the anatomic detection of heart disease. As our recent understanding has improved, so has our detection of disease and our ability to reduce the amount of radiation our patients receive and that which we receive secondarily. Seventy-five years after Blumgarts original work, we have peered through the uncertainty of our equipment and the limitations of our old methods. Today, we can truly detect heart disease and utilize it to improve the care provided to our patients and be confident of our diagnoses and treatment. We have replaced the "Gold" standard of coronary angiography which can only provide anatomic information of coronary (Figure 36) lumen disease (Fleming 2000f, 2001) with a "Platinum" standard providing both anatomic and physiologic information required for the better detection and treatment (Figure 37) of coronary artery disease.

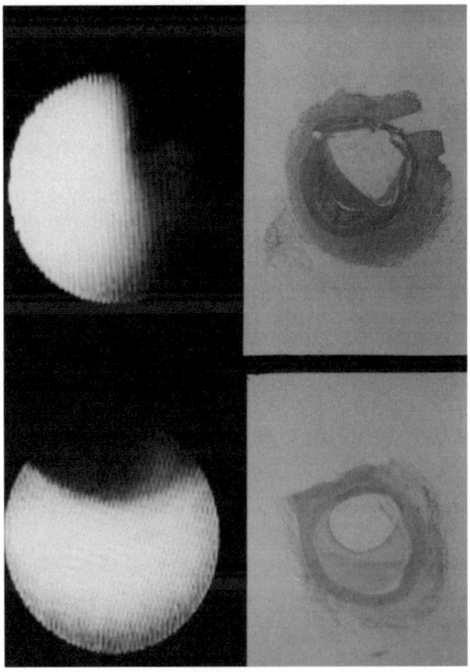

Fig. 36. Coronary angiographic detection of disease

Coronary angioscopy with tissue specimens show immediately to the right of each following death of the individual. The upper panels show an individual with plaque intruding into the coronary lumen. The bottom panels represent a patient without visible lumen disease. As evidenced by the pathology specimen, the inflammatory plaque laid beneath the endothelial layer and was not detectable by visual inspection of the coronary lumen either by angioscopy or conventional cardiac catheterization and contrast injection. Nonetheless, this inflammatory plaque (Fleming 1999c-d, 2000g, 2002f, 2003d-f, 2008a, 2009b) is physiologically responsible for angina and plaque rupture leading to death. Such individuals may be easily missed by the angiogram and stress-rest approaches; but, can be unmasked by FHRWW stress-stress imaging (Fleming 2009b) as demonstrated in this chapter.

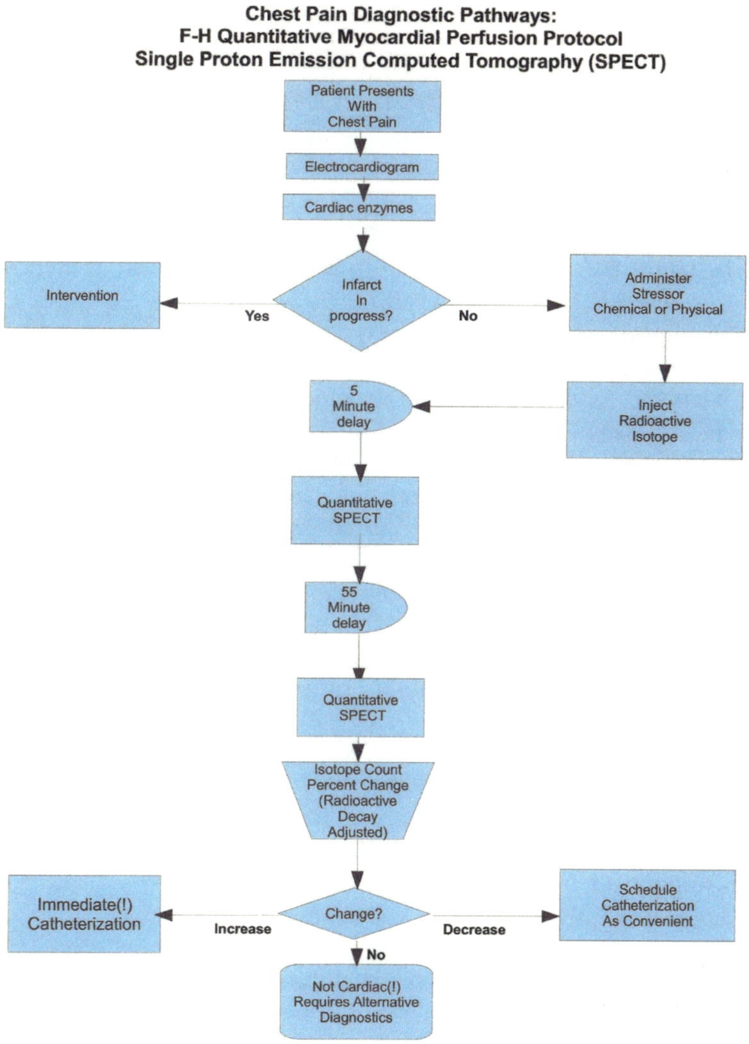

Fig. 37. Chest pain algorithm[11] using FHRWW

Efforts to improve acute chest pain analysis employing FHRWW can be used to distinguish between the most critically ill individuals who will have critically narrowed arteries or arteries with vulnerable inflammatory plaques by virtue of wash-in findings defined by reduced isotope at 5 minute post pharmacologic stress imaging and normal appearing isotope concentrations at 60-minutes post-stress from those without such critical disease.

8. References

Ahmad M, Logan KW, Martin RH. (1979) Doughnut pattern of technetium-99m pyrophosphate myocardial uptake in patients with acute myocardial infarction: A sign of poor long-term prognosis. *Am J Cardiol* 44:13-17.

Anger H. (1957) A new instrument for mapping gamma-ray emitters. *Biology and Medicine Quarterly Report UCRL*, 3653: 38.

Aodah B. (2007) "Nuclear Medicine and Gamma Camera" Instructional Course from the King Saud University College of Applied Medical Science, *Biomedical Technology DeSectionment*. 2007.

Ayalew A, et al. (2000) A comparison of the overall first-pass kinetics of thallium-201 and technetium-99m MIBI in normoxic and low-flow ischaemic myocardium. *Eur J Nucl Med* 27:1632-40.

Ayalew A, et al. (2002) 201 Tl and 99m Tc-MIBI retention in an isolated heart model of low-flow ischemia and stunning: Evidence of negligible impact of myocyte metabolism on tracer kinetics. *J Nucl Med* 43:566-74.

Beller GA, Sinusas AJ. (1990) Experimental studies of the physiologic properties of technetium-99m isonitriles. *Am J Cardiol* 16:5E-8E.

Blumgart HL, Yens OC. (1926) Studies on the velocity of blood flow: I. The method utilized. *J Clin Investigation* 4:1-13.

Calnon DA, et al. (1997) Effects of dobutamine stress on myocardial blood flow, 99m-Tc sestamibi uptake, and systolic wall thickening in the presence of coronary artery stenoses: implications for dobutamine stress testing. *Circulation* 96:2353-60.

Calnon DA, et al. (1999) Myocardial uptake of 99mTc-N-NOET and 201 Tl during dobutamine infusion. *Circulation* 100:1653-9.

Crane P, et al. (1993) Effect of mitochondrial viability and metabolism on technetium-99m-sestamibi myocardial retention. *Eur J Nucl Med* 20:20-5.

Dahlberg ST, Leppo JA. (1994) Physiologic properties of myocardial perfusion tracers. *Cardiol Clin* 12:169-85.

Everett DB, et al. (1977) Gamma-radiation imaging system based on the Compton effect. *Proceedings of the IEEE* 124:995-1000.

Fallahi B, et al. (2008) Single Tc99m Sestamibi injection, double acquisition gated SPECT after stress and during low-dose dobutamine infusion: a new suggested protocol for evaluation of myocardial perfusion. *Int J Cardiovasc Imaging* Jun 18. [Epub ahead of print]

Fleming RM, et al. (1990a) Feasibility of SPECT Perfusion Imaging with Technetium 99-m Teboroxime: Comparison to Thallium- 201 and Quantitative Coronary Arteriography. *5th World Congress of Nuclear Medicine and Biology, European Journal of Nuclear Medicine*, Montreal, Canada.

Fleming RM, et al. (1990b) Tc-99m Teboroxime SPECT Imaging: Comparison to Thallium 201 and Quantitative Coronary Arteriography. *Circulation* 82(4):III-652.

Fleming RM, et al. (1990c) Nuclear Cardiology and Imaging - Myocardial Scintigraphy II on the Feasibility of SPECT Perfusion Imaging with Technetium 99-m Teboroxime: Comparison to Thallium-201 and Quantitative Coronary Arteriography. *XIIth European Heart Journ*al 11:277.

Fleming RM, et al. (1991a) A Comparison of Technetium 99-m Teboroxime Tomography to Automated Quantitative Coronary Arteriography and Thallium - 201 SPECT. *J Am Coll. Cardiol.* 17:1297-1302.

Fleming RM, et al. (1991b) Patterns in visual interpretation of coronary arteriograms as detected by quantitative coronary arteriography. *J Am Coll Cardiol* 18:945-51.

Fleming RM, Gibbs HR, Swafford J. (1992a) Using Quantitative Coronary Arteriography to Redefine SPECT Sensitivity and Specificity. *Am J Physiol Imag.* 7:59-65.

Fleming RM. (1992b) Detecting Coronary Artery Disease Using SPECT Imaging: A Comparison of Thallium-201 and Teboroxime. *Am J Physiol Imag* 7(1):20-23.

Fleming RM, Harrington GM. (1994) Quantitative coronary arteriography and its assessment of atherosclerosis. Section II. Calculating stenosis flow reserve from percent diameter stenosis. *Angiology* 45:835-40.

Fleming RM, Rose CH, Feldmann KM. (1995) Comparing a High Dose Dipyridamole SPECT ImagingProtocol with Dobutamine and Exercise Stress Testing Protocols. *Angiology* 46(7):547-556.

Fleming RM, Feldmann KM. (1998) Comparing a High Dose Dipyridamole SPECT Imaging Protocol with Dobutamine and Exercise Stress Testing Protocols. Section II: Using High-Dose Dipyridamole to Determine Lung-to-Heart Ratios. *Intern J Angiol* 7:325-328.

Fleming RM. (1999a) Chapter 31. Nuclear Cardiology: Its Role in the Detection and Management of Coronary Artery Disease Textbook of Angiology. John C. Chang Editor, Springer-Verlag New York, NY. pp. 397-406.

Fleming RM, Feldmann KM. (1999b) Comparing a High Dose Dipyridamole SPECT Imaging Protocol with Dobutamine and Exercise Stress Testing Protocols. Section III: Using Dobutamine to Determine Lung-to-Heart Ratios, Left Ventricular Dysfunction and a Potential Viability Marker. *Inter J Angiol* 8:22-26.

Fleming RM. (1999c) Chapter 64. The Pathogenesis of Vascular Disease. Textbook of Angiology. John C. Chang Editor, Springer-Verlag New York, NY. pp. 787-798.

Fleming RM. (1999d) Chapter 29. Atherosclerosis: Understanding the relationship between coronary artery disease and stenosis flow reserve. Textbook of Angiology. John C. Chang Editor, Springer-Verlag, New York, NY. pp. 381-387.

Fleming RM. (2000a) The Clinical Importance of Risk Factor Modification: Looking at Both Myocardial Viability (MV) and Myocardial Perfusion Imaging (MPI) *Intern J Angiol* 9:55-69.

Fleming RM. (2000b) The Natural Progression of Atherosclerosis in an Untreated Patient with Hyperlipidemia: Assessment via Cardiac PET. *Intern J Angiol* 9:70-73.

Fleming RM. (2000c) The Fleming Unified Theory of Vascular Disease: A link between atherosclerosis, inflammation and bacterially aggravated atherosclerosis (BAA). *Angiol 51:87-9.*

Fleming RM, Boyd L, Forster M. (2000d) Unified Theory Approach Reduces Heart Disease and Recovers Viable Myocardium. *42nd Annual World Congress - International College of Angiology*, San Diego, California, USA, June 29, 2000.

Fleming RM., Boyd L., Forster M. (2000e) Angina is Caused by Regional Blood Flow Differences - Proof of a Physiologic (Not Anatomic) Narrowing, Joint Session of the European Society of Cardiology and the American College of Cardiology, *Annual American College of Cardiology Scientific Sessions, Anaheim, California*, USA, 12 March 2000, 49th (Placed on internet www.prous.com for physician training and CME credit, April 2000.)

Fleming RM. (2000f) Shortcomings of coronary angiography. Letter to the Editor. *Cleve Clin J Med* 67:450.

Fleming RM, Boyd L, Forster M. (2000g) Reversing Heart Disease in the New Millennium - The Fleming Unified Theory, *Angiology* 51(10):617-629.

Fleming RM. (2001) Coronary Artery Disease is More than Just Coronary Lumen Disease. *Amer J Card* 88:599-600.

Fleming RM. (2002a) High-Dose Dipyridamole and Gated Sestamibi SPECT Imaging Provide Diagnositic Resting and Stress Ejection Fractions Useful for Predicting the Extent of Coronary Artery Disease. *Angiology* 53(4):415-421.

Fleming RM. (2002b) A Tate-en-Tate Comparison of Ejection Fraction and Regional Wall Motion Abnormalities as Measured by Echocardiography and Gated Sestamibi SPECT. *Angiology* 53:313-321.

Fleming RM. (2002c) Breast enhanced scintigraphy test demonstrates improvement in breast inflammation in women consuming soy protein. *The Journal of Nutrition* 132:575S.

Fleming RM. (2002d) Mitochondrial Uptake of Sestamibi Distinguishes Between Normal, Inflammatory Breast Changes, Pre-cancers and Infiltrating Breast Cancer. *Integrative Cancer Therapies* 1(3):229-237.

Fleming RM, Dooley WC. (2002e) Breast Enhanced Scintigraphy Testing (B.E.S.T.) Distinguishes Between Normal, Inflammatory Breast Changes and Breast Cancer. A Prospective Analysis and Comparison with Mammography. *Integrative Cancer Therapies* 1(3):238-245.

Fleming RM. (2002f) The Effect of High, Moderate and Low Fat Diets On Weight Loss and Cardiovascular Disease Risk Factors. Preventive Cardiology V(III):110-118. [http://www.medscape.com/viewarticle/438769]

Fleming RM. (2003a) What effect, if any, does soy protein have on breast tissue? *Integrative Cancer Therapies* 2:225-8.

Fleming RM. (2003b) Are there differences in breast tissue as a result of hormone replacement therapy? Can BEST imaging distinguish these differences? *Integrative Cancer Therapies* 2:229-34.

Fleming RM. (2003c) Do women taking hormone replacement therapy (HRT) have a higher incidence of breast cancer than women who do not? *Integrative Cancer Therapies* 2:235-7.

Fleming RM. (2003d) Angina and coronary Ischemia are the result of coronary regional Blood Flow Differences. *J Amer Coll Angiol* 2003;1:127-42.

Fleming RM. (2003e) Using C-Reactive Protein as a Marker of Bacteriallly Aggravated Atherosclerosis in Acute Coronary Syndromes. *J Amer Coll Angiol* 1:165-71.

Fleming RM. (2003f) Stop Inflammation Now! with Tom Monte. Published by Putnam Books and Avery Books. December 2003.

Fleming RM, Harrington GM. (2008) What is the Relationship between Myocardial Perfusion Imaging and Coronary Artery Disease Risk Factors and Markers of Inflammation?, *Angiology* 59:16-25.

Fleming RM, Harrington GM, Baqir R. (2009) Heart Disease in Men. Chapter 3. Using Multiple Images Post-Stress to Enhance diagnostic Accuracy of Myocardial Perfusion Imaging: The Clinical Importance of Determining Washin and Washout Indicates a Parabolic Function between Coronary Perfusion (Blood Flow) and Cellular ("Uptake/Release") Function. Alice B. Todd and Margo H. Mosley Editors, Nova Publishers pp. 75-100. (https://www.novapublishers.com/catalog/product_info.php?products _id=8409)

Fleming RM, et al. (2009b) The Evolution of Nuclear Cardiology takes Us Back to the Beginning to Develop Today's "New Standard of Care" for Cardiac Imaging: How Quantifying Regional Radioactive Counts at 5 and 60 Minutes Post-Stress Unmasks Hidden Ischemia. Methodist DeBakey *Cardiovascular Journal* (MDCVJ) 5(3):42-48.

Fleming RM, et al.(2010a) Renewed Application of an Old Method Improves Detection of Coronary Ischemia. A Higher Standard of Care. *Federal Practitioner* 2010;27:22-31.

Fleming RM (2010b) Innovations in myocardial perfusion imaging reveal potential life-saving strategy. By: Brian Ellis, Cardiology Today, *Feature story*. 13(9). (http://www.cardiologytoday.com/view.aspx?rid=68069).

Fleming RM, Harrington GM. (2010c) FHRWW Stress SPECT Protocol Reduces Radioactive Dosage and Increases Ischemia Detection. *ANZ Nuclear Medicine* 41:24-32.

Fukushima K, et al. (2007) Myocardial kinetics of (201) Thallium, (99m) Tc-tetrofosmin, and (99m) Tc-sestamibi in an acute ischemia-reperfusion model using isolated rat heart. *Ann Nucl Med* 21:267-73.

Fujiwara S, et al. (1998) Prediction of functional recovery in acute myocardial infarction: comparison between sestamibi reverse redistribution and sestamibi/BMIPP mismatch. *J Nucl Cardiol* 5:119-27.

Giubbini R, et al. (1995) Evaluation of technetium-99m-sestamibi lung uptake: correlation with left ventricular function. *J Nucl Med* 1995;36:58-63.

Glagov S, et al. (1987) Compensatory enlargement of human atherosclerotic coronary arteries. *N Engl J Med* 316:1371-5.

Glover DK, et al. (1995) Comparison between 201Tl and 99mTc Sestamibi uptake during adenosine-induced vasodilation as a function of coronary stenosis severity. *Circulation* 91:813-20.

Goldstein RA, Fleming RM, et al. (1991) SPECT Imaging with Tc99m-teboroxime (TEBO). Japan Society of Nuclear Medicine. *Jap J Nucl Med* 28:937.

Gorlin R, et al. (1959) Effect of nitroglycerin on the coronary circulation in patients with coronary artery disease or increased left ventricular work. *Circulation* 19:705-18.

Gould KL, Kirkeeide RL, Buchi M. (1990) Coronary flow reserve as a physiologic measure of stenosis severity. *J Am Coll Cardiol* 15:459-74.

Heart (2011) http://www.theheart.org/article/1176107.do

Heisenberg, W. (1927). Ueber den anschaulichen Inhalt der quantentheoretischen Kinematik and Mechanik, *Zeitschrift für Physik* 43:172-198.

Hurwitz GA, et al. (1993) Pulmonary uptake of sestamibi on early post-stress images: angiographic relationships, incidence and kinetics. *Nucl Med Commun* 14;15-22.

Hurwitz GA, et al. (1996) Stress/injection protocols for myocardial scintigraphy with sestamibi and thallium-201: implications of early post-stress kinetics. *Nucl Med Commun* 17:400-9.

Hurwitz GA, et al. (1998) Pulmonary uptake of Technetium-99m-Sestamibi induced by dipyridamole-basedstress or exercise. *J Nucl Med* 1998;39:339-45.

Husain SS. (2007) Myocardial perfusion imaging protocols: Is there an ideal protocol. *J Nucl Med Tech* 35:3-9.

Ikawa M, et al. (2007) Evaluation of respiratory chain failure in mitochondrial cardiomyopathy by assessments of 99mTc-MIBI washout and 123I-BMIPP/99mTc-MIBI mismatch. *Mitochondrion* 7:164-70.

Kern MJ, et al. (2006) Physiological assessment of coronary artery disease in the cardiac catheterization laboratory: A scientific statement from the American Heart Association committee on diagnostic and interventional cardiac catheterization, council on clinical cardiology. *Circulation* 114:1321-41.

Khaw BA. (1999) The current role of infarct avid imaging. Semin Nucl Med 29:259-270.

Kodavanti UP, et al. (2008) The role of Particulate matter-associated zinc in cardiac injury in rats. *Environ Health Perspect* 116:13-20.

Kumita S, et al. (2002) Assessment of myocardial washout of Tc-99m-sestamibi in patients with chronic heart failure: comparison with normal control. *Ann Nucl Med* 16:237-42.

Lenzi P, et al. (2003) DNA damage associated with ultrastructural alterations in rat myocardium after loud noise exposure. *Environ Health Perspect* 111:467-71.

Liu Z, et al. (2001) Detection of myocardial viability in ischemic-reperfused rat hearts by Tc-99m sestamibi kinetics. *J Nucl Cardiol* 8:677-86.

Love WD. (1965) Isotope Technics in Clinical Cardiology. *Circulation* 32:309-15.

Maddahi J. (2001) Myocardial perfusion tracers in the detection and evaluation of coronary artery disease. *48thannual meeting of the society of nuclear medicine* 2001.

Matsunari I, et al. (20010Comparison of Sestamibi, Tetrofosmin, and Q12 Retention in Porcine Myocardium. *J Nucl Med* 42:818-23.

Matsuo S, et al. (2007) A novel clinical indicator using Tc-99m sestamibi for evaluating cardiac mitochondrial function in patients with cardiomyopathies. *J Nucl Cardiol* 14:215-20.

Maublant JC, Gachon P, Moins N. (1988) Hexakis (2-methoxy isobutylisonitrile) technetium-99m and thallium-201 chloride: uptake and release in cultured myocardial cells. *J Nucl Med* 29:48-54.

Meerdink DJ, Leppo JA. (1990) Myocardial transport of hexakis(2-methosyisobutyl isonitrile) and thallium before and after coronary reperfusion. *Circulation Research* 66:1738-46.

Meissner K, et al. (2002) Expression and localization of P-glycoprotein in Human Heart: Effects of Cardiomyopathy. *J Histochem Cytochem* 50:1351-6.

Ono S, et al. (2002) Rest delayed images on 99mTc-MIBI myocardial SPECT as a noninvasive screen for the diagnosis of vasospastic angina pectoris. *Kaku Igaku* 39:117-24.

Ono S, et al. (2003) Enhanced regional washout of technetium-99m-sestamibi in patients with coronary spastic angina. *Ann Nucl Med* 17:393-8.

(Oregon 2008) Researchers make case for standardized analysis of cardiac imaging. Oregon Heart & Vascular Institute, University of Oregon and L.A.'s Cedar-Sinai. March 13, 2008. http://pmr.uoregon.edu

Pace L, et al. (2005) Washout of [99mTc] sestamibi in predicting response to chemotherapy in patients with multiple myeloma. *Q J Nucl Med Mol Imaging* 49:281-5.

Parameswaran RV, Purantharan N, Prasad RD. (2006) Comparison of nitrate augmented 99mTc-Sestamibi infusion with nitrate augmented 99mTc-Sestamibi bolus injection for the detection of myocardial viability. *IJNM* 21:36-40.

Parkey RW, et al. (1976) Pathophysiology of myocardial infarct scintigraphy with Technetium-99m Pyrophosphate, Tecnnetium-99m Diphosphonate and thallium-201. *Invest Radiol* 11:395.

Poiseuille JLM. (1840) Reherches experimentales sur le mouvement des liquides dans les tubes de tres petits diametres. *Comptes Rendus Acad Ac* 2:961-1041.

Richter WS, et al. (1995) Washout and redistribution between immediate and two-hour myocardial images using technetium-99m sestamibi. *Eur J Nucl Med* 22:49-55.

Saha M, Forrest TF, Brown KA. (1994) Lung uptake of technetium-99m-sestamibi: relation to clinical, exercise, hemodynamic, and left ventricular function variables. *J Nucl Cardiol* 1:52-6.

Sattari A, Dadashzadeh S, Nasiroghli G. (2001) Urinary excretion and external radiation does from patients administered thallium-201 and technetium-99m methoxy isobutyl isonitrile. *Radait Prot Dosimetry* 95:59-61.

Sheikine Y, Berman DS, Di Carli MF. (2010) Technetium-99m-sestamibi redistribution after exercise stress test identified by a novel cardiac gamma camera: Two case reports. *Clin Cardiol* 33:E39-E45.

Shin WJ, et al. (1995) Reverse redistribution on dynamic exercise and dipyridamole stress technetium-99m-MIBI myocardial SPECT. *J Nucl Med* 36:2053-5

Sinusas AJ, et al. (1994) Redistribution of 99m-Tc-sestamibi and 201-Tl in the presence of a severe coronary artery stenosis. *Circulation* 89:2332-41.

St. Goar FG, et al. (1991) Intravascular ultrasound imaging of angiographically normal coronary arteries: An in vivo comparison with quantitative angiography. *JACC* 18:952-8.

Sugiura T, et al. (2006) Usefulness of Tc-99m methoxyisobutylisonitrile scintigraphy for evaluating congestive heart failure. *J Nucl Cardiol* 13:64-8.

Takeishi Y, et al. (1996) Reverse redistribution of technetium-99m-sestamibi following direct PTCA in acute myocardial infarction. *J Nucl Med* 37:1289-94.

Takahashi N, et al. (1996) Myocardial uptake of 99m Tc-tetrofosmin, Sestamibi, and 201 Tl in a model of acute coronary reperfusion. *Circulation* 94:2605-13.

Taki J, et al. (2001) 99mTc-Sestamibi retention characteristics during pharmacologic hyperemia in human myocardium: Comparison with coronary flow reserve measured by Doppler flowire. *J Nucl Med* 42:1457-63.

Tanaka R, et al. (2006) Clinical implication of reverse redistribution on 99mTc-sestamibi images for evaluating ischemic heart disease. *Ann Nucl Med* 20:349-56.

Toriyama T, et al. (2005) 99mTc-sestamibi scintigraphy in the prediction of cardiac events in patients with congestive heart failure. *7th International conference of Nuclear Cardiology-European Society of Cardiology* 2005.

VanBrocklin HF, et al. (2007) Mitochondrial avid radioprobes. Preparation and evaluation of 7'(Z)-[125I]iodorotenone and 7'(Z)-[125I]iodorotenol. *Nucl Med Biol* 34:109-16.

Walsh WF, et al. (1977) Assessment of diagnostic value of technetium-99m pyrophosphate myocardial scintigraphy in 80 patients with possible acute myocardial infarction. *Br Heart J* 39:974-981.

Part 6

Computed Tomography

14

Diagnostic Value of Multisliced Computed Tomography in Coronary Arteries Atherosclerotic Lesions Detection in the Patients with Coronary Heart Disease – a Comparative Study

Maryna N. Dolzhenko, Sergey V. Potashev and Natalia N. Nosenko
The P.L.Shupik National Medical Academy Of Postgraduate Education/Cardiology And Functional Diagnosis Department
Ukraine

1. Introduction

Today method of X-ray conventional coronary angiography (CCA) is a "golden standard" in diagnosis and evaluation of severity of coronary vessels atherosclerosis (Fleisher et al., 2007; Scanlon et al., 1999). But being invasive, this method has certain limitations, and cannot be suitable for stratification the patients with coronary arteries disease (CAD) suspicion in order to decide the necessity of revascularization (Laissy et al., 2007 ; Leschka S. et al., 2008; Mahmarian, 2007).
On the other hand, promising data regarding high correlation of non-invasive evaluation of left ventricle (LV) ejection fraction (EF), for instance, between resting echocardiographic EFs and single photon emission computed tomography (SPECT) resting gated sestamibi images in patients with single-vessel disease, and a moderate correlation in patients with 2- and 3-vessel disease, respectively (Fleming, 2002), as well as pharmacologically induced stress acquired from gated SPECT sestamibi images, providing a valuable diagnostic marker as to the number of significantly diseased coronary arteries (Fleming&Boyd, 2002), give only indirect information, being inappropriate for a surgeon prior to myocardium surgeon revascularization.
That is why a significant influence today is paid to design of newer methods of coronary pathology diagnosis, especially non-invasive. Among the demands to up-to-date examination methods high specificity, sensitivity, accuracy and safety should be mentioned, as well as high repeatability and economical suitability (Hamon et al., 2006). All these features are attributes of multislice spiral computed tomography (MSCT) (Abdulla et al., 2007; Achenbach, 2006; Kyung-Jong et al, 2003), what explains constantly growing interest to this method. Over the past years there has been a large quantity of works discussing value of contrast MSCT in diagnosis and evaluation of severity of coronary arteries atherosclerosis in the patients with CAD as an future alternative to CCA (Hamon et al., 2006; Kyung-Jong et al, 2003; Meijboom et al., 2006; Mollet et al, 2005; Mozaffarian, 2005).

In Ukraine there has been no attempts to compare informative and diagnostic value of invasive and non-invasive methods of left ventricle (LV) structural anomalies and coronary arteries lesions in the patients with CAD and after acute myocardial infarction (AMI).
The aim of this study was to compare the efficacy of contrast MSCT coronary angiography in diagnosis and severity of coronary vessels lesion in the patients with CAD compared to the "golden standard" CCA.

2. Methods

The study was approved by local ethics committee.
In the study we prospectively included 116 patients after AMI with LV postinfarction aneurism (LVA) without significant valvular dysfunction eligible for CABG combined with LVA resection. Exclusion criteria were a history of recent myocardial infarction (4 weeks before pre-operative angiography), atrial fibrillation, significant valvular heart disease or previous CABG. During and after the CABG, standard laboratory markers for myocardial infarction were obtained and none of the patients was diagnosed with perioperative myocardial infarction. Medication treatment in all the post-infarction patients included aspirin, statin, beta-blocker, ACE inhibitor and nitrates, if indicated. All patients underwent MSCT prior to the operation. Fourty age-matched subjects with CAD and without AMI history, who underwent CCA, and contrast MSCT for coronary revascularization decision, served as controls. Program of the study included X-ray contrast CCA and MSCT with chambers and coronary arteries contrast.

2.1 Coronary angiography

Coronary angiography with ventriculography was conducted and interpreted by trained physicians 1 week preceding CABG+AE. A 50% or more reduction of the luminal diameter in 2 orthogonal projections of a major coronary artery or one of its major branches or a bypass graft was considered to be significant for CAD[3,10,15]. Severity of coronary atherosclerosis were evaluated as coronary artery narrowing to 30% (grade 1), 50% (grade 2), 75% (grade 3), 90% (grade 4) of diameter or full occlusion (grade 5), respectively (Mollet et al, 2005; Scanlon et al., 1999).

2.2 Multislice computed tomography

MSCT was performed on tomographer «Light Speed-16» («General Electric Company», USA) using cardiological «Advantage Workstation 4.2» («General Electric Company», USA). Spiral mode of tomography with 2,5 mm thick slice and retrospective ECG synchronization was intravenous ed with 6-8 seconds scanning time and 360^0 rotation. Study was performed at breath held after infusomat "Omnipac" intravenous infusion. Exposure dose constituted 2,2 mSv per one study at 16 slices per 200 frames. Severity of coronary arteries stenosis was evaluated, as well as coronary calcium index (CI) by A.S. Agatston, as a general coronary atherosclerosis and calcinosis marker, was quantified (Achenbach, 2006).

2.3 Statistics

Comparison of different methods was performed using multiple regression analysis with 95% confidence interval and correlation analysis (Petry & Sabin, 2003; Rebrova, 2002). In comparison of diagnostic value of the studied methods we evaluated the following

characteristics: accuracy (diagnostic efficacy) - percentage of correct test results out of general quantity of both positive and negative results; sensitivity (Se) - percentage of subjects with positive test results in the population with the studied pathology; specificity (Sp) - percentage of subjects with negative test results in the population with the studied pathology; positive predictive value (+PV) - probability of symptom or disease in case of positive test result; negative predictive value (-PV) – case of negative (normal) test result.
The above numbered indices were calculated by formulas:

$$Se=N(TP)/(N(TP)+N(FN))x100\%;$$

$$Sp=N(TN)/(N(TN)+N(FP)x100\%;$$

$$+PV=N(TP)/(N(TP)+N(FP)\ x\ 100\%;$$

$$-PV=(TN)/(N(TN)+N(FN)x100\%;$$

where N is the quantity of studied patients; TP – truly positive diagnosis; FP – false positive diagnosis; TN - truly negative diagnosis; FN - false negative diagnosis[12,13]. The results are expressed as the mean and 1 standard deviation. The parameters of patients and healthy subjects were compared using an unpaired t-test. A paired t-test was used to compare results within the same group. A P-value of <0,05 was considered significant.

3. Results

The main clinical features of the study group patients are presented in Table 1.

Index	Abs.	%
LV EF (%)	37,1±12,4	-
LV EDI (ml/m^2)	112,4±28,2	-
LV ESI (ml/m^2)	73,8±27,6	-
Diabetes mellitus (n)	14	12,1%
Hypertension (n)	75	64,7%
Angina pectoris	107	92,3%
Functional class I	15	12,9%
Functional class II	23	19,8%
Functional class III	64	55,2%
Functional class IV	14	12,1%

Heart failure (NYHA functional class)		
I (LV > 45%)	17	14,7%
II (LV < 45%)	86	74,1%
I (LV < 45%)	13	11,2%
Lesions localization (by CCA)		
3-vessels disease and/or left main (n)	41	35,4%
2-vessels disease (n)	39	33,6%
1 -vessel disease (n)	35	30,2%
No significant lesions	1	0,8%
Coronary atherosclerotic lesions localization (by CCA)		
Main left coronary artery (LCA)	15	12,9%
Anterior descending left coronary artery (AD LCA)	112	96,6%
Diagonal LCA	7	6,0%
Circumflex (Cx) LCA	62	53,5%
Right coronary artery (RCA)	79	68,1%
*Data are presented as total (n) or M±SD (n=116)		

Table 1. Clinical features of the patients studied

As it is seen from the table, according to CVG data there were predominantly patients with 2- and 3-vessels disease of left main coronary artery lesion.

According to contrast MSCT results data, main LCA lesion was found in 8 (6,9%) patients (46,7% false negative results), AD LCA lesion – in 89 (76,7%) patients (20,5% false negative results), diagonal LCA lesion – in 0 cases (100% false negative results), Cx LCA lesion – in 32 (27,6%) patients (48,4% false negative results), and RCA lesion – in 48 (41,4%) patients (39,2% false negative results). Therefore, in approximately one third to one half of the patients contrast 16-slice MSCT was unable to reveal significant trunk coronary arteries stenosis.

Data of contrast MSCT results still significantly correlated with CCA data. Like this, quantity of stenotic arteries significantly correlated with CCA data ($r=0,50$, $p<0,0001$). High enough correlation was found in main LCA stenosis diagnosis ($r=0,75$, $p<0,0001$), proximal segments of RCA ($r=0,61$, $p<0,0001$) and Cx LCA ($r=0,49$, $p<0,0001$). Still, there was weak correlation between MSCT data and CCA in diagnosis of AD LCA, especially its distal segments ($r=0,33$, $p=0,0002$). Besides, contrast MSCT wasn't able to diagnose significant stenosis of diagonal LCA and a. intermedia (9 false negative results).

On the other side, we found significant, not very high, though, correlation between value of CI by A.S. Agatston and quantity of stenotic coronary arteries both by contrast MSCT results data (r=0,45, p<0,0001) and CCA (r=0,39, p=0,0004) (Fig. 1 and 2).

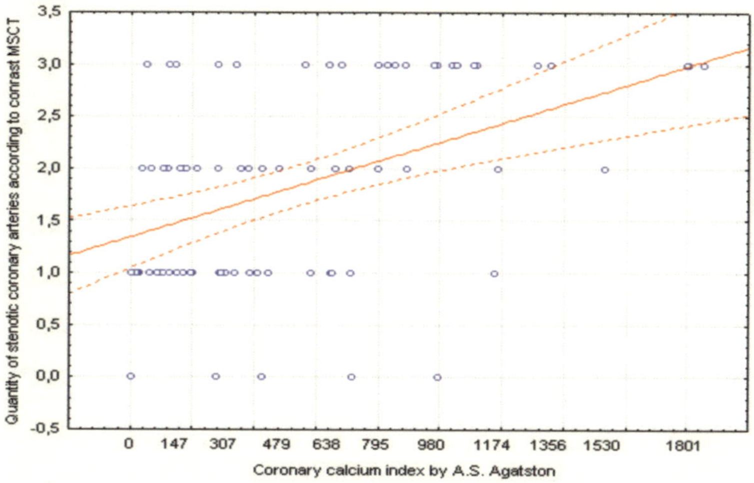

Fig. 1. Correlation between coronary calcium index by A.S. Agatston and quantity of stenotic coronary arteries according to contrast MSCT results data

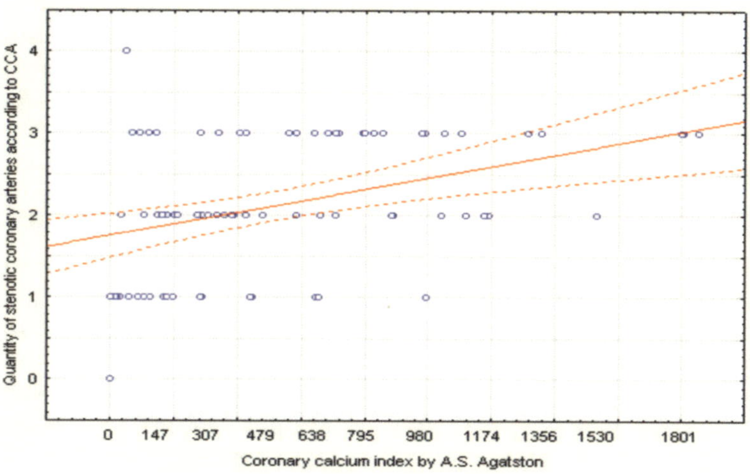

Fig. 2. Correlation between coronary calcium index by A.S. Agatston and quantity of stenotic coronary arteries according to CCA results data

At estimation of general diagnostic value of contrast MSCT compared to CCA the accuracy of the method (percentage of correct results in general quantity of positive and negative results) constituted 80,1%, p<0,0001. Still, overall sensitivity of 16-slice contrast MSCT was rather low (66,1% p<0,0001) with rather high specificity (94,75%, p=0,013) and positive presictive value of the method (91,7%, p=0,0017). Overall negative presictive value of MSCT was 76,1%, p<0,0001. We also found significant discrepancies in diagnostic value of contrast

MSCT compared to CCA depending on localization and level of atherosclerotic coronary lesions (Table 2).

Main LCA	AD LCA	Cx LCA	RCA
Se = 53,3%, p<0,0001	Se = 79,5%, p<0,0001	Se = 51,6%, p<0,0001	Se = 60,8%, p<0,0001
Sp = 96,0%, p=0,031	Sp = 50,0%, p<0,0001	Sp = 87,0%, p=0,0001	Sp = 91,9%, p=0,002
+PV = 66,7%, p<0,0001	+PV = 97,8%, p=0,11	+PV = 82,1%, p<0,0001	+PV = 94,1%, p=0,0085
- PV = 93,3%, p=0,005	- PV = 8,0%, p<0,0001	- PV = 61,0%, p<0,0001	- PV = 52,3%, p<0,0001

Table 2. Diagnostic value of 16-slice contrast MSCT in diagnosing coronary atherosclerosis compared to CCA

4. Discussion

Results of our study showed rather low sensitivity and negative predictive value of contrast MSCT, at relatively high high specificity and positive predictive value of the method campared to CCA. This data is relevant to results of many later foreign studies, dedicated to comparison of diagnostic value of MSCT and CCA (Abdulla et al., 2007; Kyung-Jong et al, 2003; Mollet et al, 2005; Mozaffarian, 2005). According to results of our study, indices of diagnostic value of contrast MSCT were significantly higher in diagnosis of more proximal segments of coronary arteries, which is confirmed by higher correlation indices between MSCT and CCA in examining main LCA (r=0,75, p<0,0001) and RCA (r=0,61, p<0,0001), with rather low rates of diagnostic value in diagnosing distal segments and minor coronary arteries lesions. For instance, according to our data, MSCT wasn't able to show lesions of diagonal LCA and intermedia, and showed rather low correlation with CCA in diagnosing Cx LCA stenosis (r=0,49, p<0,0001) and AD LCA (r=0,33, p=0,0002). These results coincide with relevant references (Abdulla et al., 2007; Hamon et al., 2006; Mollet et al, 2005). Therefore, our data allows to view 16-slice MSCT as a attractive safe non-invasive method for screening, primary diagnosis and decision about invasive methods necessity in the patients with high suspicion of significant coronary atherosclerosis, especially taking into account significant correlation between values of CI by A.S. Agatston and extent of coronary atherosclerosis regardless of the method of coronary arteries contrast visualization (Leschka S. et al., 2008; Mahmarian, 2007; Mozaffarian, 2005). On the other hand, in evaluating the extent of coronary atherosclerosis in the patients with CAD prior to the planned surgeon revascularization 16-slice MSCT could not be trusted enough to replace CCA.

4.1 Study limitations

Latest publications show results obtained from newer generations of MSCT using 32 or 64 slices per 200 frames, which explains higher resolution and better quality of coronary arteries visualization (Abdulla et al., 2007; Mollet et al, 2005), while we used only 16 slices per 200 frames, which surely influenced results of our study (Mollet et al, 2005; Romeo et al, 2005).

5. Conclusion

Contrast 16-sliced MSCT is unable to diagnose the distal and medium-to-minor coronary lesions and cannot be viewed as an alternative to CCA in the patients with verified CAD before planned surgeon revascularization due to shortcomings difficult to overcome in daily practice. Still, significant correlation between estimating coronary CI according to MSCT with results of multi-vessel coronary atherosclerosis by contrast MSCT (r=0,45, p<0,0001) and CCA (r=0,39, p=0,0004) allows to view 16-slice contrast MSCT as an attractive and trustworthy screening method in low-symptomatic patients with high risk of CAD for primary diagnosis, stratification and decision about reasonability of invasive diagnosis and revascularization.

6. Acknowledgment

Authors thank Prof. Anatoliy Rudenko, Head of Coronary Heart Disease Surgeon Treatment Department of The N.M.Amosov Institute Of Cardiovascular Surgery Of AMS Of Ukraine, and Dr. Oleg Sharayevskiy, Head of MSCT Department of NSC "The N.D.Strazhesko Institute Of Cardiology" Of AMS Of Ukraine, for the provided CCA and MSCT results data for the studied patients.

7. References

Abdulla J., Abildstrom S.Z., Gotzsche O. 64-multislice detector computed tomography coronary angiography as potential alternative to conventional coronary angiography: a systematic review and meta-analysis. *Eur. Heart J.*, Vol. 28 (December 2007), pp. 3042 - 3050.

Achenbach S. Computed Tomography Coronary Angiography. *J. Am. Coll. Cardiol.*, Vol. 48 (November 2006), pp. 1919 - 1928.

Fleisher Lee A. et al. ACC/AHA 2007 Guidelines on Perioperative Cardiovascular Evaluation and Care for Noncardiac Surgery: A Report of the American College of Cardiology/American Heart Association Task Force on Practice Guidelines (Writing Committee to Revise the 2002 Guidelines on Perioperative Cardiovascular Evaluation for Noncardiac Surgery. *Circulation,* Vol. 116 (October 2007), pp. e418 - e500.

Fleming R.M. A Tate-en-Tate Comparison of Ejection Fraction and Regional Wall Motion Abnormalities as Measured by Echocardiography and Gated Sestamibi SPECT. *Angiology*, Vol. 53, 3 (May 2002), pp. 313-321.

Fleming R.M., Boyd L.D. High-Dose Dipyridamole and Gated Sestamibi SPECT Imaging Provide Diagnositic Resting and Stress Ejection Fractions Useful for Predicting the Extent of Coronary Artery Disease. *Angiology*, 53, 4 (July 2002), pp. 415-421.

Hamon M. et al. Diagnostic Performance of Multislice Spiral Computed Tomography of Coronary Arteries as Compared With Conventional Invasive Coronary

Angiography: A Meta-Analysis. *J. Am. Coll. Cardiol.*, Vol. 48 (November 2006), pp. 1896 - 1910.

Kyung-Jong Yoo, Donghoon Choi, Byoung Wook Choi, et al. The comparison of the graft patency after coronary artery bypass grafting using coronary angiography and multi-slice computed tomography. *Eur. J. Cardiothorac. Surg.*, Vol. 24 (July 2003), pp. 86.

Laissy Jean-Pierre et al. Comprehensive evaluation of preoperative patients with aortic valve stenosis: usefulness of cardiac multidetector computed tomography. *Heart*, Vol. 93 (September 2007), pp. 1121 - 1125.

Leschka S. et al. Combining dual-source computed tomography coronary angiography and calcium scoring: added value for the assessment of coronary artery disease. *Heart*, Vol. 94, (September 2008), pp. 1154 - 1161.

Mahmarian J.J. Computed Tomography Coronary Angiography as an Anatomic Basis for Risk Stratification: Déjà Vu or Something New? *J. Am. Coll. Cardiol.*, Vol. 50 (September 2007), pp. 1171 - 1173.

Meijboom W.B. et al. Pre-Operative Computed Tomography Coronary Angiography to Detect Significant Coronary Artery Disease in Patients Referred for Cardiac Valve Surgery. *J. Am. Coll. Cardiol.*, Vol. 48 (October 2006), pp. 1658 - 1665.

Mollet N.R. et al. High-Resolution Spiral Computed Tomography Coronary Angiography in Patients Referred for Diagnostic Conventional Coronary Angiography. *Circulation*, Vol. 112 (October 2005), pp. 2318 - 2323.

Mozaffarian D. Electron-Beam Computed Tomography for Coronary Calcium: A Useful Test to Screen for Coronary Heart Disease? *JAMA*, Vol. 294 (December 2005), pp. 2897 – 2901.

Petry A., Sabin K. (2003). *Demonstrable statistics in medicine*, GAOTAR-MED, Moscow

Rebrova O.Y. (2002). *Statistical analysis of medical data*, Media Sphere, Moscow

Romeo G. et al. Coronary Stenosis Detection by 16-Slice Computed Tomography in Heart Transplant Patients. *J.Am.Coll.Cardiol*, Vol. 45 (June 2005), pp. 1826-1831.

Scanlon P.J. et al. ACC/AHA Guidelines for Coronary Angiography: Executive Summary and Recommendations. *Circulation*, Vol. 99 (May 1999), pp. 2345-57.